THE ART OF VINYASA

Also by Richard Freeman

The Mirror of Yoga

Also by Mary Taylor

What Are You Hungry For? Women, Food, and Spirituality
New Vegetarian Classics: Soups
New Vegetarian Classics: Entrees

THE ART OF VINYASA

Awakening Body and Mind through the Practice of Ashtanga Yoga

RICHARD FREEMAN
& MARY TAYLOR

SHAMBHALA
BOULDER
2016

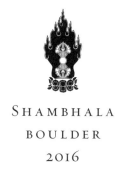

Shambhala Publications, Inc.
4720 Walnut Street
Boulder, Colorado 80301
www.shambhala.com

9 8 7 6 5 4 3 2 1

FIRST EDITION

Printed in the United States of America

♾ This edition is printed on acid-free paper that meets the American National Standards Institute Z39.48 Standard.
♻ Shambhala Publications makes every effort to print on recycled paper.
For more information please visit www.shambhala.com.

Distributed in the United States by Penguin Random House LLC
and in Canada by Random House of Canada Ltd

Designed by Steve Dyer

LIBRARY OF CONGRESS CATALOGING-IN-PUBLICATION DATA

Names: Freeman, Richard, 1950– author. | Taylor, Mary (Yoga teacher)
Title: The art of vinyasa: awakening body and mind through the practice of ashtanga yoga / Richard Freeman and Mary Taylor.
Description: Boulder: Shambhala, 2016. | Includes index.
Identifiers: LCCN 2016002192 | ISBN 9781611802795 (paperback)
Subjects: LSCH: Aṣṭāṅga yoga. | BISAC: HEALTH & FITNESS / Yoga. | PHILOSOPHY / Hindu.
Classification: LCC RA781.68 .F74 2016 | DDC 613.7/046—dc23
LC record available at https://lccn.loc.gov/2016002192

To Sri K. Pattabhi Jois and his wife, Ammaji.
And with deep gratitude to Sarasvathi, Manju, and Sharath,
who continue to inspire us all in this practice.

This book is designed to shed light on establishing an internally rooted yoga practice that can last a lifetime. It also looks deeply at āsana practice as an external expression of the internal forms that give a profound and direct experience to the awakening of body and mind through the practice.

CONTENTS

Introduction 1

PART ONE

Foundation: The Roots and Depth of Yoga

1. Natural Alignment: The Internal Forms of the Practice 7
2. Aligning Intention and Action: Where the Rubber Meets the Road 33
3. Fluid Movement: Alignment, Form, and Imagination 51
4. Mechanics: Essential Anatomical Perspectives 82

PART TWO

Āsana: Movements and Poses Strung Together Like Jewels on the Thread of the Breath

5. Building Sūrya Namaskāra 99
6. Standing Poses 127
7. Forward Bends 157
8. Backbends 202
9. Twists 230
10. Balancing Poses 245
11. Finishing Poses 275

Acknowledgments 299
Appendix 1. Ancient Wisdom, Contemporary Circumstances 301
Appendix 2. Invocation 303
Appendix 3. Sequencing 305
Appendix 4. Illustrations of Mūlabandha, Kidney Wings, and Cobra Hood 313
Appendix 5. Sūrya Namaskāra A and B 316
Index 319
About the Authors 326

THE ART OF VINYASA

INTRODUCTION

YOGA IS A LIVING ART. IT IS A MEANS OF MOVING, breathing, thinking, expanding and contracting, evolving and interacting within the complex, ever-changing landscape of the world within and around us. As with any art form, yoga nurtures seeds of aesthetic satisfaction that stimulate flashes of understanding and compassion. For many practitioners, a keen truth and meaning spontaneously arise as insight into the vast, interconnected nature of all things.

When embodied, these aesthetic sparks and seeds of insight are experienced as feelings of resonating with our surroundings. They occur in yoga when we're not looking for them—just as they may when we're standing in front of a great work of art or enjoying the perfect sunset. Somehow (possibly by chance) our perception of self is released just long enough for us to feel intimately connected to everything and everyone else, and the underlying field of kind, openheartedness that is our true nature naturally arises. Clarity or conscious awareness is the fallout—the residue—from practicing yoga in this way, as an art rather than as a means of attaining this thing or that.

This approach to practice requires a willingness to invite and *be with* not knowing. It encourages us to show up ready and eager to meet whatever arises. Perhaps most important, it demands the mental and emotional agility to be comfortable with the paradox of simultaneously holding two or more points of view with equal attentiveness.

We learn to be focused and disciplined while letting go, surrendering the ego while steadying the mind, and all the while remaining tuned in to the complexity of whatever is arising. By cultivating open-minded states of inquisitiveness and acceptance in the controlled structure of a practice, encountering paradoxes and the unknown begins to feel safe, interesting, and exciting rather than tedious or frightening. Gradually habitual patterns of behavior and thinking dissipate as preconceptions dissolve and freedom unfolds.

This isn't what most of us sign up for when we walk into our first yoga class, but at some point in our practice, it happens: that seed within is awakened. As if by accident, the art in the form is revealed, along with a glimpse of what it is like to be satisfied and fully awake. Of course this arising of free or conscious mind, like so many mysterious and important things in life, is illusive. The moment we recognize how wonderful it is, how we feel liberated and free as if swimming effortlessly in an ocean of equanimity, the mind grabs hold of the idea of feeling good and tries to package it, make a formula that will ensure we can hold on to it, or concoct a plan to duplicate (and possibly profit from) the state. And already it has vanished.

With time—possibly many years—we may realize that the awakening of this seed of reality is not something we can create but something we invite; we can simply do the work required to arrange things so that perhaps it arises again. The "work" we must do is to practice with dedication, consistency, and an open mind. We practice as a means of waking up to and seeing clearly the process of whatever is presented. At the same time we constantly remind ourselves to let go of our expectations about what we may attain or acquire through our efforts. The work is never done. It is as if, again and again, we prepare a meal and set the table for honored guests who may or may not arrive. Whether they do or not, the next day we set the table again with unyielding enthusiasm. When yoga is approached in this way, as an art form and an offering containing an endless mixture of complementary, interwoven oppositions, then the practice itself is fully satisfying. Any residual benefits we may feel or insights we may happen upon as a result of the practice are icing on the cake.

Yoga practice can take the form of *āsanas* (poses), *prāṇāyāma* (breathing), meditation, chanting, or philosophical inquiry. Each of these methods grows from an understanding and a trust in relationship. Everything that comes up in practice is a reflection of the interaction of oppositions, interactions, and contexts both within and without. To adapt, respond, and find balance in this web of relationship is the key to practicing yoga in a contemplative manner. The practice of *vinyāsa* reframes our perception of any particular thing by equalizing the relational background in which it exists.

The Sanskrit word *vinyāsa* can be broken down into its two components. *Nyāsa,* meaning to sanctify and draw one's full attention into a particular meditative focus and then release the content of the focus. *Vi* means to arrange or sanctify in a specific way in response to context or a lack of context. This implies a sequence of steps and countersteps. Vinyāsa, then, means the focused, intentional sequence of form, thought movement, and breath that frees the mind by recontextualizing the body, sensations, form, and all objects of attention. It can be a specific form of yoga practice, but in a broader sense, vinyāsa is the mindful process that naturally occurs when we arrange any circumstances correctly.

Most of the time, in our attempts to focus the mind (vinyāsa on its way to nyāsa), the chosen pattern is incomplete. Normally a large part of the intelligence in the rest of the body rises up in the background as a distraction. For example, if you are meditating with attention on feeling the relaxed upper portions of the sinuses, it can be a very exciting and luminous experience. But soon, some parts of your body are likely to become tense, and your thoughts will scatter; these changes in composition seep in quietly and unseen, gradually coming into full bloom. The vinyāsa process is to allow the arising of oppositional forces, contexts, and perspectives, and at just the right moment—before a story line or movement pattern is allowed to fully manifest and wander off—to consciously introduce the balancing counterstep to harmonize the field. In this way, the current focus and action merge with and digest the residue of the previous step.

Perhaps the most obvious example of vinyāsa is the constant movement of our breathing: inhaling and exhaling. This pattern is one that has been with us since we drew that initial breath during the first moments after birth and will remain as a consistent, background sensation until our final exhalation at the time of death. We all share the oppositional patterns associated with the breath—the constant rising and falling, ebbing and flowing, spreading and contracting, stimulating and relaxing union of opposites within breath, body, and mind. The fluctuation of breath is a natural manifestation of a complete and pristine intelligence that is always there, if we choose to pay attention. When we carefully observe and feel our breath, eventually both patterns—the inhalation and the exhalation—remain simultaneously awakened in our nervous system and our awareness, the embodiment of paradox. With practice, we experience a singular focus within the field of awareness, and our thoughts settle effortlessly as the mind becomes calm and steady—the result of paying attention to composite, opposing, and paradoxical patterns as they arise. This is the essence of vinyāsa.

In this book, we will be exploring the idea of yoga as an art form and as an interlacing of opposites—a vinyāsa—within the context of what is known as the Aṣṭāṅga Vinyāsa system of yoga. Aṣṭāṅga Vinyāsa yoga is a form of āsana codified by Sri T. Krishnamacharya and his student, Sri K. Pattabhi Jois, in the early twentieth century. In this form, specific series of poses are practiced in a dynamic, flowing sequence that coordinates movement with the gaze and the breath. The Aṣṭāṅga Vinyāsa form also includes breathing and meditation practices and the union and synthesis of perspectives within each of the eight limbs of yoga described by Patañjali in the Yoga Sūtra. In Aṣṭāṅga Vinyāsa yoga, four underlying threads are always at play, harmonizing relationships through vinyāsa to bring balance, depth, and integrity. These threads, or "internal forms," are breath, *bandha* (bonding), *mudrā* (sealing), and *dṛṣṭi* (gazing) (discussed in Chapter 1). They are woven together in a seamless stream of form, movement, and awareness that automatically awakens the intelligence.

Here we focus on vinyāsa as it relates both to the external forms of the practice, such as correct alignment within poses, and to the sequencing of subtle movements within the postures that truly ignites and liberates the mind. We explore the idea of vinyāsa and yoga as relationship: sometimes joining, sometimes separating; interpenetrating, communicating, or merging together. Through practice, this sense of interconnectedness gradually becomes familiar within every field of experience—inhalation with exhalation, focus with horizon, text with context, foreground with background, inner world with outer world, given or physical world with creative or imaginary world. On the deepest level then, we can see that yoga is relationships with other beings, with friends, family, coworkers, pets, bugs, the world at large, our community, and the environment. Though the struggle to balance rotations in our hip joints so we may sit effortlessly in Lotus Pose may seem important at times, it is clear that most important is relationship with others because that's where the emotions—our ability to use and see through self-image and those things we value and that give life meaning—come into play. Half the world is given to us, but the other half is created by how we frame it.

PART ONE

FOUNDATION

The Roots and Depth of Yoga

As modern yoga practitioners we find ourselves in an exciting though sometimes confusing time, as long-standing yoga lineages and traditions are coming face to face with modern interpretations and spin-offs inspired by individuals and cultural waves of style. It's easy to treat your own school of yoga as the final word and then ignore the wonder and variety of other traditions and perspectives. Juxtaposing different metaphors and images is a great way to let go of our rigidity and to slide into a more open-minded experience of yoga in our search for truth.

In the next three chapters we explore subtle internal techniques and forms traditionally used in classical systems of yoga to transmute emotions and to wake up creativity and our imagination into the joy of relationship. We explore different types of images that blend together the concentration of attention with movements of Praṇa and sensation into an unfolding of embodied form. Visualization and imagery help us to harmonize our internal experiences with other beings and with the entire world around us. Finally, in Chapter 4 we take an introductory look at a more classical anatomical perspective that also underscores the necessity of good form, alignment, and imagination within a healthy and balanced yoga practice.

1

Natural Alignment

The Internal Forms of the Practice

IMAGINE THAT YOU GET A JOB AS A MODEL FOR AN artist who's going to carve a statue of Avalokiteśvara, the buddha of infinite compassion. Avalokiteśvara is to be seated holding the wish-fulfilling gem in front of the lotus flower (*padma*) of the heart, and your alignment must be perfect! All you have to do is sit in that pose and not move.

It takes extraordinary focus to picture what Avalokiteśvara looks like, bringing your attention again and again to rest along the plumb line of your body. Releasing the palate in silent contact with a softening tongue and feeling a smooth, steady breath unfold, you begin to experience all the physical patterns associated with inhaling. You then drop even more deeply in, observing as the breath effortlessly turns around; the exhalation dissolves all those endless forms back to their roots, like petals falling from a flower. The centers of your ears are directly over the centers of the shoulder joints, so they're aligned exactly on the coronal plane of the body; your hip joints are centered in that same precise line. The back of the diaphragm spreads, and you notice that right around the twelfth thoracic vertebra, a radiant point of awareness is forming a warm, vibrant circle. You envision yourself having four arms, but you know not to pinch any of the shoulder blades together or the artist will kick you out and hire someone else as the model. So you drop back into the breath and feel more arms growing—just a few at first, but then an infinite number sprout and reach up out of that warm, vibrant area in the middle of your lower back. The center of each palm tingles, and you realize you can actually *see* through the palms as you reach out to all other sentient beings, but you're not distracted by this visual stimulation. It's hard work and you start to sweat, but if you release the palate and the muscles in the back of the tongue, your mind clears; you feel an extension along the spine, out through sides of your body, and then up through the crown of the head as if you are growing bigger and taller. The pose feels easy, steady, and buoyant. You cultivate a vivid sense of concentration and form and, at the same time, the ability to dissolve and let go.

This is how alignment was taught in ancient times before the study of anatomy and theories of biomechanics and postural alignment became the norm. In those days, alignment was embodied through visualizing deity forms, which brought the finer qualities of the emotions, sensations, and thought patterns into the breath and body. Artists trained for generations in a highly disciplined manner to reproduce in their sculptures and drawings exactly what sages had discovered to be, through lifetimes of practice and visualizations, optimal forms of alignment. Forms that would facilitate a physiologically awake and open, integrated, and finely tuned state of being that is perfectly suited for contemplative practice. Symbolic representation of this kind of esoteric knowledge followed prescribed patterns and proportions that were described in minute detail so that one could meditate on a deity form and *feel* correct alignment. In those days, teachers didn't bother describing the alignment of joints or any of that dry, boring anatomical stuff. Instead, they went right for the source—the deity form—and breathed right into it.

Visualizations would often start with simple geometric forms like squares, circles, and triangles—something easy to imagine. Using the sequences of a vinyāsa, practitioners gradually would learn to interface simple forms with sensation patterns in their own bodies; this trained the imagination-body to link sensation points throughout the physical body with patterns of breath and movement. This method of learning alignment is still extraordinarily viable and valid today when studying yoga and yoga anatomy. Of course, visualization and the study of classical anatomy are by no means mutually exclusive; in fact, they inform and complement each other well. Studying anatomy gives a tangible context for the intuitive, internal feelings and sensations that fine artistic representations of breath and movement can stimulate within. With practice, you can visualize the deities in endless detail and begin to experience the inner sensations of waking up and harmonizing your own internal awareness as a means of balancing the nervous system and the subtle body. Then when you check an anatomy text, you learn why certain movements feel better than others. Visualization helps you to organize sensations and perceptions so you can release habitual, self-centered perspectives on these sensations and relate to the world as a composition of interconnected parts. Diety visualization (or any symbolic deity construction, such as a maṇḍala) follows the step-by-step process of vinyāsa. At a certain point of balance, contextualization, and harmony the visualization or construction is placed down as an offering to the whole world as pure consciousness. We then let it go. In placing the content of the mind down, or nyāsa, insight arises into the impermanant nature of all gross and subtle structures.

Deity visualization can, of course, be taken too literally by the ego. A student may become infatuated with a deity as a true independent entity—thinking, for example, that the forms and mythology of Gaṇeśa or Garuda actually exist as absolute and separate. At this point, the student's own ego absorption has gotten in the way of truly deepening insight through study. When these kinds of challenges arise, they are a sign to smile softly and lighten up so as not to lose balance. The key to visualizing a deity is to foster the trust that at the right moment you will look at the deity, embody it, and just "get it." This takes patience and an open, inquisitive mind. Deity visualization is akin to abstract thought, such as exploration of the idea of infinity, but visualizations can be embodied to give direct, visceral experience of what otherwise might be a complex construct.

Yoga alignment can be and usually is approached from the point of view of classical anatomy, physical form, and biomechanics. And this is good. We look at similarities and differences in the structure of bones, muscles, and interconnected patterns of breath and movement. Visualization bridges a gap in understanding movement between what happens in the mind and what happens in the body. As we breathe and move in and out of postures, we simply allow a visualized form to rest in the background as a subconscious context from which to experience whatever actually arises as feeling, sensation, or thought. The visualization provides a reference point for our experience so we can be there with full attention.

Between the externally oriented perspective of studying form and movement from a classical anatomical perspective and the more abstract perspective of visualization lies another method for insight into alignment and form. That is an understanding of the internal forms of the practice. Each of these perspectives is important and may be an effective means of establishing a context for understanding our practice. Merging visualization, abstract thought, and classical anatomy through an embodiment of the internal forms gives a full understanding of form and alignment. This really is what the Aṣṭāṅga Vinyāsa system of yoga is all about: taking a multidimensional view of what happens when we practice yoga. Cultivating the simplest of circumstances in a context of open-minded awareness and a full range of movement, we invite the yoga practice to unfold like a flower in bloom.

This blossoming naturally occurs through the consistent practices of meditation, prāṇāyāma, and āsana, each of which has specific external forms that serve as gateways to understanding. We gradually learn to focus the mind by sitting straight and cultivating a stable base in the body while practicing meditation and prāṇāyāma; we move with attention to the actions and counteractions within the muscular and skeletal systems while practicing āsana. As the practice deepens, more subtle levels of movement and awareness (what we call the internal forms) emerge, providing depth and insight. These forms are integral to practicing yoga as a meditative art rather than as a gymnastic exercise or an uninspired, autopilot-directed ritual.

We define the internal forms of the practice as breathing, dṛṣṭi, bandha, and mudrā. Although they are all intimate parts of our physical experience, unlike the more external forms of practice, the internal forms are initially less obvious. It takes time and patience to tune in to their subtle physical cues, but when we do, they provide an opportunity for insight into the threshold between the outer world of experience—our physical body—and the internal, intuitive, sometimes even mystical experience that arises as we practice yoga. When we open our imagination enough to consider what internal forms are, we may—on rare occasion—spontaneously feel the alignment of a deity as a representation of the interpenetrating nature of all things.

Cultivating an understanding of and connection to the internal forms is a paradoxical practice. It is at once elusive and simple, abstract and extraordinarily clear, impossible to "do" yet simple to experience. Due to their subtle nature, we begin to explore the internal forms from the most familiar—the breath—and work our way to the subtlest form—the mudrā—so we can experience their interrelationship as well as their profound impact.

The internal forms can be revealed through visualization, but it is also important to study them by establishing an embodied context for them. We call this context internal or "subtle body" anatomy, and the most direct route to understanding it is through an interfacing of the breath (*Prāṇa*) and imagination (*citta*). Just as we might imagine ourselves to be Avalokiteśvara and then suddenly find that we are sitting in perfect physical alignment, so too we may start wherever we can with internal alignment, imagining—and therefore *feeling*—something that is already in the nervous system as a pattern sensation. Through mindful attention, the pattern unfolds in the imagination and the understanding. We start with whatever is present and build from there.

We construct and embody the internal forms by imagining that we have a central channel, the *suṣumṇā nāḍī*. It runs from the area between the pituitary and pineal glands down through the "heart center" and the core of the body to open at a point about the width of two fingers above the middle of the pelvic floor. This channel of awareness can also be imagined as extending in both directions (even beyond the top and lowest boundaries of the body). The pelvic floor, also called the pelvic diaphragm, is the fanlike muscular structure that lies along the bottom of the pelvis and immediately above the urogenital triangle. Its flat, toned surface supports, coordinates, and completes the larger muscular movement patterns of the abdominal wall, hip joints, and urogenital triangle in combination with the complementary breathing patterns of inhaling and exhaling. When feeling and visualizing the pelvic floor, an area of particular interest and importance is immediately in front of the anus, behind the genitals, and above the perineal body. This area is called the *mūla* (root). It is the center of the sacred maṇḍala or circle of the pelvic diaphragm.

All of the internal forms of yoga practice are generated through the intricate, internal core structures embedded in the mūla. Over time and with a great deal of practice, we become familiar with the core root pattern that allows the internal forms to awaken and expand outward endlessly. We can then experience our practice as vast and unbounded without becoming ungrounded or disembodied.

BREATH

Yoga practice, like life itself, begins with the breath. Breath, or Prāṇa, provides an endless, all-pervading background, a continuous ebb and flow of sound and perception that unifies, sustains, and informs us on the physical, mental, and emotional levels. Prāṇa (with a capital P) refers to the internal breath as a whole. We experience it as a vibratory quality of pure sensation and perception within every nook and cranny of the body. It is often referred to as "life breath," or the immediately distinguished characteristic of sensations, in particular the awareness of touch—what you feel within your body as the tissues expand and contract. Prāṇa is the perception of temperature or texture through the skin or the feeling of a flow from one group of sensations to another. It is associated with the visual sense of light and darkness that we comprehend as part of our visual perception, just as it is associated with the immediate quality of sound and the sensations of smell and taste. Prāṇa is perceived in all fields of perception and, like intelligence, reveals and creates context for patterns that arise. A basic axiom of yoga is that Prāṇa and citta (the mind) move together like two fish swimming in tandem. Move one, and the other automatically follows.

The broad category of Prāṇa, or breath, has many subcategories but five major subdivisions. The first is *prāṇa* (with a lowercase p), which refers to the breath as it rises and spreads and is based in the heart. *Apāna*—based in the pelvic floor—goes down, contracts, and squeezes things out of the body. *Samāna* is based in the navel; it spreads out evenly and is related to the digestive process and assimilation of everything—absorbing food as well as subtleties of awareness on all levels of perception. When awakened, the seed-point of samāna is said to shine like the sun at the root of the navel. *Udāna* is based in the throat and rises up the middle of the head and out through the top. The all-pervasive form of breath known as *vyāna* is felt throughout the body, most notably in the skin.

The most immediate and workable patterns of breath are apāna, which controls the exhalation pattern, and prāṇa, which controls the inhalation pattern. Awareness of these complementary patterns of breath opens a door to a direct experience of the sacred nature of all perceptions and mental patterns. When we inhale, it is easy to feel the characteristic expanding, blossoming, and rising sensations that spread throughout the body. The ribs naturally expand as we draw in the breath; the heart floats; and there is an ascendant, alert feeling. At the peak of the inhalation—in the gap before the exhalation begins—there is a sense of limitlessness, interconnectedness, and perhaps even joy at the unfolding of endless forms. When we exhale, it is easy to feel the grounding, squeezing-out, and dissolving pattern of the apāna as the edges of the diaphragm automatically drop and the ribs contract to accommodate the reduction in the size of the lungs. At the end of an exhale, the pelvic floor naturally tones. When the pelvic floor tones the mind easily turns inward as we experience the visceral sensations associated with the dissolution of forms—which for some may cause feelings of fear or panic to arise.

Most people tend to prefer one of these phases of the breath; there are those who love inhaling and those who favor exhaling. Some of us are too *prāṇic,* avoiding the sensations associated with exhaling and getting lost in imagination, floating off the face of the earth in our minds. Others favor the exhalation and become too *apānic,* with a rigid, boring, or depressed point of view. After some practice, we are able to enjoy the entire breath by inviting the opposite physical patterns of inhaling and exhaling to support one another within the body and mind; in this way, we can experience their interdependence.

In the Aṣṭāṅga Vinyāsa system of yoga, breath is the foundation for the internal forms of the practice. We begin with *ujjāyī* breathing, which serves as the basis for practice whether you're a beginner or an advanced practitioner. In fact, Aṣṭāṅga Vinyāsa yoga *is* just this: simple ujjāyī breathing with a little movement tossed in. More advanced practitioners can also learn Ujjāyī Prāṇāyāma, which is a very concentrated form of ujjāyī breathing and in which there is breath retention and complete internal focus.

To learn what ujjāyī breathing is, sit really straight so the belly is happy and not compressed. Bring your awareness internally. Imagine the central line of the body as vividly as possible like an imaginary plumb line running from the crown of the head down through the middle of the chest and abdomen, through the center of the pelvic floor, all the way down to the earth's core. The plumb line serves as a reference point for balance and stability within the body and may also be imagined as any stabilizing configuration within the body's core, say as breath, a shaft of light, or a pattern of energy. To establish the ujjāyī breath, imagine that the heart floats on this central axis like a lotus flower floats in a pool of still water. The base of the plumb line is stabilized as the sitting bones, coccyx, and pubic bone drop, causing the pelvic floor muscles to tone. If you are grounded through the root of the body this way and the heart area feels free and open, then breathing is easy. If you are disconnected at any point along that central line—if the heart is constricted, tense, or closed, or if the pelvic floor is asleep—then ujjāyī breathing is not happening.

Keeping the lips lightly closed, simply begin to breathe in and out. By closing your lips, the breath moves through the nose, and the mind can focus more clearly. At this point, the eyes become steady in dṛṣṭi (gazing). This automatically releases the palate and softens the tongue, so it is easy to focus on sensations in the mouth and the stream of breath going in and out through the nostrils. The waves of the breath start the process of alignment, which is merely the intelligence waking up in the center of the body. Just keep listening, allowing the breath to unfold.

Ujjāyī breath is characterized by a sound that results from closing the vocal cords a tiny bit while continuing to keep the tongue quiet and the lips softly closed. The breath makes a smooth, aspirate sound both as you inhale *and* as you exhale. It sounds almost as if you were whispering the word *ah* with your lips closed. As we know, whispering can be intimate. When you're close to someone, you don't shout, and the ujjāyī breath has that same intimate quality, as if you were whispering to your beloved.

Listen for that sound and strengthen the breath—directing it with intention to be smooth, easy, and even. It is not simply a matter of letting the breath come and go in whatever pattern it happens to take; correct ujjāyī breathing depends on a nonforced effort that, like a metronome, keeps the pace and tone of the breath consistent. This resonance of the breath is the mantra of ujjāyī breathing and Ujjāyī Prāṇāyāma, and 99 percent of this breathing technique is opening the ears and listening to that sound. It sounds very much like gas leaking through a valve—which technically it is. You could imagine the sound to be water running through pipes, wind in the trees, or the distant breaking of ocean waves on the shore.

Ujjāyī means an upwardly triumphant or victorious breath. Esoterically, ujjāyī is when the internal Prāṇa wakes up—*ut*—and victoriously shoots up the central channel of the body to stand on the crown of your head as in Samasthitiḥ (Equal Standing). That's true Ujjāyī Prāṇāyāma, which may come to you one day. In the meantime, just make some noise with your breath.

Every time we inhale, we concentrate on the residue of the exhalation, and every time we exhale, we focus on the essence of the inhalation. The heart is the radiant point of the inhaling breath, and the overall physical pattern of the inhalation is an upward, spreading, and floating pattern. The exhaling pattern is perceived in the body as a downward, contracting, grounding feeling—like water running to earth—with its seed-point at the center of the pelvic floor. When we inhale, we pull the attention of the mind like a thread up through the seed of the exhalation at the middle of the pelvic floor. When we exhale, we release the upper back of the palate to keep the heart open. We concentrate on the smooth, whispering sound and the physical feelings and sensations associated with each phase of this pattern of breath, in addition to the moments of transition—the gaps—as we move from in-breath to out-breath and back again. Feeling the pouring of the apāna into the prāṇa and the prāṇa into the apāna is contemplative, subtle, and wonderful. This is prāṇāyāma practice; the whole thing is right there.

During our āsana practice, having established the form, flow, and sound of the ujjāyī breath, we learn to move in conjunction with the breath. While transitioning in and out of āsanas, we consciously practice the inhalation during expansive movements like lifting the arms overhead or moving up and out of a pose. Conversely, we practice more rooted and contracting movements like folding forward, curling the spine, or twisting in conjunction with the exhalation. After getting into a pose, we typically hold it for five full rounds of breath (though for finishing poses and under certain circumstances, we may hold for longer) before again moving on the wave of the breath to initiate a smooth shift as we inhale into the next movement within the vinyāsa of the pose and sequence. After practicing āsanas for some time in this manner, the patterns of breath and the physical movements associated with both inhaling and exhaling deep within the body become intuitively felt, and these flowing patterns reflexively manifest in our external movements. The effect is astonishing. As we move in and out of poses in union with the breath, we may experience a sense of seamlessly joining our inner world of experience with the external world of perception and our interactions with others. As we do, the practice takes on a deeply meditative quality.

SUPERIMPOSING MANTRA ON BREATH

To intensify the mind's ability to focus on the breath, we may superimpose a mantra on the aspirate sound. Using a mantra gives the mind, which sometimes needs to be employed, a task that reminds it of the bigger job at hand—to concentrate on listening—so that its natural tendency to wander is quelled. After some practice, the mantra can then fall away, and the underlying mantra—the actual sound of the breath itself—can capture and eventually liberate the mind.

Probably the most famous mantra associated with the breath within the yoga traditions is the SĀ- HAṀ mantra. You may imagine the sound *sā,* a seed sound for the apāna, as you inhale—as if whispering inside your head so only you can hear. There is a natural pause at the top of the inhalation; at that moment you can imagine or silently whisper the seed sound for the prāṇa, *haṁ,* as you exhale. In the gap at the end of the out-breath, the mind can again return to thinking the sound *sā,* and so on. This mantra is sometimes referred to as the swan mantra because *haṁsa* means "swan" in Sanskrit, and if you try to superimpose SĀ- HAṀ on the breath, you'll notice that after a few rounds it starts to sound like HAṀ -SA.

The mantra can also be considered divine sound associated with the *paramātman* (pure consciousness beyond any individual or particular being) and it may be whispered internally as either SĀ-HAṀ (feminine "I am she") or -SO'HAṀ (masculine "I am he"). She or he is the paramātman, which is experienced as the openness of the central channel. So through this mantra we remind ourselves that "I am she/he," or "I am the paramātman, the goddess or the god who is pure consciousness." The idea that you are the beloved other, the paramātman, and are located in your own central channel and heart is usually enough of a conundrum (a self-reference paradox) to stun an active mind and make it willing to just listen to the background of the sound of the breath.

Whatever meaning you choose to associate with the mantra, placing it on the breath is pretty simple—make the sound *sā* as you breath in and *haṁ* as you breath out. Now you may wonder, "Who is saying SĀ-HAṀ? Is it me, or is it the breath?" Or it may cross your mind to ask, "If I am she/he, does that mean I am divine? After all, what do I mean by the word *I*?" These are the types of things people who think a lot can't help fretting over. It's natural. Don't worry about it. It becomes clear after a few breaths.

With practice focusing on the breath, a smooth tone and an even extension of the breath unfold effortlessly. This causes all of the little pockets in the sense fields to become filled with Prāṇa so the mind can rest, and the body and mind can become integrated rather than splintered. In this manner, we can perceive feelings, thoughts, and sensations clearly and respond to them with kindness and equanimity. Bringing awareness to and cultivating the sound of ujjāyī breathing is a vital, underlying thread of the internal practice of Aṣṭāṅga Vinyāsa yoga. It trains the mind to listen and become absorbed by sound so that movement is transformed from a self-directed, formulaic effort into a moving meditation.

DṚṢṬI

Another internal form that facilitates a deepening of the practice is the dṛṣṭi, or gaze. The term *dṛṣṭi* refers both to a particular place on which the eyes rest during practice and to a quality or feeling-sense associated with the gaze. The eyes are fully alert while resting on a specific point. At the same time, unlike many other situations in life when we look attentively at a particular thing, the quality of dṛṣṭi is steady, calm, and spacious—there is no physical or mental tension; no sense of drawing a conclusion with the mind; no grasping, avoiding, or naming the object upon which we gaze. No strain is created within the sensory or mental fields in proper dṛṣṭi, in spite of the fact that we look with a clear gaze and not a sleepy or dreamy gaze.

Of course, this is much easier said than done. Releasing the palate, softening the tongue, and listening to the sound of the ujjāyī breath can facilitate proper dṛṣṭi. Good dṛṣṭi is awake, innocent, and attentive. Think of how a young infant looks intensely at something: he does not identify himself as being separate from the rest of the world, and he has few if any "names" for objects, so he is just looking. Dṛṣṭi may feel as though we are gazing from a place of perception that lies behind the eyeball, somewhere along the line of the temples within the skull, and there is a felt sense of "nobody looking at nothing."

You may notice that the quality of your own gaze, even in everyday situations, can affect your state of mind. When your eyes scan or dart around the room, attention tends to be on alert, and the mind may be either highly attentive and agitated or unfocused and distracted. If the gaze is too soft or the eyes feel drowsy, attention is usually foggy. The context and content of our thoughts form patterns of tension and movement in and around the eyes. Throughout the day, the mind is naturally dragged along behind or interfaced with the quality of our gaze and the movement of our eyes. It is quite natural when we subconsciously want to avoid something (thinking too deeply about it or moving to the edge of sensation) for the eyes to flicker, causing our concentration to shift. This lets off just enough of the mental or emotional pressure so we don't actually have to examine whatever is about to arise.

Within the āsana practice, we cultivate dṛṣṭi, training the eyes to stay steady, clear, and focused while we move in conjunction with the breath, no matter what is arising. Each movement during transitions between poses is associated with a particular breath and a specific dṛṣṭi, and each pose has a specific gazing point. This helps to focus the mind. For example, while practicing Sūrya Namaskāra (Sun Salutation), during Ekam (the first movement of Sūrya Namaskāra), we lift the arms overhead as we inhale and remember something more important we're "supposed" to be doing. Rather than dashing out of the room to take care of it, we open the ears, gaze up at our thumbs, and ride the breath like a wave of sensation and thought as the exhalation draws our awareness, gaze, and sensations back down to earth, and we fold into Dve (the second movement of Sūrya Namaskāra). Moving in conjunction with the dṛṣṭi and the breath provides a powerful environment for the mind to release its presuppositions, conclusions, and opinions, allowing us to concentrate on whatever arises moment to moment so that opposite patterns of movement, thought, feeling, and sensation can be woven together intelligently.

There are eight traditional dṛṣṭi or gazing points used during an Aṣṭāṅga Vinyāsa practice—or nine if you include the internal one called *antara* dṛṣṭi. The eight are *aṅguṣṭha* (the middle of the thumb); *bhrūmadhya* (between the eyebrows); *nāsāgra* (the end of the nose); *hastāgra* (the tip of the hand); *pārśva* (the side—right or left); *ūrdhvā* (upward); *nābhi cakra* (the navel); and *pādayoragra* (the tip of the foot). Each pose has a prescribed dṛṣṭi that is sustained throughout the five counts of breath during which the pose is held. The practitioner or teacher may modify the dṛṣṭi for particular circumstances or desired effects in a pose. By holding steady to a particular gazing point and reducing physical and mental tension, we create an underlying, unifying field of experience within which mind, breath, and body can naturally adjust to accommodate the specific mental, emotional, and physical circumstances that arise.

Dṛṣṭi also means "view," as in a philosophical view that extends even to our moment-by-moment propositions about ourselves, others, and the world. The type of gazing, or dṛṣṭi, that we practice during āsanas will eventually give you a correct view—one that is kind and compassionate. Since you are just gazing, there's no strain, no aggression, no need to formulate ideas or pull out from the background of perception as separate any one particular object in your visual field. Your view (both actual and theoretical) is crystal clear, and the mind is suspended so it is only gazing. When you're not practicing dṛṣṭi, the mind will establish a gazer (you) and then make up something (an individual field or object) to identify as separate and the object of the gaze. Once this separation starts, the process of wandering mind is triggered.

Physiologically, we feel dṛṣṭi as a softening tension in and behind the eyeballs while we release the palate. Releasing the palate invites the dṛṣṭi to become integrated into the entire structure of the body, because the root of the palate is the kingpin of all the Prāṇa movements—that is, all the sensations throughout the body. Releasing the palate is a true art in that it corresponds to the letting go of technique. To begin to release, you can subtly smile, listen closely as if to a distant sound, or imagine that you feel the palate and nasal septum as pleasantly luminous. Releasing the palate is also simply suspending the language-making function and the unencumbered flooding of the sense fields with Prāṇa. During breathing practices or āsana practices, while practicing dṛṣṭi, or in everyday life situations, if you get confused, feel tension or anger, become lost in thought, or doubt yourself, simply release your palate. See what happens.

Symbolically, releasing the palate can be thought of as the act of allowing the nectar of compassion to penetrate every cell of your body. From a yogic perspective, the root of the palate, just behind the pituitary gland, is called the *candra* (moon). This moon is visualized as lying at the base of the thousand-petaled lotus flower, the *sahasrāra,* that rests in the crown of the head. Like a mirror, the moon has a pure, reflective openness with no form of its own—a selfless, discriminating awareness. It serves as a reservoir for the nectar generated by the mind when intelligence is finally applied. The nectar is called *amṛta* (literally, "no death"), truly the nectar of immortality. Its main ingredient is *karuṇā* (compassion). We each have a limitless stash of this nectar at the root of our own palate, if only we knew how to access it!

BANDHA

Bandhas are sometimes referred to as points of contraction, binding, or bonding within the body; however, thinking of them as merely some muscle squeezings can stimulate subtle levels of tension. Instead, it is better to consider bandhas as areas within the body where complementary patterns join or bond. Bandhas are specific areas where we focus on the concentrated organization of opposing patterns that flow throughout the whole body. In a manner of speaking, bandhas serve as internal gazing points; they are seed-points of clear attention from which integrated movement, thought, emotion, and Prāṇa unfold all around.

As with correct ujjāyī breathing and proper dṛṣṭi, the cultivation of bandhas is a powerful way of setting the flow of Prāṇa into patterns that pull the mind toward meditation. Bandhas involve distinct muscular patterns and equally distinct patterns of sensation that are organized as a background to the area of focus. When the bandha is perceived as the linking together of complementary patterns, then the foreground and background come into full relationship. The sense of effort and tension initially involved in the production of the bandha melts away, and the bandha transforms into a whole-body pattern and movement.

Three interrelated bandhas are most frequently associated with Aṣṭāṅga Vinyāsa yoga: *Jālandhara*, *Uḍḍīyāna*, and *Mūlabandhas*. When learning about and beginning practices that allow you to cultivate the bandhas, it is important to be attentive, calm, and patient and—particularly when first starting—to visualize muscular patterns that you associate with the specific bandha. Closely tuning in to the general area of the body that is related to the bandha is the first step, and imagining that you are doing the bandha correctly (even if you're not sure) is an excellent place to start. Over time, your familiarity with the individual areas of the body associated with each of the bandhas and your ability to tune in to and control muscular patterns in these areas will improve. Keeping the palate empty and released, the tongue quiet, the breath smooth with a clear gentle sound, and the dṛṣṭi steady helps to create an internal environment in which the bandha may manifest. In addition, it is vital to weave the appropriate phase of the breath into the bandha practice—paying attention to the physical and mental impact of both inhaling and exhaling flow patterns, as well as noticing shifts in thought and sensation that arise during any gap at the transition when one breath turns into the next.

Jālandhara Bandha

In some ways, Jālandhara Bandha, which is usually practiced in a seated position, is the easiest of the bandhas to approximate and therefore is a good starting place for bandha practice. It is the only one of the three classic bandhas that has a blatantly obvious external form.

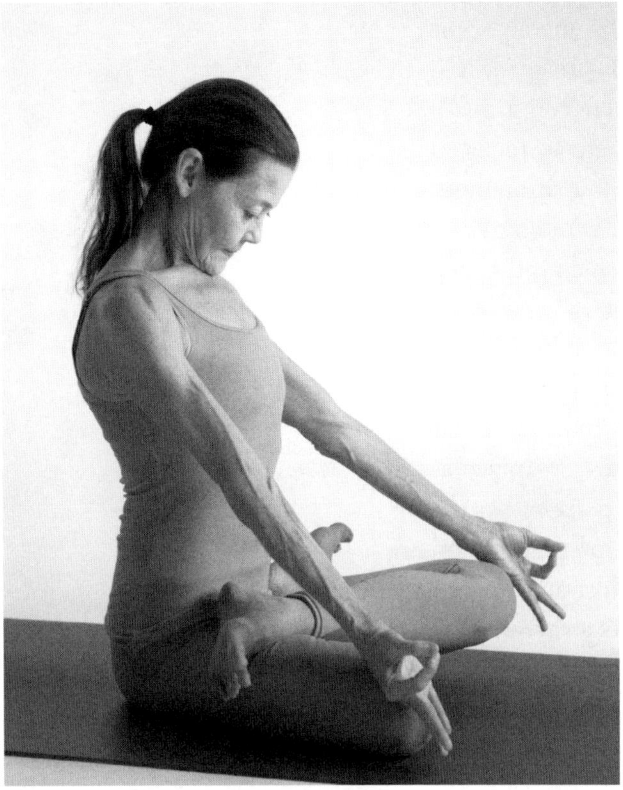

1. To begin experimenting with Jālandhara Bandha, sit straight in a comfortable position either on the floor or in a chair. Bring awareness to the central axis of the body and the sensation of being grounded by focusing on the parts of the body that touch the floor or the chair.
2. The spine should be elongated, with no strain in the muscles that support it. Notice how easily the heart area floats upward on an inhalation. In the gap at the top of the inhalation, lower the head forward, bowing so that the chin nestles down into the sternum. If dropping the chin to the sternum is not possible, a small scarf or washcloth may be rolled up and tucked under the chin to allow for support.
3. There is a feeling of spaciousness and softness in front of the throat—almost as if the chin were being lifted gently over and around a small, soft ball placed in front of the Adam's apple. Do not draw the chin back toward the cervical spine or press it down to make it touch the sternum. The buoyancy of the heart is so bright and distinct that the chin comes adoringly down as if to crown the heart.

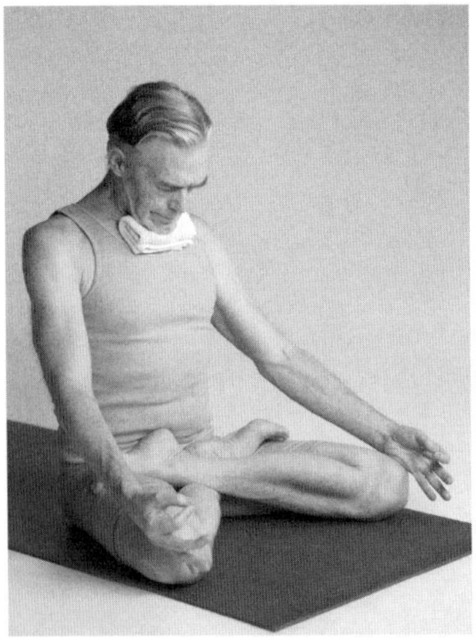

4. The middle line of the palate feels bright and high within the head. Although the lower portion of the neck is flexed, the upper cervical area near the head is not. Sitting this way is called "Jālandhara Bandha position," but it is not yet the actual bandha just as ujjāyī breathing is not quite full Ujjāyī Prāṇāyāma. Both of these distinctions can cause some confusion for beginning students. The position serves as the physical scaffolding for Jālandhara Bandha itself, and the position may be practiced while doing smooth ujjāyī breathing in Padmāsana (Lotus Pose), Daṇḍāsana (Staff Pose), and other seated poses.

5. Jālandhara Bandha holds all of the physical and breathing patterns associated with the Jālandhara position, but it has the additional element of retaining the breath at the crest of the inhalation and, occasionally (during the full Uḍḍīyāna Bandha), at the end of the exhalation. When you are first learning to practice Jālandhara Bandha, you should hold the retention for just a few seconds. After much practice, you may carefully extend the length of the retention.
6. In correct Jālandhara Bandha, the muscles in front of the neck are toned, the palate is released, and there is absolutely no strain in the tongue or jaw. The gaze is downcast along the nose, either internally or with the eyes half-open. The ears are open, and the body is quite still. The key to this bandha is in the throat, where the exaggerated, full, and expansive prāṇa pattern is allowed to meet the full forward-curling pattern of the apāna. This makes the shape of the upper body, when practicing Jālandhara Bandha, resemble that of a swan sleeping with its head resting peacefully on its large chest.

Mūlabandha

On the other end of the spine, the pelvic floor (which by no coincidence, is related reflexively to the palate) is the territory of Mūlabandha. Although Mūlabandha is talked about frequently, it is possibly the most misunderstood and difficult of the three bandhas to practice. For this reason, Chapter 3 explores it in detail. Simply stated, Mūlabandha is a subtle toning and lifting at the center of the pelvic floor. It is not something that can be grabbed and held by contracting the pelvic floor muscles, although you can start there to bring awareness to the correct general area of the body. Instead, Mūlabandha is invited to appear. It is the contracting pattern of the apāna that pulls into a seed-point at the center of the pelvic floor, ignited like a flame, and lifted by the process of Uḍḍīyāna Bandha. The muscular contraction pattern of the pelvic floor becomes a meditation on sensation flow patterns as the pelvic floor muscles fluctuate from strong to subtle and the bandha is cultivated.

Working to perfect Mūlabandha is key to enhancing an āsana practice (and to beginning and deepening your prāṇāyāma and meditation practices), because all poses ground through the seed-point of Mūlabandha and, on a more external level, the pelvic floor. Mūlabandha is the core of the core of all integrated movement. It is the process of communication across the pelvic floor from side to side and from front to back, and it becomes the platform for an engaged, meditative flow of poses. For most of us, Mūlabandha is initially understood through the practice and development of Uḍḍīyāna Bandha.

Uḍḍīyāna Bandha

Uḍḍīyāna Bandha, which literally means the "flying up bandha," comes in two forms. The full form is used on retention of the exhalation and involves passively drawing the entire abdomen, above and below the naval, back and up by contracting the auxiliary muscles used for inhaling.

1. Stand with the feet about hip-width apart. Place the hands on the upper thighs and exhale as you bend the knees slightly to fold forward.
2. As the groins deepen, push with the hands and elongate the spine slightly, but do not give in to the temptation to overly arch or overly straighten the spine. The arms should be fairly straight as you push into the femurs, with moderate pressure.
3. Placing the hands farther down near the knees tends to favor the prāṇa pattern, making the lumbar spine extend more. Placing the hands near the tops of the thighs is more effective, allowing the addition of Mūlabandha and other patterns in the abdomen.
4. At this point, after completing the exhalation, the auxiliary muscles that normally fire when inhaling—*but not the respiratory diaphragm*—are engaged. No air is drawn into the lungs. The result is that the muscular pattern associated with inhaling manifests: the ribcage expands and the abdominal cavity is automatically sucked up and back without effort. Hold this for just a few seconds. (The time of the retention, *kumbhaka,* can be extended very gradually over many months of practice.)
5. Maintain this position and the retention of the exhalation as you release the muscles associated with inhaling. This will allow the belly to drop. Give a slight puff to punctuate the end of the exhalation. Slowly begin to inhale smoothly as you return to standing.

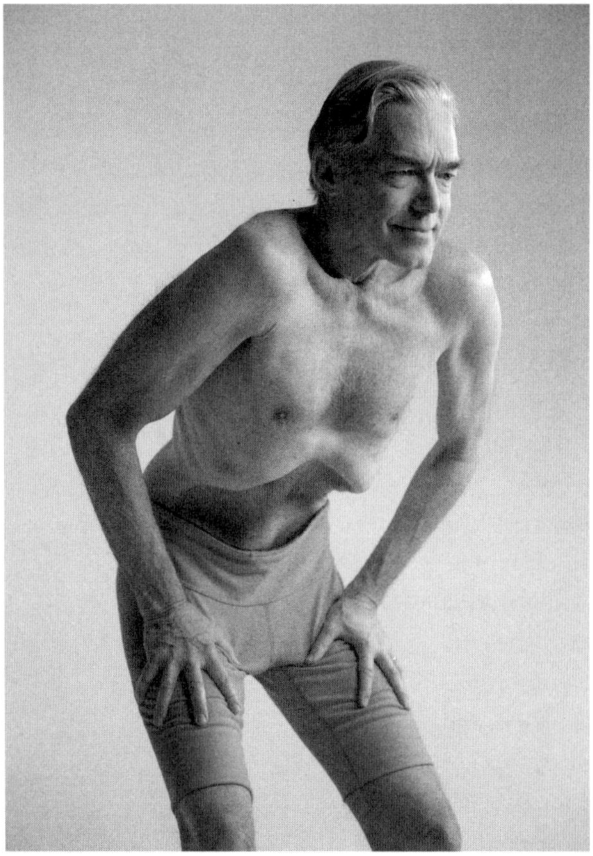

This same action can also be practiced while lying on your back and eventually while sitting. In full Uḍḍīyāna Bandha, we can imagine that we're scooping out the entire abdominal cavity with the spoon of the mind, as if we are cleaning the front surface of the iliopsoas muscles and the pelvic floor itself, as well as hollowing out the area around the diaphragm. This is both stimulating and balancing to these myofascial structures.

Mini Uḍḍīyāna Bandha

Once you have developed the full Uḍḍīyāna, a more subtle and profound form eventually manifests. It is like a miniature version of this full form. The "mini" Uḍḍīyāna Bandha takes time to cultivate and is therefore considered more advanced than the full form already described. Mini Uḍḍīyāna Bandha is practiced during prāṇāyāma and while working in āsana by distinctly toning the myofascial structures that lie deep within the body beneath the pot of the belly. The pattern of Uḍḍīyāna Bandha comes up no higher than two inches below the naval and is practiced during the course of inhaling and the retention of the breath at the top of the inhalation. It creates a space above the pelvic floor in the cave of the sacrum and allows you to feel that the center point of the perineum is being drawn up and back. This muscular pattern stimulates the appearance of Mūlabandha. Mini Uḍḍīyāna Bandha is accomplished by keeping the lowest horizontal band of the transversus abdominis muscle toned and, at the same time, keeping the psoas and quadratus lumborum (QL) muscles relaxed throughout the inhaling movement. The action is part of a scooping pattern in the front of the body that causes a feeling of a cobra hood pattern on the back of the body. It induces a distinct drawing together and ascension at the mūla, or the center of the perineum.

This description of the mini Uḍḍīyāna Bandha is not used by most surviving lineages of hatha yoga; its action is taught as part of Mūlabandha alone. Because mini Uḍḍīyāna and Mūlabandha are central to the teaching of Aṣṭāṅga Vinyāsa yoga, this distinction has been a source of confusion for many practitioners who have tried to learn from books rather than personal instruction from a teacher—which is the preferred method for learning the bandhas.

Bandha practice stimulates an internal focus and is a good place to start as you develop the skill of contemplating the central channel of the body. Within this contemplation and when all three bandhas are practiced in the correct manner, the prāṇa and apāna fully unite. When this happens, you may perceive the whole body and the entire world as balanced, empty, or open, like a flower in full bloom.

NAULI

From the practice of full Uḍḍīyāna Bandha, there gradually evolves an ability to add some distinctly opposite and complementary movements that balance the patterns of the pelvic floor, the respiratory diaphragm,

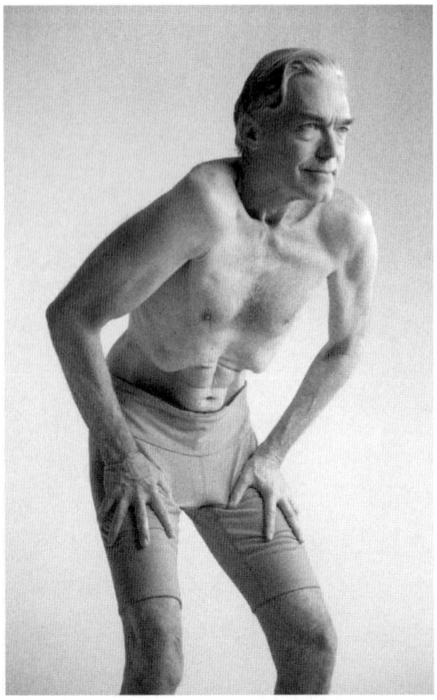
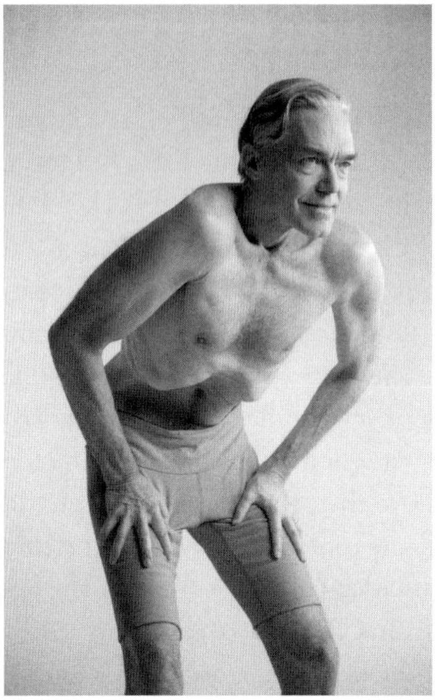
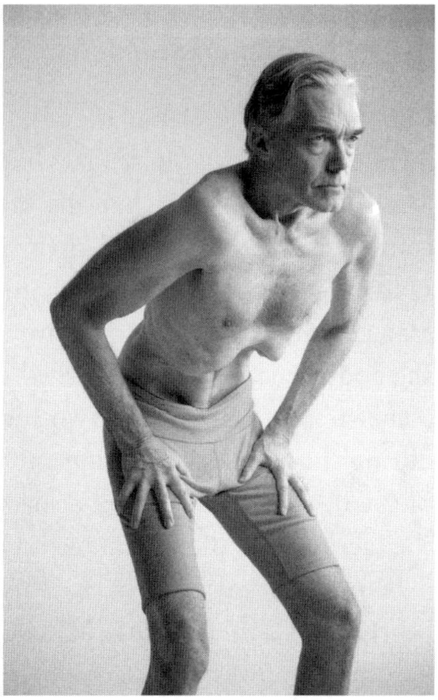
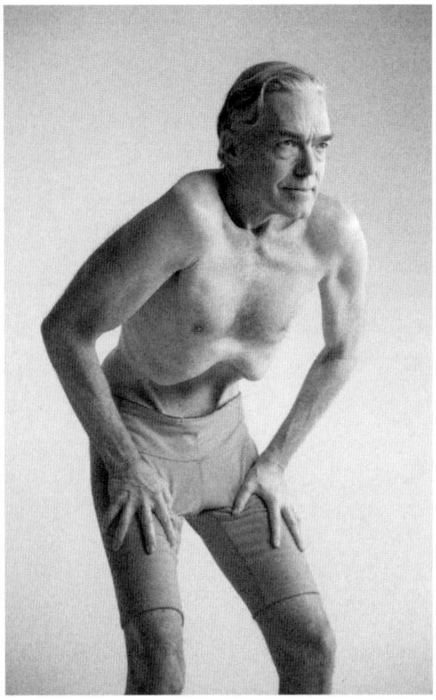

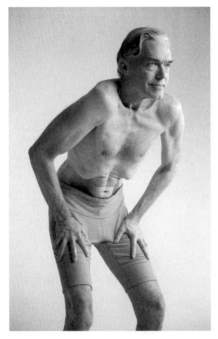

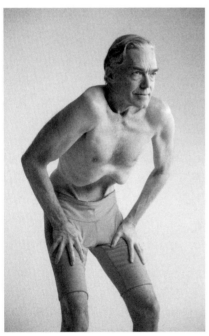

and the abdominal wall. These abdominal movements are called *nauli,* a rolling wave in the abdomen:

1. While standing, lean forward after a full exhalation, placing your hands on the upper thighs. Suck the entire abdomen back toward the spine. (See the earlier instructions for Uḍḍīyāna Bandha.)
2. Holding the well-developed and clean Uḍḍīyāna Bandha, press the hands down on the thighs to contract only the rectus abdominis muscle in the abdominal wall. This paired muscle will stand out as two parallel columns. After some weeks of practice, when the form is distinct, move on to the next step.
3. Start releasing the pressure from the hands, and then press harder with one hand than with the other hand. This will cause the muscles on that side only to stand out, and the oblique muscles on the same side will start to tone. Practice this until you can contract both sides independently.
4. Next, practice rolling the contraction from side to side by alternating the pressure of the hands on the thighs. One direction is usually easier than the other, but practice rolling in both directions diligently.
5. Further practice allows you to isolate the oblique muscles. At that point, more precise patterns of rolling can evolve.
6. Whenever you release Uḍḍīyāna Bandha and/or nauli, first relax the auxiliary inhaling muscles that created the full Uḍḍīyāna Bandha. This allows the belly to fall (like jelly) to its soft, normal, ball-like

form. Then exhale a little puff of air to reset the perineum to its end-of-exhalation seed of apāna tone. Inhale as smoothly and evenly as possible, using the underbelly scooping of Mūlabandha.

7. Fill up to the brim with breath, release the palate, and enjoy keeping the center of the heart open throughout the next exhalation.

MUDRĀ

The most subtle internal form of the practice is mudrā. *Mudrā* can have many meanings, including a seal, a mark, a ritualized gesture of joining together, or specific hand or finger positions used to focus the mind. In the context of this yoga practice, mudrā is the internal pattern that occurs within the body when a bandha is practiced flawlessly, and like bandhas, mudrās must be carefully, patiently attended to and invited to appear.

Two classic mudrās associated with an āsana practice are *Khecarī Mudrā* and *Yoni Mudrā,* both of which are points of union at opposite ends along the central channel of the body—the tongue and the pelvic floor, respectively. As we work toward these two mudrās in our yoga practice, we initially begin by exploring bandhas. As the bandhas become more established, the mudrās appear. But at first we're just practicing and trying to get some stream of sensation that grabs our attention in the general physical areas associated with the mudrās. After years—if not lifetimes—of practice, the bandhas may transmute into the deeper level of experience we call mudrā.

Khecarī Mudrā

At the top of the central channel where we find Khecarī Mudrā, we allow the energy of the tongue—the tip of which is placed near the root of the palate—to move into open space or emptiness. In this mudrā, all the fluctuations of the tongue and Prāṇa cease, and Prāṇa is then established in the central channel. Of course, true Khecarī Mudrā position—placing the tip of the tongue way back and up behind the soft palate right under the sphenoid sinus—is nearly impossible. Some extreme practitioners work at it by stretching the tongue muscle and slowly, over time, severing the frenulum (the tendon beneath the tongue) to achieve this position. Others consider those measures to be extreme, because you can attain the benefits of Khecarī Mudrā without actually cutting the tendon and placing the tip of the tongue against the sphenoid sinus behind the palate. Such zealous efforts are likely to carry negative consequences that make "achieving" the mudrā ineffective. For most people, it is better to find Khecarī Mudrā in a more subtle way.

One method is by practicing what is called *Jihvā Bandha*. Open your mouth wide, while firmly pressing the tip of your tongue into the hard palate. This action stretches the frenulum, and if you can make scary noises or demonic faces while you do this bandha, then you're doing it right. With practice, Jihvā Bandha can stimulate the same internal response as Khecarī Mudrā: complete concentration and absorption of mind, emotion, and thought, as well as a feeling of clarity into the top part of the central channel. Another approach to Khecarī Mudrā is to focus on the feeling of compassion or the experience of aesthetic satisfaction and simply feel how the tongue is already in natural contact with the palate as if there were a slight electrical current or magnetic attraction at the area of contact. Combined with soft dṛṣṭi, a release at the root of the palate occurs, and the Khecarī Mudrā practice is well under way.

Yoni Mudrā

> **pādamūlena sampīḍya gudāmārgaṁ suyantritam**
> **balādapānamākṛṣya kramādūrdhvaṁ sucārayet**
> **kalpito 'yaṁ mūlabandho jarāmaraṇa nāśanaḥ**
> **apānaprāṇayoraikyaṁ prakarotya vikampitam**
> **bandhenānena sutarāṁ yonimudrā prasiddhyati**
> **siddhāyāṁ yonimudrāyām kiṁ na siddhyati bhūtale**
>
> Completely press the anus with the heel. Slowly and strongly pull the apāna up in steps. This Mūlabandha destroys the decay of old age and death and insures a firm union of apāna and prāṇa. By means of this bandha the perfection of Yoni Mudrā comes without effort. What in this world cannot be achieved with the accomplishment of Yoni Mudrā.
>
> —*Śiva Saṁhitā,* ch. 4, v. 64–66

At the other end of the central channel, we have Yoni Mudrā, or the perfection of Mūlabandha and the bonding together of prāṇa and apāna in the epicenter of the pelvic floor—the mūla. These two complementary patterns, which are two ends of the same stick, can be represented as male and female; the prāṇa governing inhalation creates certain expansive body patterns that we associate with the feminine, and the apāna governing exhalation creates flexion in the spine that we associate with the masculine. Once you begin to fully understand this union of opposites on all different levels, you may begin to feel it in every pore of the skin, and that's when Yoni Mudrā starts to work. You feel a sort of humming in the pelvic floor that is almost a short-circuiting of logical thought, a paradoxical feeling of two complementary opposites arising simultaneously and conjoining across the pelvic floor.

When you practice (and practice and practice) Mūlabandha and Yoni Mudrā, and you start to feel them in relation to the structure of the whole body—even through the head, shoulders, hands, feet, front and back, inner body and outer body—you begin to experience how all of those patterns flow into and back out of the pelvic floor. This experience is illusive, especially if you think about it too much, and that is why many practitioners find visualization practices powerful; these practices are not directed by the mind, but arise spontaneously. All of the patterns of Prāṇa in the body bounce off of or root into the pelvic floor and come back out, just like a tree roots into the earth in order to grow. This happens moment by moment within the field of Prāṇa. When you start to feel that union of rooting and expansiveness and add to it the quality of compassion that comes from Khecarī Mudrā, *then* Mūlabandha can be called Yoni Mudrā.

Tāḍāgī Mudrā

Tāḍāgī Mudrā, the pond mudrā, is one of a number of little-known almost-secret gems. It is like a very pleasant stiffened Corpse Pose and is used within a number of Vinyāsa sequences.

1. Lie down flat on your back with the legs together. Lightly press the sides of the big toes together as if holding a coin between them. Turn the palms down so the entire thumb and index finger of each hand is on the floor. This broadens the back to enhance the apāna pattern.
2. Tilt the chin down slightly, as if the skin on the back of the head were being spread and pulled up like a cobra's hood. In this form, smooth, high-quality ujjāyī breathing is initially used to produce full breath waves with natural gaps at the ends of the breaths.
3. Keep the dṛṣṭi steady, soft, and downcast to release the palate, allowing the proper rhythms and proportions throughout the body.
4. At the top of each inhalation, notice that the prāṇa pattern lightly pushes the head back into the floor. If you choose to add full Uḍḍīyāna Bandha at the end of an exhalation, notice the same slight pushing back of the head during the retention of the breath. Remember to relax the abdomen and exhale a tiny puff more before inhaling smoothly.

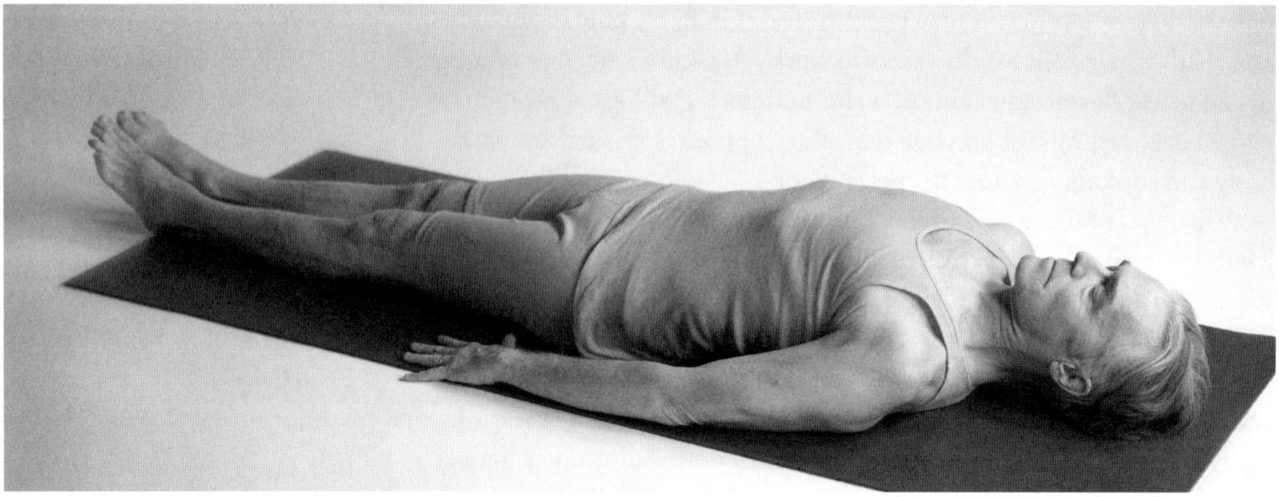

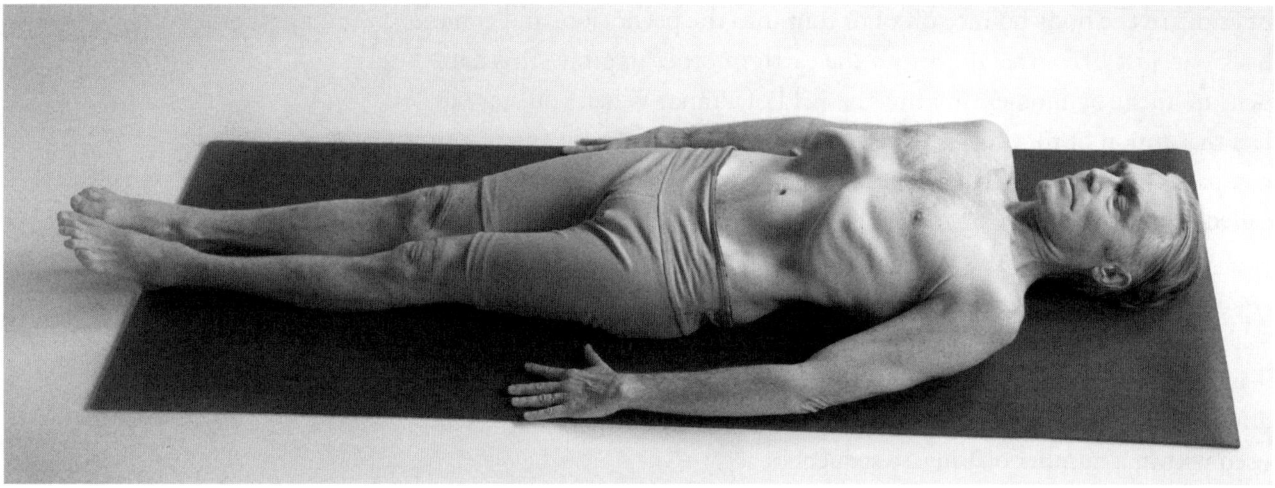

These classic mudrās demonstrate why *mudrā* means "seal," or the perfection of bandha, and cannot be achieved through force, but require strong, focused, and consistent practice. Bandha (and eventually mudrā) practice *must* be carried out for the sake of the practice itself, with no sense of striving, if it is to evolve into full form—there must be no attachment to the fruit of the practice. Otherwise the mind gets involved, makes overly simple reductionist formulas, and then tries too hard. Ego slips in and co-opts the situation. Bandha and mudrā practice is what a vinyāsa practice really is: the sequential joining together and separating of complementary opposites as a means of staying present, mindful, and alert to the feelings, thoughts, sensations, and insights that may—or may not—arise.

This joining together might seem an abstract and confusing task, yet it is actually something we do all the time, whether or not we're even aware of it. For instance, you may think, "I want to be wide awake and eager, and I want to be relaxed too." For most of us, these mind states are total opposites. So throughout the week you drink coffee, and Friday night you drink beer! Through yoga, we learn to manifest both mind states simultaneously.

INTERNAL CHANNELS: THE NĀḌĪS

By bringing awareness to the nuances of alignment that are revealed through the internal forms of practice, we discover a gateway to understanding the *nāḍī* system, part of the innermost structure and scaffolding of the practice. *Nāḍī* means "channel" or "little river" in Sanskrit, and from a yogic perspective, the nāḍīs are an intricate system of rivulets of Prāṇa and energy that flow through and penetrate every area of the body. From a Western perspective, the nāḍī system could be considered somewhat parallel to the combination of the nervous and circulatory systems. The nāḍīs bring a vibratory quality of breath and awareness to every point of sensation within the body.

As mentioned earlier, there is one central nāḍī, the suṣumṇā nāḍī, from which all other smaller nāḍīs (or rivers of Prāṇa) flow. Again and again in our yoga practice, we bring awareness into this central channel of the body so there is gradually a feeling of the practice spontaneously arising as an internalized perspective from this area of the subtle body. When we begin practicing yoga, the imagination wakes up and we may envision actually *having* a central channel. Whatever image sparks a sense of something vibrant in the core of the body will do—a hollow reed, like you might see growing up out of a glassy pond; a beam of light; or even an amorphous yet somehow contained feeling of spaciousness in the core of the body up through the heart area. Anything that helps you cultivate inner awareness along what you perceive as a "central channel" is what you're after.

In more esoteric forms of practice, practitioners also imagine that Prāṇa is behaving as the serpent (*Kuṇḍalinī*) that coils, sleeping on the pelvic floor at the base of the suṣumṇā nāḍī. It is said that until the serpent is awakened and begins to move in the central channel, the entire system of nāḍīs is unbalanced, with some nāḍīs being overstimulated and others blocked. But as beginners, we are content to imagine a simple central channel into which we may occasionally find the capacity to tap.

In addition to the suṣumṇā nāḍī, there are two other large, accessible nāḍīs. Both are said to connect to and open into their respective side of the pelvic floor alongside the suṣumṇā nāḍī. They ascend through the head and cross behind the eyes (not unlike the optic nerves) to join the sides of the *ājñā* (command/understand) cakra, behind the middle of the eyebrows. They correspond directly to the flow of the breath in the nostrils, and they wax and wane in relation to each other as different moods and thoughts come and go. Some systems of imagery cross them or channel them into the sides of whatever cakra is to be contemplated, while other systems keep them parallel to each other on opposite sides of the suṣumṇā. Paying attention to the streams of sensation associated with breath flow in these channels is initially an excellent way to calm and focus the mind for meditation.

The right channel, or sun channel, is called *piñgālā,* which means "bright, hot, warm, or sun." Piñgālā has a fixed, confident quality associated with the solar attitude of "Yes, I know the way. I know what to do!" You need to have this quality to function throughout the day and take practical actions. But this piñgālā quality can create anxiety in situations where you cannot know what something ultimately is, like the beauty of a butterfly or the intentions of another. An overly dominant piñgālā can make it difficult to rest in a state of not knowing. Of course in terms of questions like "Should I eat now or later?" you want to be able to make a decision and so piñgālā energy serves an important, perfectly divine function. In a way, waking up the energy of this channel is somewhat like pouring courage into your right nostril. But we all know that the downside of being too confident is that you may start to skip over the plurality, the multiplicity, the depth of what is going on; you cease to appreciate all the different viewpoints and different levels and gradations of beings that are participating in this entire process of life.

The moon channel on the left is called the *idā.* It cools you off and leaves you stunned at the beauty of multiplicity. The two channels, the piñgālā and the idā, are just like day and night. In the day, one star called the sun takes over, a single story line, a dominant point of view. Ah, but then night comes, other stories, other viewpoints and contexts gradually appear. Soon a million stars fill the sky and *you* disappear in the starry night. You start to contemplate enormous distances and spans of time, intuitively understanding the relativity of everything. You feel tiny, and you realize that even our solar system is in the middle of nowhere; you disappear into the vastness of that plurality, that multiplicity. It's beautiful, but of course it can also be dysfunctional at the wrong time of day.

Within the nāḍī system, there is a clear oscillation between opposites, two things that are interdependent: the singularity of structure and the plurality that reveals the openness of that structure. In the center, when the channels are balanced and the invitation for awareness (or Kuṇḍalinī) to move in the central channel is received, there is brilliance as well as balance.

CAKRAS

Another brilliant aspect of traditional imagery that invites an internalized, contemplative mind, is the cakra system; through this, we meditate on various stations along the central channel that correspond to distinct sensation patterns and perceptual modes. Cakras (wheels) are usually represented and felt as lotus flowers or *padmas.* They are strung together like a garland along the suṣumṇā nāḍī. They are imagined to be sacred spaces ranging in detail from simple geometrical yantras to elaborate maṇḍalas, temples, islands, and whole worlds populated with gods, goddesses, and (potentially) all beings. Cakras or padmas function to capture and absorb our attention fully and then to balance and deepen our insight into the actual nature of what we are experiencing. Each petal or segment of every cakra needs to be interlinked with its complementary opposites and then with its deeper background.

Smooth ujjāyī breathing introduces the natural vinyāsa of the attention to balance and illuminate the cakras. Evenly illuminated, brought to life and vibrancy, they open into the middle path of the suṣumṇā nāḍī at the center of each padma where the nectar from the root of the palate can be felt. In normal distracted breathing, it is likely to feel as though half the petals are wilted while others are overinflated. But with mindful ujjāyī breathing practice, there is a sense of calm alertness within the body and mind, and the garland along the central channel feels alive, awakened, and evenly innervated.

TRUSTING THE PROCESS

We may harbor a lot of resistance toward dropping in and practicing from an internal perspective. The fear of feeling—deep inside the body—certain things like infinity, impermanence, emptiness, or the fact that there is no ultimate frame of reference, can be terrifying. Yet it is for this very reason that the practices emphasizing the internal forms are so important and why we must take them slowly and work at them with great patience and kindness toward ourselves. This is why a teacher encourages beginning students simply to have a direct experience within their own bodies of what it actually *feels* like to take a full, deep inhale and a smooth, long exhale, and why approaching these internal forms directly through āsana practice is vital.

As an eager student, you may start with Mūlabandha practice and then sometime later realize there is more subtlety to the practice than just squeezing the anal sphincter muscle. Over the course of years and years, you finally realize that it's really just a matter of paying attention to a process that is already there. With even more time, you find yourself back at the beginning, and you see that prāṇa and apāna (or Śiva and Śakti) are already united at the center of the pelvic floor. Then Mūlabandha—experienced as a flame of pure *cit,* pure attention, or pure intelligence—spontaneously arises. It's not a contraction or the release of a contraction. It's not a noncontraction, it's not both, and it's not neither. It's just pure intelligence, and it refuses to reduce the goddess to a theory of the goddess. The internal forms, particularly Mūlabandha, support the practice inside and out and are awakening and transformative.

There are basically two approaches in hatha yoga. One is the approach that works on Mūlabandha and tries to collect and control everything. This approach is called *bindu dhāraṇa,* or a single-pointed focus on a specific seed or droplet (bindu) of awareness. In this practice, you hold the bindu still. Many schools of hatha yoga are based on this approach, and in fact, Aṣṭāṅga Vinyāsa yoga is initially presented this way. Fortunately a little of the opposite approach to hatha yoga can be mixed into a seasoned Aṣṭāṅga Vinyāsa practice to offer even deeper insight. This second approach is called the *amṛta plavana,* or the flooding of the whole system with nectar, and this is what eventually occurs when we practice bandha and mudrā. All of the minor canals, nāḍīs, and rivers of Prāṇa throughout the body are awakened and balanced. It's a flood of compassion. Actually you can't do a complete yoga practice without embracing both bindu dhāraṇa and amṛta plavana. You have to work with form, discipline, and the tight interweaving of reductionist theories of technique. And you must then also be able to let go, loosening so that a whole living reality can flow between them.

2

Aligning Intention and Action

Where the Rubber Meets the Road

MANY OF US FIND OUR WAY TO YOGA IN A SEARCH for reality—looking for answers to questions such as "Who am I?" and "What is the meaning of life?" As we tune in again and again to the ends of the breath or the vastness of the gaze, a flash of insight may occasionally arise and reveal the interpenetrating nature of all things: *everything* relates to everything else and consequently is in constant flux. That is the nature of reality, of who we are and why we're here. Understanding this, we see that many important questions are ultimately unanswerable. That doesn't mean they are not worth asking; in fact, quite the opposite. A steady and stable practice shows us how vital it is to maintain a sense of inquisitiveness so that we remain inspired by posing and re-posing questions to which we think we already know the answers. As we patiently stay the course and practice for the sake of practice, the boundless joy that resides deep within each of us spontaneously arises. This is what it means to practice yoga and to experience the cohesive nature of reality.

The view of relationship as the essence of life and reality is something we have all intimately experienced firsthand. We enter this world tied to our mother through the umbilical cord. Shortly after birth, that deepest of all bonds—the primordial physical relationship of literally being tied through a lifeline to another human being—is severed. So in some ways, from that moment forth, we might say that as we navigate our way through life, there is an instinctual interest in regaining our natural homeostasis of being intimately in relationship. We are programmed to connect and reconnect, to form bonds with other beings on a core level. Breathing—as if from the root of our navel—becomes a means of unscrambling the puzzle of how all the working parts of this world come together to make sense.

UMBILICAL BREATHING

Being connected to life and the universe through the navel is an image that figures prominently in Indian mythology and iconography. It is said that Brahmā was born from the navel of Viṣṇu, and Viṣṇu is often pictured reclining on Ādiśeṣa (the primodial residue, the serpent of infinity) with a lotus flower—symbolizing unbounded creation and clear mind—growing out of his navel, the *nābhi cakra* which is also called the maṇipūra cakra. A visualization practice that can awaken this primal sense of connection is to imagine yourself, in exquisite detail, as Viṣṇu; relaxed, content, and happy, you recline on the comfortable sofa of support offered by your loyal attendant and vehicle, Ādiśeṣa. Deep in the core of the body, between your belly button and your spine, there is a warm, solidly rooted feeling that pulsates smoothly up and down the central channel and also radiates out. As you breathe, this feeling gently penetrates your skin, and delicate extensions of creative energy, like the petals of a lotus flower, bloom and automatically connect, as if through a strong magnetic attraction, to the world's vast and intricate web of existence. The feeling is organic and deeply emotional. It could be called "umbilical breathing." Resting with such an image for a moment, you might experience a feeling of connection unfolding, dissolving, re-forming, and disappearing, an ever-changing sense of relating to others from deep within your own core. Of course, like other visualization practices, this is one to visit and release, since you know full well that if you did find yourself with a lotus flower growing out of your navel (or worse yet, believed and proclaimed such a thing in its absence), you'd be rushed to an emergency room for immediate attention!

You can also feel this depth of connection by simply *visualizing* that the yoga practices actually work, that you have insight into relationship as the core of existence, and that you celebrate the opportunity to ask the important questions again and again. Through this practice, we find that even though we repeatedly ask the difficult questions with our intellect and emotions, we're also inquiring on a deeper, embodied level.

This means we keep the experience of the "other" in the foreground of our awareness, and although we draw conclusions, we continuously let go of even those theories and techniques that seem useful and contextually correct, as if the root of the navel is the unfolding ground for the intense radiance of true relationship and the actual nature of being.

In a yoga practice inspired from this depth within our core, we can step down off the cloud of illusion that pictures self as separate from other and walk around *seeing* everything and having insight into the true nature of things. We are able to trust in not knowing exactly what we are encountering, comfortable in upgrading our methodology and understanding. Without a deep, visceral rooting (as if from our own navel), yoga and relationships gradually break off from reality and float away as disembodied, abstract stories and dreams.

Through practice, we find that focal points consciously selected for meditation pass through the window of awareness and are met with an inquiring mind. In this way, each time they arise, they are brand-new, yet there is always something familiar about them that we know to be true, and it becomes clear that everything is built on this open awareness.

THE YAMAS AND NIYAMAS

We practice in an intelligent and disciplined manner in the service of truth. This ensures that the practices remain in the practical realm of relating to the world and other sentient beings in a joyful and unselfish way. In texts such as the Yoga Sūtra, the Upaniṣads, and the *Haṭha Yoga Pradīpikā,* ethical underpinnings or guidelines for behavior on which other practices rest are called the *yamas* and the *niyamas.* The precise list and number of yamas and niyamas vary from text to text, with some identifying fifteen yamas, and others fewer. In the Yoga Sūtra, the yamas and niyamas are identified as the first two limbs of the eight-limbed path of Aṣṭāṅga yoga, indicating their importance and their underlying purpose of providing a grounded and non-self-centered context based on relationship with others, from which our practice may grow.

The Yamas

Having a taste of the nature of reality and our intrinsic intimacy with all other beings, certain imperatives, or yamas, present themselves. From a truly yogic perspective, each of the thousand and one choices we must make every day has to be based on the necessity of love and relationship and a clear perception of reality. Many of the major choices we face must be calculated around our self-interest or the interests of our family, friends, or community. Consequently, conflicts and ethical dilemmas are inevitable, and poor choices at these times can have deleterious effects on many fronts.

The yamas address the issues that arise in difficult situations that cause suffering and confusion. They provide guidelines for decision making and actions that not only allow us to consider our self-interest but also set a context for understanding the impact that our choices and behaviors may have on others. When, in our everyday perspective, we embrace the notion that everything we do is in relationship and therefore has some impact on others, then all our choices—especially those that have ethical nuances—hit us deeply on the visceral, subtle levels of the body that are designed to inform us when we are acting in alignment with what we know to be true (our "gut" feelings). The yamas offer a full, wholesome context within which we learn to act ethically from a place of truth, kindness, and compassion. Equally, we see that if the yamas are taken as steadfast rules and regulations, if they are applied blindly or with our own self-interest in the forefront, then they may cause harm.

Ahiṁsā, the first of the yamas, means to not kill or harm. On a simpler level, ahiṁsā just means to be nice. This refers to being nice to ourselves as well as to other beings. Because of the nature of biological life, we are largely unaware of the effect of our actions on many species, so we do the best we can, seeing ourselves in all beings and acting accordingly.

Like everything else, the yamas are embedded in an understanding of relationship and, in fact, have a special link with one another—as each is built on and stems from this first yama and the notion of nonharming. So even if you are a dedicated and sincere yoga practitioner, if you apply ahiṁsā (or any of the other yamas) without considering the bigger picture within which the specific situation has arisen and how your actions may affect yourself and others, then you run the risk of acting unskillfully or harmfully. Many ethical dilemmas arise from strict rules around nonviolence. Imagine the difficult choices made when having to protect one being from another, from having to protect innocent children from aggressors like germs, psychopaths, or even terrorists. You might have to strike or even kill the aggressor (or pay someone to do it for you). A strict nonviolence rule will have to be violated. We must choose the least harmful way and forgive all involved. Often there is little time to make calculations before having to act in situations where inaction will bring huge suffering. Similar ethical dilemmas can arise in the field of medicine in emergency rooms and in situations where life and death lie in the balance. Dilemmas can even arise when we are dining with others—faced with dietary choices different from our own.

Just as we constantly refine yoga āsanas (hopefully in a way that is nonaggressive and nonharmful to our own body and noncompetitive with others), we have endlessly subtle aspects to practice in all the yamas. Ahiṁsā, when approached with a clear and kind mind, must be practiced while carefully weighing all aspects of any situation. The point is that you see the context of the situation, and considering all the available information, you make the best, kindest, least harmful choice of what action to take. When practiced in this way, ahiṁsā serves as the foundational yama from which all others unfold. Skillfully practicing ahiṁsā allows us to apply it and all of the yamas deftly rather than robotically.

The next yama, *satyam,* means honesty, though it is often translated as "truthfulness." Satyam asks us to face things as they are and to honestly assess the nature of how we *know* things to be "as they are." It also requires a willingness to make adjustments when we see our assessment is incorrect. When practicing satyam, we do not pretend to know what we don't know, taking action on the pretense of knowledge. By the same token, we do not plead ignorance and step aside when, in fact, we have enough information to allow us to act skillfully.

Honesty may be differentiated from truthfulness by an insight into how our actions may impact others and, given this insight, whether or not we should take action; this is how satyam builds on ahiṁsā. Practicing satyam is mostly a matter of common sense, though sometimes the appropriate choice can be unclear. Obviously, if a friend with an unfortunately large nose asks how he looks, we don't practice "truthfulness" by telling him his nose is huge. Instead, we practice honesty in the face of kindness and nonharming. When we practice satyam, we can face our own and others' suffering. It is particularly important in terms of satyam to keep questioning ourselves and our motives.

Asteya, the next yama, means to not steal. This, of course, means not forcibly taking from others that which they believe to be their own. But there are different degrees of stealing, and sometimes the mind is all too eager to rationalize why this or that isn't really "stealing." Taking something that is not rightfully our own can take many forms and may also cause varying degrees of damage. Asteya may be blatant, like stealing a car, or it can be subtle, like allowing your insecurity and greed to drive your actions within a friendship. It can also be more theoretical, like stealing ideas—plagiarism—or taking credit for thoughts that are not really your own.

The next yama, *Brahmacarya,* literally means "to act within Brahman," or to treat all beings as sacred or Brahman. By practicing Brahmacarya, we cultivate respect for others and maintain the perspective of not knowing, not assuming, and not introducing ego (even in the form of preconceptions) into conclusions, behaviors, and all forms of relationships. Traditionally Brahmacarya means to approach life as a student or a monk, someone who follows a disciplined and austere routine. Being a monk, of course, includes celibacy, and that is another sense of the word *Brahmacarya.* Esoterically, Brahmacarya means to move in the *Brahmā nāḍī,* which is the subtle channel inside the suṣumṇā nāḍī. Moving Prāṇa in the Brahmā nāḍī precludes the object-making reductionism created by an inflated ego and cancels any need or desire to seek satisfaction in exploitive relationships.

In a practical sense, Brahmacarya means that we do not separate ourselves from the rest of the world and the universe; rather, we experience ourselves as living, breathing organisms that are part of the bigger whole. We practice Brahmacarya as a demonstration of our desire to live in harmonious relationship with others. In terms of sexual activity, it is practiced within the context of nonharming, truthfulness, and not taking what is not ours. Brahmacarya implies that we never treat the sexual act or our partner from an egocentric perspective as an object for our personal gratification.

Brahmacarya is a particularly important yama to be addressed and carefully considered by any good yoga teacher. Sexual intimacy is an incredibly powerful act of sensation and emotion (not to mention relationship). Under these circumstances, the ego-driven mind has a powerful attraction to the pleasure involved in the act as well as the ego boost that results from being found attractive. So the ego is prone to overlook, warp, or rationalize a person's own belief system, or ethical standards, to experience the gratification of the sexual act. It is imperative that we be aware of the complexity of this specific yama, because those of us who are yoga teachers are in a position of power and trust in relation to our students. A teacher may claim that the sexual act with a consenting student is not outside the bounds of ethical behavior. However, just like with a priest, gang leader, or politician—anyone in a position of power—consent from someone who looks to you as a leader is not coming from a free, autonomous, integrated being. That form of consent is from an actor in the circle of the teacher's narcissism.

Aparigraha, the last of the yamas put forth by Patañjali, means not grasping, whether inside, outside on the gross level, or on the subtle levels. This is the constant discipline of cutting through desire and misappropriation in everything we think and all that we do. It is the ability to let go of our comparisons between self and others that can result in jealousy and instead to remain deeply rooted in the internal experience of being part of the vibrant, interpenetrating matrix of relationship called life. Contrary to what the ego-based mind thinks, our ability to let go of everything within the fabric of our experience by seeing it as empty of separate self provides true satisfaction.

The Niyamas

The niyamas are disciplined ways of taking action that facilitate our interaction within the world. They set a tone for understanding our own experiences and providing insight into relationship.

The first niyama, *śauca,* means purity or cleanliness. Not only does this refer to the obviously important act of cleaning our living space, but it also refers to cleaning our own bodies, both in terms of washing and caring for the body itself and eating a clean diet and maintaining good mental habits.

Purity or cleanliness on all levels is really a matter of taking care of loose ends. We resolve our misperceptions and unskillful actions so we can perceive everything in the world around us or inside us as part of life's background rather than pulling things out and giving them an emotional charge that perpetuates patterns of attachment and avoidance. In the language of yoga, this is the arising of *sattva,* or the harmonized, luminous state of intelligence that allows us to see things as they actually are. "Cleaning up" when taken literally, as in mopping the floor, or figuratively, as in improving our attitude, will often resolve ambiguous feelings of confusion or anxiety.

Saṁtoṣa, or contentment, is a pure and excellent form of happiness that spontaneously arises when we free ourselves from the mind's constant nagging about unfulfilled desires. This niyama allows us to appreciate things as they are rather than being disappointed, frustrated, or angry about our current circumstances. This is really the secret to moving on with our lives rather than being stuck in and trapped by a specific situation. Saṁtoṣa arises when the mind lets go of its iron grip of a situation long enough to let us simply observe with great interest but without drawing conclusions or making judgments and assumptions. Letting go, we automatically tap into an endless reservoir of kindness and compassion that lies within.

Tapas, which is usually translated as "austerity," really means to burn or to shine. It is the ability to reflect on and contemplate what is actually arising in our experience and to stay with the immediate experience, repeatedly returning to it with a state of open-mindedness. This role of a deeply engaged observer prevents us from slipping into the mental habit of projecting our fears, unconscious doubts, and shadows out onto the world and onto others. Negative thoughts and emotions as well as the positive ones are experienced without going along with their story lines. It is like sealing a container or pot when you're cooking. Cultivating the role of fully engaged observer is the basic technique used in any contemplative practice, including that of tapas.

As a result of tapas, the deeper and brighter intelligence is awakened. This creates the perfect environment to nourish the next niyama, *svādhyāya,* or self-inquiry. Svādhyāya is the willingness to make an open-minded exploration and assessment of our own desires, mental habits, and ultimate nature. Of course, to actually practice svādhyāya rather than the often much more comfortable acts of rationalization, denial, and self-delusion, we must always practice satyam—we need to remain unflinchingly honest and truthful with ourselves.

One good beginning step when cultivating the practice of svādhyāya is to start to notice without laying blame or trying to change, when we justify our actions or twist our thoughts to make a situation or interaction fit more comfortably with our self-image or preconceptions. Svādhyāya can seem brutal—having to admit (to ourselves, no less) our shortcomings and mistakes and to stop covering up our imperfections. However, once we watch closely, looking past our presumptions, judgments, actions, and feelings, it is not harsh at all. A deeply satisfying feeling of living in alignment with ourselves, as if we've come home, emerges. It is said that svādhyāya culminates in a yoga, or union, with our *iṣṭa devatā,* or beloved deity—or the truth that lies in the core of each of our hearts and connects us to the seed of truth in others.

The final niyama is the surrender to Īśvara, or God, and is called *Īśvara-praṇidhāna.* Īśvara must be understood not in the normal theistic sense as a God separate from or above all else, but as that which is the true being and the true nature of all beings. So in relation to the yamas, surrender can constitute an active giving or rendering of service to Īśvara or the interpenetrating pattern of the world by perceiving the true nature of all beings (ourselves included) and then by contributing in whatever way possible that we and others may awaken.

The yamas and niyamas afford us a context in which to practice yoga both on and off the mat. They provide an underlying framework that the wandering mind can use as a reference point for clear thinking when doubts, questions, and complicated situations arise. Working with them over time, we move from their literal application to their more subtle aspects.

THE KLEŚAS

> Although you may not always be able to avoid difficult situations, you can modify the extent to which you can suffer by how you choose to respond to the situation.
>
> —Dalai Lama XIV, *The Art of Happiness*

Why is it that so much of this world seems to be about suffering? Of course we see the obvious roots of suffering: injustice, hatred, killing, and domination of one person or group by another (which from a geopolitical perspective seem endless). But equally, for many of us, every day seems to present infinite opportunities for suffering: not getting what we "need" or want; being in the company of others who contribute to our unhappiness; having our bodies forsake us with the aging process or illness; or, the worst insult of all, doing everything "right" and dying anyway.

The First Noble Truth of the Buddha, *sarvam duḥkham,* or "all is suffering," reflects this and, on first pass, sounds dismal at best. In fact, for many beginning students of yoga and Buddhism, this tenet causes alarm, if not the perfect excuse to abandon their studies and head straight for the door! But a second look reveals the teaching (both in Buddhism and yoga) that there is a cause for suffering, there can be an end to suffering, and there is a path out of suffering.

In the Yoga Sūtra, the *kleśas* are identified as the causes of suffering, all of them arising from the first, which is *avidyā,* or ignorance. This ignorance is our confusion when faced with the paradox of existence—being a distinct, individual human being with emotions, thoughts, and sensations that seem to be encased within our "own" sack of skin that separates us from everything else but at the same time, understanding intuitively that we are somehow nonseparate from everything else. For beginners, learning to feel both separate and nonseparate at the same time may feel rather like wrapping the mind in sandpaper.

Yet as we have seen, the ability to be comfortable in the face of paradox is foundational to a liberating yoga practice. In yoga, we learn to experience the seemingly distinct patterns of inhaling and exhaling by returning to the breath when the mind wanders. Through this practice, we gradually absorb and assimilate the nature of paradox into the subtle layers of body and mind. According to the Yoga Sūtra, losing sight of this paradoxical perspective is the first cause of suffering. Over and over we have a flash of insight into the true nature of things, and perhaps just as quickly the story of "we" returns, encapsulated by our own separate little universe, and we lose sight of the union of opposites.

The second kleśa, *asmitā,* or "I am-ness," stems directly from avidyā. In a modern or psychological sense, asmitā would be the formation of ego or the concept of separate self in which image is confused with what it represents. To complicate matters, cultivating a healthy ego is an essential skill if we are to navigate through the world and through our yoga practice. The ego function keeps us safe; noticing the boundaries between ourselves and a mountain lion is essential for obvious reasons. Ego helps us to function in society—to work, play, love, and grieve in the context of others. But when it is not softened by intelligence and compassion, an unhealthy ego derails our understanding and happiness. So again, a paradoxical comprehension is imperative: we must see the ego's construction of our self-image as an amazing organization of the mind so it can make sense of things and work efficiently, but we must constantly be alert, eager, and ready to dissolve and update the images and stories the ego spins out.

When the ego function kicks in without an ability to merge into the unknown, it leads us to believe that we are indeed separate, special, and independent from others. This quickly sets up an opportunity to feel either better or worse ourselves—smarter, richer, more timid, or more miserable. The mind leaps at these kinds of extreme comparisons with others and conclusions about self based on the misbelief that we (as an ego) are the center of the universe. This is a natural deduction, since everything we know and all of our perceptual fields are uniquely processed through our individual body and ego structure. The mind must be gently and repeatedly reminded to let go of this conclusion, which is exactly what we do when we practice yoga.

Once we've fallen prey to the ego and the belief that we are separate, then the next two kleśas quickly arise. We find things we like, "need," or want and immediately have a great attraction to them; this is called *rāga.* Or *dveṣa,* an aversion to things we hold to be unpleasant or disdainful, surfaces. The natural response is to grasp at the things we find pleasant and push away those we find unpleasant; both of these mind states cause suffering. We suffer because it seems we can never get exactly what we want, or things we don't want are forever bombarding us. Our dreams and expectations don't live up to what's happening—the perfect recipe for suffering.

The last kleśa is called *abhiniveśa,* which is usually translated as "fear of death." In the Yoga Sūtra, Patañjali says that abhiniveśa is something that every living being experiences—from a tiny bug being swept away by a flood to the most practiced yogis and learned sages facing death. As a living organism, there is an instinctual fear of death, so in what we perceive to be threatening situations, we cling to life and also resist change.

Another way to look at abhiniveśa is as the fear of the ego dissolving—which is somewhat the same thing and possibly as scary as death; in both cases, we disappear. Or we might even say that abhiniveśa is a fear of yoga itself, because a natural by-product of a consistent practice is that longer and longer periods of dissolution—letting go of who we believe ourselves to be and annihilating the ego—naturally occur.

THE FOUR BOUNDLESS ABODES

Keeping the yamas, niyamas, and kleśas in the wings of our awareness, kindness and compassion begin to manifest. At some point, the question naturally arises, "What good is it for me to have these insights and become filled with joy, if others around me still suffer?" Compassion leads us to see clearly that since we are not separate from the fabric of the world, we are not truly liberated and happy until all beings are free. This is the bodhisattva vow: to forego our own liberation and keep helping others until all sentient beings have become enlightened (and if you've looked around recently, you know there are a *lot* of sentient beings).

The Yoga Sūtra and other yoga texts offer practices that help us to fulfill this desire to help others skillfully and perhaps endlessly. These texts teach us how to stay in healthy relationship with others while we follow the path on which we ourselves may awaken from this dream state we call life. Many traditions of Buddhism also offer the same basic practices, which are called the four boundless abodes. They are a means of reining in our emotions so we may see clearly and act intelligently and kindly within the construct of our own emotional and mind states.

The boundless abodes may be practiced whenever we observe certain states of mind and of being arising in ourselves or others. The first is that when we meet someone who is *sukha,* or happy, we practice *maitrī,* which is friendliness or kindness—essentially, we demonstrate love. Unless you're in a really bad mood, this one is easy. If you're open to the presence of someone who is happy, it's difficult not to feel the same. Think of a baby, so full of enthusiasm and busting with excitement as she wiggles and kicks and coos while being cradled in her mother's arms. Or imagine a kitten or puppy or baby chimp and notice how hard it is not to, at least momentarily, feel an inward smile!

When we practice maitrī, there is a noticeable impact on our own nervous system that allows the mind and emotions to clear (even if ever so slightly) and our innate sense of happiness to radiate out to others. In a situation where maitrī or love is arising, it is good to notice the tendency for the mind and ego to jump in and immediately become attached to the circumstances or feelings, or to become fearful or unhappy when the situation changes. So just as it is important to practice maitrī, it is equally important to release attachment to the residue so the mind and emotions remain clear and open.

On the other hand, when we encounter a situation where someone is *duḥkha* (suffering), we do not reflexively run away from the situation, nor do we dovetail onto the suffering, becoming somber and depressed ourselves. Instead, we practice karuṇā (compassion), the second of the boundless abodes. Compassion is a complex state of being that arises naturally when, in the face of suffering, we tap into our own nature as loving beings and tune so deeply in to another's suffering that our own ego function begins to dissolve. In this state, we can *feel* the suffering of the other without confusing the boundaries that separate us from the other. By dropping into our own physical experience, checking in on deep visceral levels within ourselves as to who we are and what we perceive the other to be, we are able to offer the necessary level of clarity of intention to help without our ego function—and our own needs—interfering. If we detach ourselves from the situation, we cannot connect to our intelligence and see what action needs to be taken. Compassion arises naturally in the face of suffering when we are in a state of complete presence and open-mindedness, skills we hone in our yoga practice.

The third boundless abode is called *muditā,* which may be called sympathetic joy. We practice this when we are in the presence of someone who is *puṇya.* Puṇya is often translated as "pious" or "holy," but it is better to consider it as virtuous, clear, and truthful. Someone who is truly puṇya radiates a sense of wholeness, clarity, and great presence. This stimulates a similar feeling within others. It is said that when we meet someone who is puṇya, we respond with sympathetic joy—delight in their experience, even if we are not quite able to feel the extent of it fully. Experiencing sympathetic joy is partially dependent on your own attitude and state of mind. If you feel that things are limited or limiting, that there is never enough to go around, or that others are out to best you, then fear and aversion get in the way of connecting fully to the joy that resides within each of us as the basis of life, that which is felt in the presence of someone who is puṇya.

The fourth boundless abode is practiced in the presence of someone who or a situation that is *apuṇya,* or in a traditional translation is "non-holy." Someone who is apuṇya is not virtuous, clear, or truthful and may even be toxic. To varying degrees, we run into people and situations that are apuṇya on a regular basis. A tyrant would be considered apuṇya, and we encounter less vile versions of tyrants in those who manipulate or have a total disregard for others. The yogic advice for dealing with apuṇya is to act with what is called *upekṣā,* which can be translated as "indifference," "nonattachment," or "equanimity." A vivid metaphor for such nonattachment (pure *vairāgyam*) is in the *Aparokṣānubhuti*:

> **brahmādisthāvaranteṣu**
> **vairāgyaṁ viṣayeṣvanu**
> **yathaiva kāka viṣṭhāyāṁ**
> **vairāgyaṁ tad dhi nirmalam**
>
> The indifference with which one treats the excreta of a crow—such an indifference to all objects of enjoyment from the realm of Brahmā to this world (in view of their perishable nature) is verily called pure vairāgya.
>
> — *Aparokṣānubhuti,* v. 4

Crows are notorious for eating the worst of the worst—decaying flesh, garbage, sewage-laden scraps, and so on. So the excrement of a crow is considered to be particularly disgusting and foul. Nonetheless, from the yogic perspective, *everything* that manifests, including crow excrement, is regarded as Brahman or God. Instead of rejecting the excrement, we see it in a level-headed, neutral way, with equanimity. This graphic description powerfully demonstrates the vision of interconnectedness with godliness at the center of every manifestation. It points to the necessity, when searching for truth, not only of seeing God in all beings, situations, and manifestations, but of seeing all beings in God. The example demands we see through concepts of mind, not making one thing more "holy" than another (our concept of God, for example) or making something of lesser value (the excrement). This is the same as discriminating awareness or enlightenment, and it is absolutely necessary for true relationship and happiness to occur.

VIVEKA KHYĀTIḤ

Viveka khyātiḥ is a term used to describe the skill of discriminating awareness, or the ability to see the truth clearly. It is the capacity to cut through the illusions of mind. Viveka khyātiḥ is the fruit of the practice of meditation, when the mind stays with its content long enough to see the subject matter in context and as part of its background. The content of mind is then observed in its open, sacred, irreducible form, which gives us the insight that everything exists within relationship. Viveka khyātiḥ allows us to use the ability of the mind to make symbols, categories for perceptions and thoughts and games out of concepts, conclusions, and goals without mistaking the symbol for the thing symbolized or the map for the territory. With this clear vision, we begin to see through the ego function and can experience, in an embodied way, the emptiness and "nonabsoluteness" of our beliefs—the importance and incompleteness of theory in finding reality or true relationship.

Viveka khyātiḥ is an essential skill for any serious yoga student to cultivate and maintain. Due to the abusive ways in which some people in this world discriminate against one another, a beginning student may misunderstand the term "discriminating awareness" and think of it as a bad thing. Discriminating without a sense of truth and compassion, without taking full account of the context of a situation or the relationship of another, or discriminating through a lens of prejudice or preconception is when the process of discernment goes wrong. But discriminating awareness is the ability to remain fully aware as we determine the relative truth of a given situation. It is the capacity to see through preconceptions, illusions, and prejudices. Viveka khyātiḥ is a direct path to seeing the essence of situations—even those that are difficult, complex, or distasteful—and experiencing compassion.

EMBODIMENT, SAṀSKĀRA, AND AWARENESS OF PRĀṆA

Prāṇa links what you're thinking and perceiving into its background. As embodied beings, all that we experience is processed through Prāṇa (breath) and citta (mind). These two distinctly different layers of our experience are inseparable, though we are prone to separate them in our mind's eye. Sometimes they are joined in our awareness into one powerful experience. Most of the time, however, the citta wanders around, and the physiological background (Prāṇa) is less apparent in our awareness. In a contemplative practice, we take the attention (citta) and turn it straight to Prāṇa. It is said that Prāṇa and citta move together like two fish swimming in tandem; where Prāṇa goes, citta follows, and where citta goes, so too flows Prāṇa. When we are aware that they move together like this, we experience our whole body (from subtle to gross) as unified, alert, and harmonious, giving us a tangible, embodied understanding of healthy relationship. When our experience of breath and mind is fragmented, so too is our embodied state and our visceral understanding of healthy relationship.

Tapping into the internal forms of the practice stimulates the subtle layers of body and mind in a profound trust of this process of vinyāsa, or the joining together of Prāṇa and citta. It is impossible to separate mind from Prāṇa on the subtle level, and the inner forms of practice gradually awaken an awareness of this unity. This deep level of experience is rooted in what is traditionally called the subtle body. Mind and Prāṇa serve inseparable functions in the process of perception, but the immediate perception is embedded in Prāṇa (sensation). Due to the overlaying of Prāṇa and mind, the subtle body is not a matter of pure abstraction and data processing but a virtual storehouse of deeply rooted clumps and knots of unconscious emotions, internal sensations, concepts, memories, tendencies, and stories. To affect and transform the subtle body as we practice, we use special forms, images, and ideas to take us immediately back to a pure perception of whole, balanced patterns of Prāṇa. These internal forms of embodied perception are delicate and can easily become destabilized and distorted by conclusions of the mind, even simple conclusions such as the identification of the subtle states themselves.

At the same time, without mental process, there is no understanding. The mind works by creating contingent dualisms in which symbols for things (including those we experience through our sense fields) are usually understood to be separate from the things they symbolize. Though we experience mind all the time, there is nothing in the content of our experience that we can point to as being the mind or the self, although we inevitably try. To feel or even imagine this deep experience in which our attention (citta) stays and merges with the immediate sensations (Prāṇa) is nearly impossible, yet it is so precious and important. In fact, the initial definition of yoga in Patañjali's Yoga Sūtra reflects this:

> **Yogaḥ citta vṛtti nirodhaḥ**
>
> Yoga is the suspension (nirodha) of the modifications (vṛtti) of the citta.
>
> —Yoga Sūtra, Samādhi Pāda, v. 2

In yoga, when there is a presentation, a *vṛtti,* of some content to the conscious awareness, the habitual, unconscious response is suspended. The vṛtti is not accepted, rejected, or further wrapped in concept or category, but is perceived in and of itself. This has a radical and wonderful effect on both our understanding and our deep unconscious store of memory and conditioning.

SAṀSKĀRAS

As yoga practitioners, we meditate to understand and come into Prāṇa as it is. Surrendering to this process of merging an unbiased awareness of body and mind marks the point at which the subtle body starts to be purified by dismantling what are called *saṁskāras.* Saṁskāras are old overlays of memories, emotions, and conditioning onto the sensations within the subtle body that are experienced through the senses, or Prāṇa. In other words, saṁskāras are what we would call unconscious habits, memories, and conditioning. When we unravel saṁskāras, direct perception is no longer automatically reduced to a memory, an idea, or a theory that elicits an automatic, unconscious response. Breaking the habitual loop of "knowing" what a perception is allows a fuller grasp of the content and context of the perception and possibly a glimpse of infinity. The nature of reality comes into the foreground, and we see the interdependence and relationship of all things rather than having a perception stimulate an involuntary journey into the self, memory, and imagination. These kinds of involuntary journeys are our habitual way of being in the world—the hub of the wheel of saṁsāra.

Most saṁskāras are neutral. They fuel the ways we perceive and interact day to day. Some saṁskāras are bad; they perpetuate ignorance and cause suffering. Some are initially good and later get in the way, like a good scientific hypothesis that oversimplifies. Others are profound and sometimes religious saṁskāras founded in a one-time encounter of a deep, possibly mystical experience. In this situation, it is not uncommon to subconsciously attempt to make even these deep experiences into something familiar by reducing them to a theory about the occurrence so we can hold on to and possibly reproduce it. The reductionist mind mistakes the joyous experience itself for the particular content of the mind at that moment.

Perhaps nowhere in Western literature has this experience been more beautifully and famously captured than in Marcel Proust's *Remembrance of Things Past,* in which he described his experience of a cup of tea and a petite madeleine served to him by his aunt:

> No sooner had the warm liquid mixed with the crumbs touched my palate than a shudder ran through me and I stopped, intent upon the extraordinary thing that was happening to me. An exquisite pleasure had invaded my senses, something isolated, detached, with no suggestion of its origin. And at once the vicissitudes of life had become indifferent to

> me, its disasters innocuous, its brevity illusory—this new sensation having had on me the effect which love has of filling me with a precious essence; or rather this essence was not in me, it was me.

Since the body is a sensing organism and the mind is the interpreter, what most frequently happens when we have a brief encounter with the subtle body realm (like Proust's) is that this dichotomy of understanding immediately kicks in, and the mind "understands." It labels the experience as good, bad, radical, mundane, and so on. Unless we consciously intervene, our memories and associations with the perception live encased in our story and our myofascial webbing within the subtle body. When we have an experience, like that of eating a madeleine, overlapping yet unrelated patterns of sensation and thought (saṁskāras) are established. We may have a moment of insight, but then the mind leaps back into "understanding" (its job), the ego function perks up to identify with the insight (its function), and we latch on to the story line; this process reinforces the saṁskāra. When we happen into the deep levels of experience within the subtle body, the feeling is so powerful and enticing that we may try to re-create the same situation in order to experience that unspeakable feeling again. But because the mind has reduced, identified, categorized, and codified the inexpressible, the experience is never the same. As Proust, after describing attempts to re-create his experience, put it, "The truth I am seeking lies not in my cup, but in myself."

We learn exactly this through a yoga practice. Although it is perfectly natural to look outside ourselves for the source of profound insights, the truth lies not externally but within. Once we experience and evaluate each moment fresh, there is a sense of vastness and harmony merging patterns of citta into Prāṇa.

LOOKING CLOSELY

When we perceive an external or internal object either correctly or incorrectly, our subtle body produces a vṛtti, an image or idea of that object comprising a variety of sensual and abstract categories combined with our memories and associated body patterns. This patterning of perception then resonates through the nāḍīs. In a contemplative practice, the whole phenomenon is observed through to the end and clearly exposes the phenomenon itself.

Every perception, or vṛtti, is a combination of an "external" form overlaid by internal categorization that determines our actions and the structure and form of our subtle body. If the external object is "brought closer" and held more delicately, as in meditation, we are at the borderline of internal/external name and form. The ability to be "awake" enough at this instant to consciously participate in the process of perception as it occurs and to pause—even for just a single breath—results in a moment of insight. This, of course, is an advanced skill. It is easier to become aware of the circuitry of the flow of Prāṇa as it occurs in the body and then to balance that circuitry through a natural vinyāsa to keep the perception open and hold the object with clear mind. That's a fine place to start!

Using the brilliant sword of discriminating awareness to cut through and eliminate overlays of mind and to understand what is right in front of us allows insight and compassion to spontaneously arise. The middle path allows the mind, body, and environment to come together and work in harmonious relationship. They then do their processes in a way that creates brilliant, self-manifesting truth and also reveals self-dissolving, nondual patterns.

3

Fluid Movement

Alignment, Form, and Imagination

THE BODY, BOTH SUBTLE AND GROSS, IS A STOREhouse of unconscious and semiconscious tensions, retractions, expansions, and discrete movements of Prāṇa. All these movements are based on past and current thinking—a form of misunderstood imagination that picks out objects, constructs self-images, makes goals, and charts out theories soaked in the emotions of attachment and repulsion. Through the integration of Prāṇa and citta, intelligent movement effortlessly manifests within this maze of conditions that arise, and we are slowly freed from preconditioned patterns that keep us both mentally and physically entangled.

For yoga āsanas to be a truly useful aspect of this unraveling, they must be grounded and properly aligned. Then the imagination is used intelligently so poses have an open, pleasant quality that allows meditative states of mind to arise easily and so that strong, balanced, delightful currents of Prāṇa flow effortlessly. A healthy āsana practice is liberating. It ultimately supports insight that frees us from a misunderstood imagination and its habitual patterns and suffering. However, it is essential to use the imagination with boundless creativity to understand and free ourselves from it!

In the yoga traditions, imagination has been used extensively to embody idealized forms and functions among gods, goddesses, and heroes as a way of breaking our habitual patterns of perceiving our own body and feeling required movements, attitudes, and characteristics within yoga poses. Embodiment practices have contributed to the evolution of yoga, uniting subtle and esoteric teachings within the everyday physical realities of having a body. Profound and deep insights we might access through our imagination can be gateways for understanding how to live on the practical plane—a merging of practice, tradition, lineage, and mythology into "real" life.

The viability of yoga as a living art rests in the fact that even in the imagination, it never becomes stagnant. Although we use preconceptions and formulaic thinking in vinyāsa practice, the practice is not based on them; rather, it balances, exposes, and contextualizes preconceptions. Herein lies the value of visualizing whole-body patterns that can prove more insightful than attempting to understand movement from a dry, analytical approach. Whole-body patterns of alignment are associated with deep feelings, emotions, and sensations that we perceive directly rather than patterns fragmented by conceptual ideas. Whole-body patterns unite subtle-body patterns to support and inform movements. Of course, they typically do not describe a local anatomical structure in detail, so it is important to embrace scientific forms of study along with visualization; both approaches need each other to evolve.

Mindful use of the imagination in yoga reveals that impressions and stories that come into our awareness depend on context and are therefore not absolute and exclusive of other impressions and stories. This means there are potentially unlimited brilliant metaphors and images that can be used to describe or imply a yogic state in the body. On the other hand, it does *not* mean that we should fall into a relativistic mind-set in which any metaphor or myth is an adequate (or even decent) description of alignment or yogic states. Limitless stories, forms, and metaphors correspond to deluded states of mind and can induce those unhappy states. Good metaphors are rare, like brilliant art and insight. Metaphors must be precise, expandable, visceral, and clear to really do the trick. All of them are only metaphors and must eventually be released and allowed to dissolve so they can do their job. The importance of lineage in image making is tantamount. All effective imagery shares a similar flavor, though the forms it takes may be radically diverse. Tradition is like a flame of intelligence passed on and shared by countless practitioners over centuries, using many versions of metaphor, philosophy, and technique.

Visualizations can be helpful with alignment in specific poses too, such as imagining the heart "floating," which can stimulate a full feeling of expansiveness in a pose. But where subtle anatomy is most useful is in shedding light on levels of alignment and form that govern obscure aspects of the practice, such as Mūlabandha, and whole-body patterns that connect us from top to bottom. By practicing āsana with some of these patterns in the nervous system, the poses are enhanced, and perhaps more important, the affected parts of the nervous system are primed for meditation.

OVERVIEW OF SUBTLE ANATOMY

During the Italian Renaissance, an understanding of human form came to life as great artists of the time became anatomists, peeling back the skin of dead bodies and dissecting corpses to study the intricacies of form and structure in fine detail. Some, such as Leonardo da Vinci and Michelangelo, were inspired to explore and broaden their understanding of the body in action, and their art became infused with a level of realism never before imagined. Their direct study of anatomy, merged with their innovative imaginations and artistic skill, transformed the face of art forever. As a yoga practitioner, fusing together a knowledge of anatomy with the art form of your imagination—deeply feeling movement and sensation, along with patterns of connection and breath—may not make you the Michelangelo of yoga, but it will add a uniquely clear means of inhabiting your own skin.

To begin experiencing our own subtle anatomy, it is helpful to have studied classical anatomy and artistic renderings of the body so we have a general idea of the landscape of human form. Imagining our own structure as an overlay to clear images of anatomy, while focusing on feelings and sensations as they arise, provides an embodied, broad-spectrum experience of the subtle body. In this context, it is helpful to establish a vocabulary specific to these elusive layers of understanding. Doing so is referred to as *sādhanā bhāṣā,* or practice language. Every group or school (and ultimately every practitioner) has a unique and often abstruse sādhanā bhāṣā; words, images, and myths that give us markers of understanding and serve as memory cues so we may easily return to and build on the insight that inspired the vocabulary.

As an example, to assimilate an understanding of what it feels like to sit with balanced, well-aligned posture that connects you from the crown of your head to your pelvic floor, you might visualize a detailed image of this form and then assign some words to the experience to serve as anchors within your nervous system so your body can remember the experience and reproduce it more easily. Imagine, for instance, that you can *feel* sensations (from subtle to gross) within your body of what it would be like if you were royalty—sitting up straight on a throne, wearing a pair of bright gold earrings and a jewel-studded crown with a golden feather rising out of the top. The more details you can invoke, the better; imagine what you must do to remain feeling regal. What minor adjustments do you need to make in your feet or sitting bones to establish a stable and balanced base from which your spine can feel strong, elongated, and supported so that your heart has an open, expansive feeling? How does this buoyant feeling in your upper body provide a complement to the weight of the crown and the tug of the earrings on your earlobes? Imagine how you actually *feel* open and light thanks to the sense of a feather shooting up and out from the top of the crown and your head. You notice that a steady gaze helps your tongue to quiet and soften, which automatically releases your palate and allows your mind to settle; with time, you feel fully aligned and tapped in to the central channel of your body. Even though you haven't instructed yourself to expand your rib cage, spread the skin on your lower back, or release tension in your feet, you notice that these things are indeed occurring. The natural intelligence of your body, triggered by the image, has taken a front seat to preconceived concepts about what you should be doing to achieve proper alignment. After practicing with the image for a while, you find that if you simply think, "bright gold earrings" (or another sādhanā bhāṣā), it is enough to activate the entire response in your nervous system and body.

This is how subtle anatomy works. It taps into the body beneath the level of conceptual mind and makes full use of the mind's ability and agility to connect and assimilate all echelons of information. Subtle anatomy is a way of getting our sense fields involved in the process of understanding and creating stunning moments of direct perception of what is really happening in and around us.

ASPECTS OF SUBTLE FORM

This section includes thirteen important visceral visualizations that describe internal forms of the practice. They are used as sādhanā bhāṣā instructions for various āsanas so that complex movements may be described in fewer words. They can be contemplated separately when not "officially" practicing āsanas and are also essential to certain integrating yet complex movements within poses. All of these imagination-based expressions of internal forms are related to actual anatomical structures, but they have a generous overlay of imagery to produce an experience of alignment. With practice , they will eventually produce distinct patterns within body, mind, and movement that somehow seem familiar.

These imaginary forms require attention and repetition over a long period of time, because each brings together at least two different and complementary movements as well as the feelings, thoughts, and emotions that come with them. Although they are rich with imagery, releasing all grasping and neediness triggered by them makes them more effective because they then resonate within us. At the same time, we return to the specifics of the forms repeatedly as a means of rekindling the connection of imagination and structure so we may fully embody a pose or movement.

Mūlabandha

> **yanmūlaṁ sarvabhutānāṁ**
> **yanmūlaṁ citta bandhanam**
> **mūlabandhaḥ sadā sevyo**
> **yogyo 'sau rājayoginām**
>
> That which is the root of all beings and the complete binding (cessation) of thought is Mūlabandha. It should always be served and attended to since it is fit for Rāja yogins.
>
> —*Aparokṣānubhuti,* v. 114

To some Aṣṭāṅga Vinyāsa practitioners, trying to master Mūlabandha is like attempting to grab the brass ring on a carousel ride. You "win" when you get it, but trying for it can become an obsession that ruins the ride. Grabbing the ring takes opportunity and skill, and it is a treasure worth striving for if you like merry-go-rounds because the reward is usually another ride on the carousel. On a quest for Mūlabandha, however, striving too hard can be counterproductive. Under the correct circumstances, Mūlabandha will manifest; when it does, the most glorious reward—like on a carousel—is the opportunity to try it again in another round of practice. The most appreciated gift for any yoga practitioner *is*, after all, more yoga!

In search of Mūlabandha, we may begin with some aspects of a form that are not particularly subtle yet are still observed with an open, focused mind so that deeper patterns connect through the body. It's likely you can contract your anal sphincter muscles; many organisms do this on a daily basis, and the feeling is probably familiar. You could stop right here and say, "Ah! I know Mūlabandha." As encouragement to beginners, a teacher would say, "That's good, but keep practicing." By observing those sensations and the attitudes and thoughts associated with them, you are able to isolate the supporting muscles, then the rest of the body starts responding, creating a three-dimensional map within your awareness around the focus of attention on the area of the mūla, or pelvic floor. Eventually other images emerge through which you can chart the experience. The attention becomes pure and undistracted, and the mind stops feeling compelled to draw conclusions. Like magic, all levels of the body and mind fall into line, and we then say that Mūlabandha is coming along. (See an illustration of Mūlabandha in Appendix 4.)

If you treat Mūlabandha like a trophy to be attained, it will disappear immediately. Instead, treat it with great devotion, as a deity invited to appear and rise up like a flame at the center of the pelvic floor. Take all the necessary steps and make all the proper preparations to greet an honored guest and then wait. Perhaps one day she will emerge, or perhaps not. More important than "mastering" Mūlabandha is the joyful, unending process of keeping the heart and mind connected and open for the moment compassion emerges in the form of Mūlabandha. This kind of practice is very advanced and profound, and it erases the subtext of ego striving.

Mūlabandha is a highly intimate and individualized part of any āsana practice, yet it is key to integrating the body, mind, and emotions. You must be patient. Finding images that work for you are paramount, as are constantly rethinking, reexamining, releasing, and redrawing your imagery and preconceptions about what exactly Mūlabandha is and what you are experiencing. You feel Mūlabandha in your mouth and then up and down the central line of your body, even down into its base in the pelvic floor, where it is actually occurring. In a broad sense, Mūlabandha is the basic pattern of conjoining opposites like prāṇa and apāna, expansion and contraction, or focus and horizon. These unions can take place at any station (any cakra) along the central axis of the body, facilitating meditation on that specific spot and eventually pulling in patterns of unification from all the other stations.

One method for bringing focus to Mūlabandha is first simply to *imagine* you can feel your pelvic floor. You might envision the bony structure of your pelvis and the muscles that connect from side to side and front to back to form the "floor" of the bowl. Onto this you could overlay an image that makes the territory come to life. For example, you could imagine the four corners of the pelvic floor as four distinct flower petals that make up a type of dais in the base of the body. You might imagine yourself as a deity seated right in the middle, and as you settle into your pelvic floor, you experience the perfection of integration. In this case, the deity is the Mūlabandha, and it is naturally effortless in a fully awakened state that bypasses preconceptions of Mūlabandha in which "you" have to "do" something to "make it happen."

Another of many indirect ways to feel Mūlabandha is to meditate on the seed mantra ṬHAṀ with your mind focusing on your palate. As you say the mantra repeatedly, it resonates through your nasal septum, releases the upper back of the palate, and moves down into the heart. At the same time, you can visualize the iṣṭa devatā (beloved deity) sitting in your heart and expand the image to include a nanoform of the deity in the shape of a subtle flame or mark within the various cakras. After a time, the relaxation associated with the imagery clarifies and descends through the body and the image returns through the pelvic floor in the form of Mūlabandha.

Kinesthetically we can also tap into Mūlabandha by imagining that the breath moves by being pulled up like a thread out of the fabric of the center of the pelvic diaphragm. Just as in needlepoint where the cloth must be smooth with an even tone and secured to a ring so the movement of the thread is precise, the toning of the "cloth" of the pelvic floor contributes to a detailed establishment of Mūlabandha. Then the thread of the breath can be drawn up slightly toward the back of the body as if feeding it into a straw—the central channel. As the image of the breath is pulled up and back, the center of the pelvic floor cloth lifts delicately and evenly to let the thread through. This causes a stimulation of the pelvic floor muscles in a way that isolates them from the other muscles around the hip joint area so there is an unusual sense of symmetry front to back, left to right, and up to down. The drawing up of the center of the pelvic floor corresponds to the even release of the sitting bones down toward the earth or the release of the coccyx and pubic bone down (or all four at once). Keeping this pattern and residual tone while canceling the peripheral asymmetries in the surrounding muscle area is the basis of the Mūlabandha action.

Releasing the Palate

> **ata ūrdhvaṁ tālumūle**
> **sahasrāraṁ saroruham**
> **asti yatra suṣumṇāyā**
> **mūlaṁ savivaraṁ sthitam**
>
> Above the ājñā lotus at the root of the palate is the thousand-petaled lotus in which is the root opening of the suṣumṇā.
>
> —*Śiva Saṁhitā,* ch. 5, v. 156

At the opposite end of the central channel from Mūlabandha is its complementary subtle-body form—a release of the palate. When we release the palate, the *tālu,* we feel a pattern along the entire core of the body, and that pattern penetrates out and beyond.

From an ordinary perspective, the palate, situated at the roof of the mouth, is associated with taste. Gastronomes and artists speak of having a good palate or good taste, and indeed, from a yogic point of view, the palate is associated with *rasa,* which translates as "flavor" or "taste." Rasa also means juice, and the palate deals with the juices associated with flavor as well as other fluids from deep within the body, such as tears, saliva, and mucus. Rasa is not restricted to taste sensations from food; it is also associated with refined emotional flavor.

From a more esoteric perspective, it is said that the basic emotions we all experience can be transmuted through yoga when we meditate on them as rasa, a metaphorical flavor in the palate. Once transformed through observation, the "juice" of an emotion is transformed along the central axis so the emotion is not projected out into the world. With the release of the palate, emotion can become a seed for insight and skillful action rather than a reactionary state of being. For example, anger in its raw state may feel hot, fiery, and intense. If we identify with the sensations and our associations with the feelings that arise—thereby activating the anger—we are likely to be swept away by a constellation of feeling, thought, and sensation into what is usually less than skillful action. But if we focus the mind to release the palate, observing condensed droplets of the sensations of anger dripping toward the back of the palate, we can sense the essential rasa of that emotion. It is then automatically transmuted into a powerful quality of awakened, clear mind. This process is the same for any emotion: we observe it and release the palate, and its rasa transforms into a form that is beneficial rather than a root of suffering. Awareness in the palate, therefore, is associated with the sattva, or the harmonizing mode of energy that spontaneously arises when we have the pleasure of knowing, understanding, or even allowing something to transform.

Physically the palate is like an exchange center between the inner world of the organism of the body and the outer environment. It is also a storehouse for our past and present feelings, thoughts, and sensations—an epicenter connecting the mind and physical makeup from top to bottom. As a sounding board for language expression, the palate connects our abstract and subjective thoughts into the world. It is where the input we take in from all around is quickly sorted. With a released palate, this data can be channeled into a pattern or form that frees the mind and body for meditation.

If you look at the anatomy of the palate in an anatomy book—or even better, and perhaps scarier, open your mouth and look in a mirror—it's remarkable to see that you carry such a complex combination of strange and urchin-like structures around with you all the time. With your mouth wide open, you probably first see the shape-shifting muscle of the tongue resting beneath the bony, dome-shaped hard palate. The delicate area in the back of the mouth forms the soft palate and includes the uvula. The hard palate extends up into the skull to form the nasal septum, which is not visible when you open your mouth, but you can feel the intersection of the hard palate and nasal septum because its juncture vibrates when you talk, sing, or hum. Seeing, feeling, or just imagining the anatomical relationship of these structures allows you to tune in to the sensations within them and gives you a base for subtle-body visualizations involving the relationship of the tongue to the different sections of the palate. Awareness of the palate helps you understand the sinus passages and allows you to feel how their extensions can be experienced as reaching on and on out in patterns of sensation throughout the whole body.

To release the palate, begin by relaxing the tension in your jaw and mouth as if you were ceasing all desire and effort to talk in order to fully listen. Allow the gaze to be soft and clear along the line of the nose. Relaxation of the palatal muscles creates a distinct sensation pattern that is open and full and can be felt in the back of the mouth and head, up inside the skull, and down through the tongue and throat. Eventually there is a feeling of nectar, an elixir made of kindness and compassion, dripping down to fill the nāḍīs from what can be visualized as a moon-like cup at the base of the thousand-petaled lotus flower that spreads at the crown of the head.

The simplest way to start feeling this release of the palate is to meditate on the sensations associated with the contact of your tongue with the upper part of your mouth and, at the same time, bring awareness to the sensations of the breath flow in your nostrils. This technique is similar to just listening closely to sound; gazing with gentle, empty eyes; or smiling softly while focusing on any associated feelings that arise in the head or face. Perhaps you can induce the same feeling by imagining you are looking closely at the *Mona Lisa* and tuning in to the feelings so vividly captured in her timeless smile. Contemplating the face of someone who is extremely kind or compassionate can have a similar effect. There are many ways to find compassion and to tune in to the sensation of the palate releasing.

Releasing the palate is also a reflexive physical action associated with being moved deeply by an aesthetic experience, having a great insight, being in love, or simply getting a joke. In all of these situations, our philosophical inquiry into beauty, deep thought and emotion, or an understanding of root paradoxes (as in a good joke) is the mind attempting to understand the whole of reality. Yet in instinctively "getting" paradox or beauty, we know that we will fully understand only through a moment of not knowing. In this instant of insight, the mind is stunned, and the Prāṇa stops moving asymmetrically in all the various paths to which it is accustomed. When Prāṇa stops moving, the mind stops too, and there is a spontaneous, deeply satisfying sense of release at the root of the palate that spreads throughout the body.

The objective in all of these meditations and visualizations is to create an optimal environment in your mind and body for you to be able to establish feelings associated with deep understanding and compassion. With no conscious technique of physical manipulation, when you feel kind or compassionate—or when you have an "aha" moment because you understand the interdependence of things—the root of your palate automatically begins to soften and release. While cultivating a release of the palate, or any of these subtle-body forms of alignment, we must define, redefine, and then redefine again that specific form so the ego doesn't think that it has mastered or achieved the action. Then we may go deep and disappear into the sensation patterns as they arise. The actions themselves involve dissolving the sense of ego function, and this is why they are illusive.

Psoas Line

The psoas muscles flow like ribbons on each side of the body, just to the side of the pubic bone through the groin; they are attached to the uppermost inner back edges of the femurs, or thighbone. The ribbons move out through the pelvis and up the sides of the lumbar spine, where they attach to the upper lumbar vertebrae all the way to the twelfth thoracic vertebra (T12) at the base of the rib cage (see illustration on page 92). This is where the diaphragm attaches as well. As muscles go, the psoas are among the most elegant due to their length and smooth, even fibers, as well as the fact that they are unifying muscles, connecting the top half of the body to the bottom half. Possibly because they are structurally designed to act as go-betweens, the psoas muscles seem to have an emotional quality to them. Like the "mother" muscles of the body, they often facilitate movements and make things work in a unified manner from top to bottom, even in some situations when it is structurally impossible for the muscles themselves to physically connect and work in this way.

With just a little imagination, we can extend the image of these unifying muscles and feel continuous lines that stretch on each side from the fingertips through the arms, the sides of the torso, the pelvis, the legs, and the feet. We call these lines of awareness the "psoas lines," and they become a remarkable tool for stimulating the experience of interconnectedness as we dissolve into subtle-body feelings and sensations that unify breath, body, and mind.

If we release and stretch the psoas muscle on one side while inhaling fully, it can feel as if there is an empty tube in the approximate area of the released muscle. This sense of a cylindrical shape deep in the abdomen can be imagined to extend up and down the side like a "pelvic nostril," and creates a pathway for Prāṇa to flow connecting the top half of the body to the bottom half. Maintaining a feeling of openness and release along the line, we can then stretch the psoas muscle itself, which creates a subtle-body pattern that, when properly organized, wakes up the pelvic floor. The muscles that oppose the psoas—such as the hamstrings—are also awakened by this awareness to create a sort of void or spacious feeling behind and to the sides of the belly and back in the pelvic basin. This feeling of spaciousness is a primary component used in meditation on the idā nāḍī, the piṅgālā nāḍī, and the pelvic floor.

To trace the entire inhalation in this way, while keeping associated psoas patterns awake, is challenging because the tendency of both the inhaling and exhaling patterns of breath is to break away from each other, particularly when they reach peak expression. For example, when we inhale, the expansive feeling in the core of the heart naturally occurs, yet at the top of the inhalation, it is difficult to maintain the sense of spreading and expansion of the ribs in the lower back—a primary pattern associated with the exhalation. When the physical patterns represented by the ends of the breath break apart—one becoming dominant and overshadowing the other—then the smooth flow of Prāṇa is interrupted. Disruption in the Prāṇa automatically manifests as asymmetrical tension in the psoas muscles themselves, as well as tightness in the other hip flexors and possibly an uprooting of one of the sitting bones when seated. Therefore, learning to release the psoas muscles and follow the psoas lines as they extend top to bottom in the body is extremely important, though extraordinarily subtle and illusive.

Unlike some muscles, like the biceps, that thrive on being prodded and pumped to become strong and effective, if we strive too hard to release or stretch the psoas, then misaligned muscular tension or imbalances in the pelvic floor can occur, resulting in an uneven flow of Prāṇa. An uneven flow can also occur due to a conceptual misunderstanding of or poor instruction about deep internal breathing patterns. Remember, good form and technique feel really good. Poor alignment results in a sense of holding, making it almost impossible to trace the simple psoas lines smoothly with the stream of the breath.

If our movements become confused, and the psoas muscles become habituated to trying to help us release elsewhere when they can't actually *do* anything, then the psoas muscles themselves can become chronically engaged. Though it is challenging, we should keep practicing—adjusting tiny details of uniting prāṇa and apāna at the ends of the breath, while intelligently stretching and imagining a release in the psoas muscles. Once we understand these muscles and let go of our desire for them to release, if we just breathe smoothly, they *will* let go and establish the pattern deep within that reveals the Mūlabandha.

Releasing the psoas muscles also stabilizes T12, so as we stretch from top to bottom, the vertebra will stay positioned back, allowing full, deep flow and movement of the breath. When this subtle pattern of expansion in the back of the body on the inhalation is achieved, the psoas' companions, the quadratus lumborum (QL) muscles, will also stay released. This pattern is key in protracting the shoulder blades, which facilitates the action of reaching through the entire arm and in turn feeds back into the stretch of the psoas line.

Within the practice, it is paramount to experience the fully expressive sense of reaching "as if to infinity" from foot to fingertips along the psoas line. As a pattern of movement, this psoas line stretch is key to getting the juice out of many movements and poses; it automatically begins to facilitate a release of the palate, so there is no straining or grasping at images and technique within our movements. Of course, one more element is essential in this integrating movement, and that is the dṛṣṭi. Without proper gazing, which stops the tongue and also helps to release the palate, these whole-body patterns are unavailable. If we grasp too tightly with the literal mind at any technique, then we miss the unifying quality of the whole-body pattern within a pose.

PSOAS STRETCH

1. Lie on your back in *Tāḍāgī Mudrā* (Pond Mudrā) (see page 28) and hold for five breaths.
2. On an inhalation, draw the left knee up and catch the top of the shin with your left hand. Let the leg fall out to the side at about 30 degrees from the midline.
3. Reach over your head along the floor with the right arm and gently pull the left knee toward the outer left shoulder. Already the psoas muscle on your right side is lengthening and stretching.
4. Next, firm up the right leg as you reach farther and farther with the right arm. Turn the right palm in toward the midline to protract your

right shoulder blade. Be sure to stay with the breath so that sensations around the edges of the diaphragm, the pelvic floor, and the pelvic basin are included in the pattern.

5. During the inhalation, continue to reach through the right hand and arm. The right collarbone should feel as if it is rotating slightly and falling back; the front edge of the right armpit, the pectoralis major muscle, will spread and flow back toward the floor as it continues to spread away from the midline. The outwardly spiraling line of the right shoulder blade and arm links to the inward rotation of the right leg as both stretch with no perceived limit.
6. Begin to point your right foot slightly and push the heel firmly into the floor so the quadriceps and hamstrings of the right leg engage. Keep reaching in opposite directions throughout the entire inhalation. When you exhale, release the sense of reaching and allow the awareness to dissolve into the midline of the body. Then again inhale and stretch.
7. Each time you inhale, turn on the reaching pattern through the right leg and right arm. As you do this, imagine that the twelfth rib on the right side is falling a little closer to the floor and that your whole back area is spreading as it moves up your body. At the same time as you draw the left knee toward the outer left shoulder, the pelvis automatically does a posterior tilt (rolls back). Imagining the connection of your body from fingertips to pelvic floor and foot facilitates the whole-body pattern.

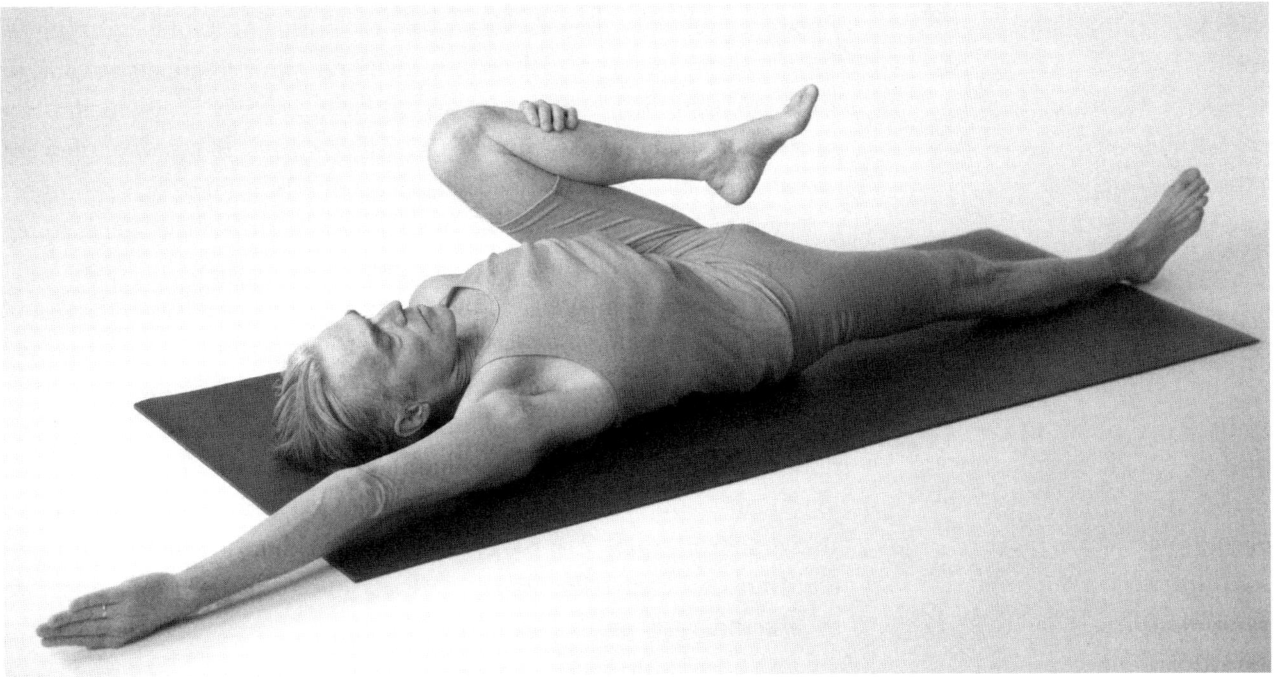

8. After stretching and releasing the whole-body pattern three to five times, on the final exhalation gradually release the stretch and let the brilliance of the psoas line pattern soften and dissolve into the subtle background layers of the breath, body, and mind. Bring the right arm down to your side, and allow the left leg to return to the floor next to the right.
9. Repeat the same stretch at least three times on the other side.

The psoas stretch allows you to embody a feeling of infinite expansiveness, reaching as if forever. An image that can stimulate this feeling is that of Viṣṇu in the *Trivikrama* ("Three Steps") myth: he reclaims the whole cosmos from the egotistical demon Bali by stretching the length of his legs infinitely in both directions to step across the entire expanse of the universe. His third step places his lotus foot on the crown of Bali's head. When you tap into the psoas line, it feels as if you might be able to do such a thing. Not only does this afford an integrating whole-body pattern to emerge top to bottom, it also lengthens the actual psoas muscle on the side being stretched while giving awareness of the participation of the pelvic floor in organizing the movement. We find that as we deepen our āsana practice, attention to the psoas line in many poses and phases of movement can be exciting and liberating because it allows the Prāṇa to flow fully and without interruption.

Cave of the Sacrum

Awareness of the *cave of the sacrum* is another way of beginning to feel the pelvic floor, Mūlabandha, and the lower underbelly version of Uḍḍīyāna Bandha. The sacrum, to which the coccyx is attached, is set in the sacroiliac (SI) joints in the back of the pelvic basin. Together, the sacrum and coccyx form a contour that resembles a deep cave—almost a separate chamber—below the overall abdominal cavity. The bladder, rectum, and uterus or prostate are housed in this area of the pelvis.

To feel and articulate the pelvic floor, we need to develop a sense of emptiness or spaciousness, a suction sensation in this cave, as if we had spooned its contents back and up toward the lower lumbar vertebrae. This feeling depends on having some feeling of tone in the pelvic floor muscles attached to the coccyx—as if we were holding the coccyx in place to provide stability so we could scoop the spoon of the mind back and up along the front surface of the coccyx and sacrum to "clean out the cave." Cultivating this cavelike feeling under the belly helps to fully integrate the internal form of nearly all poses and the movements between them.

Energetically the cave of the sacrum is the origin, the womb, and meditating there allows you to relax into the great irreducible mystery beyond thought. Be aware that clean and healthy bowels, as well as some of the less popular and strange *kriya* (practices) in hatha yoga, facilitate this ability to sense the cave of the sacrum. Most of these esoteric practices, like the ability to suck water up the anus, are actually rooted in training the same muscles of the pelvic floor that establish a sense of the cave of the sacrum. Overzealous practitioners are sometimes tempted to take the kriyas—like anything extreme or strange—too far, practicing the exercises to excess or believing they are the answer to everything when in fact they are simply another type of perspective or tool among many for connecting to the subtle layers of awareness in the body.

Kidney Wings

The *kidney wings* are initially defined by the position and movement of the twelfth ribs, the small ribs on the back of the body that are referred to as "floating" because, unlike other ribs, they do not attach to the sternum. The twelfth ribs lie directly behind the center of the kidney on each side of the back. Because they attach the back edges of the diaphragm to the QL muscles, these ribs are intimately involved in respiratory patterns.

When inhaling, you can feel not only the lifting and spreading of the twelfth ribs themselves but also a sense of expansion that originates at the level of the kidneys as this part of body opens back and up. By overlaying an image of wings on this kinesthetic pattern, when you fully inhale and reach up while engaging and spinning the arms, it's easy to imagine that this is what a bird must feel when beginning to spread its back to open its wings and fly. There is an integrating pattern all the way down the sides and back of the body to the kidney area, and the stretch extends on into the psoas muscles to create a feeling of suction in the cave of the sacrum. With the arms, hands, and back of the body awake like this, you may get the feeling of a smaller repeating pattern of this same kidney wing form occurring in the outer half of each hand (from the middle finger out through the little finger), and this image can serve to integrate the pattern throughout the entire body. Imagining the kidney wings while inhaling can encourage this particular illusive and unifying trail of sensation and movement. Normally the pattern is difficult to access and is seldom used in the nonintegrated body, but with imagery, the pattern automatically presents itself. (See an illustration of kidney wings in Appendix 4.)

Instead of visualizing wings, you might be able to access the feeling by imagining that you have multiple arms rooted in the kidney area of your back, like a deity form. The arms are reaching up and out—as if reaching with infinite kindness in all directions so that the back of the body and diaphragm are luminous, expansive, and spread. This sense of reaching is a reminder of your supportive relationship to the world, to others, to someone outside yourself.

The kidney wing pattern is difficult to find and maintain because there is a tendency, when inhaling, to unconsciously contract the hip flexors, which reflexively closes the back in the area of the kidney wings. This contraction is a natural part of the inhaling (prāṇa) pattern, when the mind is distracted and wandering in discursive thought. When this happens, the inhaling (prāṇa) pattern can break away from the complementary exhaling apāna pattern, thereby tightening and collapsing the ribs in the lower back and interrupting the kidney wing pattern. It is common, when our minds wander, for prāṇa to separate from apāna this way, allowing the sensation patterns and our thoughts to drift away from the present moment. As we inhale, if we deliberately maintain an awareness of the seed of the complementary apāna pattern—which stabilizes the coccyx, expands the kidney area, and requires that the psoas and QL muscles refrain from contracting—then the prāṇa pattern opens symmetrically from the central axis without separating and wandering off. Preserving the smooth, rising, and spreading kidney wing pattern creates this union; fully spreads and lifts the back of the diaphragm; inflates the lower lobes of the lungs; and stimulates an expansive feeling of being awake, grounded, and symmetrical.

Psoas Buttons

Psoas buttons are two of a number of points on the abdomen from which we can practice retracting or pulling in as a way of encouraging an awareness of the mechanics of inflating the kidney wings. Attention to the psoas buttons can also increase our awareness of the muscles in the pelvic floor and aid in the cultivation of Mūlabandha. We can imagine psoas buttons as small, circular areas on either side of the lower belly that root into the body and connect to the actual psoas muscles, which lie deep beneath the points. The "buttons" are located immediately in front of the medial edge of each of the psoas muscles, about four or five finger-widths below the navel, and about three or four finger-widths out to the sides. They lie a couple of finger-widths above the outer edges of the pubic bone and just in front of the medial border of the psoas muscles. The fibers of connective tissue from the lowest segments of the transversus abdominis muscles cross from one side of the lower belly to the other to form a band across the top edge of the pubic bone just at the point where we feel the psoas buttons.

Like buttons you might find on a wall when calling an elevator, you can imagine the psoas buttons as substantial and secure yet easy to push. Touch them lightly with the tip of a finger or fingernail in a way that causes them to pull back a bit. It should feel as if the tip of whatever touches the buttons is actually an irritant, causing the retraction, rather than that you must press hard on the buttons. By stimulating the psoas button points, the fibers of this lower section of the transversus abdominis are given a signal to tone in such a way that causes the abdomen to assume a kind of pot shape that floats up and out of the pelvic basin. We can use the image of touching the psoas buttons to train the muscles for an effective inhaling pattern.

1. Sit straight and bring the awareness to the breath. Place the fingertips of each hand on the low belly just over the line of the psoas muscles. The pressure on the belly when pushing the psoas button does not need to be forceful.
2. Instead of your fingertips, you could also place the tips of small dowels or chopsticks on the points to focus your attention.
3. During the course of a smooth, deep inhalation, keep touching the psoas button points as a reminder to keep this lowest part of the abdominal wall slightly retracted. This will tone the pelvic floor while keeping the apāna pattern stimulated at the same time. When you have found and activated the psoas buttons, it will feel as if the sitting bones are moving down as the floating ribs behind the kidneys spread.
4. As you exhale, lift the fingertips off the low belly, keeping the mind focused on the sensations that arise during the smooth and even breathing pattern. At the very end of the exhalation, bring particular attention to any sense of movement, toning, or activation in the pelvic floor muscles. This is like depositing the seed of the entire apāna pattern at the center point of the pelvic floor.
5. Gently place the fingertips back on the psoas buttons to stimulate an even retraction of the lower band of muscles that cross the abdomen as you inhale again.
6. Repeat this breathing pattern, using the fingers on the buttons as a reminder to contract without gripping on the inhalation, lifting the fingers on the exhalation, and cultivating the sense of the pot of the belly floating during the entire wave pattern of breath.

The image of a psoas button implies that lightly touching the button can begin this deeper and more complex process, which is actually the cultivation of Uḍḍīyāna Bandha and Mūlabandha. The line of tone in the transversus abdominis is distinct and does not go any higher than two finger-widths below the navel. If you overcontract the abdomen so that toning travels too far up the abdominal wall muscles, Mūlabandha will not manifest distinctly, and extraneous tension in the upper part of the abdomen will prevent a sense of being fully grounded. These two aspects of movement that are activated through the psoas button practice are precursors for a deep transformation of emotions that can occur as the inhaling and exhaling patterns of breath unite and spread throughout the body from the lower stations of the central axis.

For the psoas button areas to actually retract on the inhalation, the pubococcygeus (PC) muscle needs to tone distinctly as you initiate the action. To help in finding this action, you might imagine that you were shrinking the tissues of the pelvic floor, as if pulling a zipper closed from the front edge of the anus back and up the front surface of the coccyx until it reaches the middle of the sacrum. The entire area of the pelvic floor from front to back and up the inside of the cave of the sacrum will feel tidy and awake. You can augment this sensation by imagining that the action of inhaling is being initiated from the area immediately above the center of the pelvic floor.

With practice, even without actually touching the psoas buttons, you can maintain a sense of responsive toning in the pelvic floor and low belly throughout all of the phases of the inhalation. This should be true even at the crest of the inhalation when the scalene muscles of the neck tone so that the upper lobes of the lungs fill with breath. At this point, the mind tends to flicker and lose touch with the bodily sensations associated with the apāna at the root of the exhaling pattern in the central channel and pelvic floor. This unlinking of prāṇa and apāna happens all the time, so we study it from slightly different angles again and again. Using the psoas buttons is an effective method of pointing out this subtle and illusive internal form.

Gaṇeśa Belly

Imagining what we call a *Gaṇeśa belly* is an inclusive whole-body image. Gaṇeśa, the elephant-headed deity, is considered to be a loving, jolly, relaxed, and extremely intelligent holder of the mysteries of the central channel. He represents the idea of paradoxical thinking within the esoteric yogas. One of his notable features is that his abdomen is expansive, side to side and front to back, in an even and toned way at the plane of his navel. In the most beautiful and finer artistic representations of Gaṇeśa, his lower abdomen, right at the top of the pubic bone, is hollowed out slightly. Often he is depicted with a cloth wrapped around his hips, draping around his body in such a way as to suggest a convergence of energies under the floating "pot" of his belly. Often this cloth is tied in a knot in what would on our bodies be a point around four or five fingerwidths below the navel. Sometimes a fine jewel is installed there.

Gaṇeśa is definitely cued into his kidney wings, the cave of his sacrum, and his psoas buttons! He *is* the Mūlabandha. The sense of a floating, happy potbelly, which instantly stimulates an integrating pattern that loops through the entire body, is represented in immaculate detail in Gaṇeśa's form: his large elephant ears, which are tuned to the infinity of divine sound, or *nāda;* his deep, bright eyes that reflect his intelligent, humorous, and compassionate view of all circumstance and beings; and his long nose representing the complete cleansing of the nāḍīs. Of course, Gaṇeśa also has immaculate shoulder alignment, often manifesting with at least four arms, so he is clearly tuned in to the finer details that occur throughout the breath and body when one unites complementary opposites with a trusting, intelligent, open mind.

It is said that with much practice the breath can be united by drawing the apāna (the downward contracting pattern) up the middle line of the body into the roots of the navel, while at the same time allowing the prāṇa (which by nature is an expansive, spreading pattern) to be pulled down to the plane of the navel. This union comes naturally to Gaṇeśa. In our yoga practice when the two patterns of breath unite at the nābhi cakra (the root of the navel), you may experience the distinct contracting, shrinking pull of the apāna united with the expansive flower-like spreading of the prāṇa. This awakens the *samāna vāyu,* the equalizing form of Prāṇa that is in the navel. Samāna vāyu is related to digestive fire and functions to synthesize opposite patterns of sensation, which then helps in synthesizing conceptual opposites and complementary movement patterns throughout the body. Allowing yourself to imagine Gaṇeśa's embodied form of this relaxed yet intentional and unstrained union of opposites at the nābhi cakra can automatically facilitate a distinct feeling of the samāna vāyu and its penetrating form. This may take a number of lifetimes to occur.

apane ūrdhvage jāte prayāte vahnimaṇḍalam
tadā'nalaśikhā dīrghā jāyate vāyunā 'hatā (v. 65)

tato yāto vahnyapānau prāṇamuṣṇasvarūpakam
tenātyantapradīptastu jvalano dehajastathā (v. 66)

tena kuṇḍalinī suptā saṁtaptā saṁprabudhyate
daṇḍāhatā bhujaṅgīva niḥśvasya ṛjutāṁ vrajet (v. 67)

bilaṁ praviṣṭeva tato brahmanāḍyantaraṁ vrajet
tasmānnityaṁ mūlabandhaḥ kartavyo yogibhiḥ sadā (v. 68)

When the apāna, tending downward, is turned upward and reaches the circle of fire (at the navel); when the apāna touches the fire, the flames lengthens. When the apāna and the fire reach the prāṇa, which is hot by nature, the heat in the body is intensified. The Kuṇḍalinī, who has been sleeping being heated completely, wakes up like a snake that has been hit by a stick and straightens herself. Then, like a serpent she enters her hole, the Brahmā Nāḍī. Therefore the yogi should always practice Mūlabandha.

—*Haṭha Yoga Pradīpikā,* ch. 3, v. 65–68

Cobra Hood

Cobra hoods are extremely visceral and useful images for developing essential yet illusive internal movements and conjunctions that facilitate whole-body patterns of movement. If you look at a cobra from behind when it is alert or charmed, it is easy to see the importance of being fully grounded in order to have a stable, expansive, and articulated upper body. As the snake sits on the ground, lifting up and out of the nest of its coil, its upper back and neck (referred to as its "hood") spread and broaden, connecting a line of energy from the sides of its body up and out to form an acoustic band-shell shape just behind the snake's head. This image is useful to our yoga practice as it intuitively suggests the sense of joining together through vinyāsa—rooting down on the exhaling pattern in order to expand up and out through the inhaling pattern. Cobra hoods even describe the broad feeling in the back as well as the back portion of the shoulder joint when the arms are overhead in āsanas. You can feel this in many poses, from the Downward Dog Pose to Ūrdhvā Dhanurāsana. (See an illustration of cobra hoods in Appendix 4.)

If you meditate deeply on embodying this form, imagining that you are grounded, awake, and alert while listening carefully to the acoustic space at the edges of the spreading hood, you may feel a sense of broadening and lifting throughout the entire back of your body—as if you were a cobra waking up. The sense of spreading like a snake will start in the area of your kidney wings, which will stimulate the dropping apāna pattern that coils as a tail in the pelvic floor and rises to expand the back. The cobra hood pattern continues to extend evenly over the crown of the head and can come to life if you relax extraneous tension in the mouth, release the palate, and soften the eyes as if smiling. Rather than losing focus in a dream state, it is possible to stay alert—as would any snake worth its salt—by again listening deeply. The natural counteraction, the vinyāsa, is that the middle of the heart opens to become the focus of the cobra hood pattern. The cobra hood shelters and adores the precious one at the center of the heart.

Cobra hoods can be visualized in many ways, from the simple sense of something expansive that arches over the crown of the head to precise and detailed complex images. You might imagine, for example, that from the root of a single coiled tail on which you sit, there are thousands of cobra heads extending up and out across your back, curving gently over your head to form a sort of canopy. Perhaps each head of this infinitely expansive upper part of the snake is wearing a crown of effulgent jewels, and each head is singing scriptures or hymns in an endless variety of languages from infinite points of view. Meanwhile, your upper body remains stable, strong, and expansive, yet it is also fluid and firmly rooted down through the base of the snake. Your ears and the hearing function stay with the pure cacophony of sound (without the mind picking out objects) that opens, unfolds, and soothes your nervous system. With your awareness returning to focus on the geometric wholeness stimulated by the form of serpent heads arching through and above you, the integrity settles into your entire body as it softly dissolves back down to the center of the heart and all through the central axis of the body. From the core of the heart up through the crown, it feels as if the heads are sheltering and adoring this sacred space, and from the navel down, there is a feeling of rooting deeply into the earth.

> **maṇi bhrātphaṇā sahasraravighṛtaviśvam**
> **bharāmaṇḍalāyānantāya nāgarājāya namaḥ**
>
> salutations to the king of the *nagas,*
> to the infinite, to the bearer of the maṇḍala,
> who spreads out the universe with thousands
> of hooded heads, set with blazing, effulgent jewels.
>
> —*Kūrma Purāṇa,* ch. 9, v. 5

Embodying this, like other images, is important to our āsana practice because it helps elicit feelings that slow us down and suspend interruptions of mind. Rather than jumping to habitual story lines and conclusions about our circumstances, our alignment and form, or our yoga practice, there is a sense of both mental and physical spaciousness that allows us to feel engulfed by a trust in not knowing. We can stay open to the arising of fresh viewpoints and a feeling of deep respect for the process of transformation within the mind, Prāṇa, other beings, and the universe at large. Feelings of safety within a vastness are enabled through the visualization of being crowned by a cobra hood as we gently hold what is most precious in the core of the heart. If you hold the center of the heart too tightly—with a motive to get or achieve something from the precious content of that space within the heart—then you just have a cobra on the loose! To really embody and enjoy the sense of a cobra hood, there is an element of embodied nonattachment and sincerity.

Skin Flow

The skin, which develops in utero from the same layer of embryonic tissue as the brain (ectoderm), is well innervated. When we pay attention to specific areas of the skin, we switch on its sensitivity, and this can allow us to feel structural alignment as well as existing tension in the myofascial layers that lie beneath the skin. One of the hallmarks of good alignment is that the skin seems more awake and vibrant, as if it's glowing. When we talk about *skin flow,* we're really talking about a particular pattern of release or stretch in the myofascial sheathes under the skin. Real skin does not flow very far; if it did, a person with tattoos would find them moving all around the body.

To feel the sense of skin moving, you must focus on the sensation of air touching the outer layer of skin and at least an imaginary sense of the skin's ability to move and slide around on the layer of adipose tissue (fat) just beneath it. For example, when you sit or stand with good shoulder alignment, with close attention you can feel the shoulder blades and the muscles and skin that cover them spreading and descending down the back in just the right way. At the same time, you can feel the skin on the chest spreading and flowing up and out over the collarbones, as the skin on the front edges of the armpits flows up, back, and out. This requires a subtle level of awareness or toning that, when complemented by attentiveness and a relaxed feeling on the skin's surface, results in a gentle stretching of the pectoralis major muscles. The whole-body feeling of this movement is one of the skin being guided or smeared up and out across the fronts of your shoulder joints. Simultaneously the backs of the armpits feel as though they are flowing down and forward in space as they spread out. This allows the skin behind the floating ribs to expand

and releases the extraneous tension in the rhomboid and upper trapezius muscles. If you focus on these sensations, you may feel as though the skin, starting from the back of the skull, softens and flows down the sides of the spine.

In many poses, when good alignment of the head, neck, and shoulders finally manifests, extraneous tension releases in all these areas, and there is a spontaneous feeling in the front of the throat that the skin is soft and luminous. This is a great opportunity to breathe into the sensations and imagine the skin flowing upward toward the back of the throat, which automatically softens tension in the jaw and releases the root of the palate. Simply focusing on the movement of skin in this way can stimulate an integrating whole-body pattern of awareness.

The manifestation of Prāṇa, or intelligence, in the skin is one of the functions of the *vyāna vāyu.* It has no center or home of its own, but it does integrate the vast peripheral structures of the body with their environment and then back into the central core of the body, serving an all-pervading function to connect all systems. Prāṇa and the intelligence—which have no self-form—love to link systems, to support, to hold, and to communicate. Skin flow is a secret ingredient in this alignment and form.

Holding the Tail of a Serpent

An image that facilitates integrated whole-body patterns of extension via a sense of grounding through the edges of the pelvic floor is that of *holding the tail of a serpent.* In this image, holding our "tailbone" steady is the precondition to initiating the inhaling pattern of the body. When we talk about the tailbone we are referring to the coccyx, the small triangular bone that attaches to the base of the sacrum and that, in most people, naturally curls down and in slightly toward the front of the pelvic basin. We sometimes speak of the coccyx dropping or moving, and there *can* be a tiny bit of movement associated with the bone as the muscles of the pelvic floor tone. But because the coccyx is fused to the sacrum, that movement is actually very slight. So the use of visualization—imagining that instead of a little stump of a tail, we actually have a long, powerful tail like some other members of the animal kingdom—can help to bring movements associated with the coccyx to life and may be enough to initiate the patterns of Prāṇic flow we want to stimulate.

Imagine what it would feel like to have the dynamic tail of a dragon, a snake, or a monkey. Take that feeling into the patterns of movement related to the coccyx in the pelvic floor so those movements become distinct in your nervous system. Of course, for most of us, just *finding* the coccyx and muscles of the pelvic floor—the pubococcygeus, the iliococcygeus, and the coccygeus—can be difficult. You can begin to locate the general area by repeatedly squeezing and releasing the anal sphincter muscles or by doing what are referred to as Kegel exercises. With practice, you will be able to connect to the pelvic floor on a more refined and intelligent level by paying close attention to what happens in that region when you complete an exhalation—especially if at the end of an exhale you give a short puff, almost like a punctuation mark. A connection to the pelvic floor makes it easier to use the imagination to refine movements and to map out that area of the body. Imagining that you have a tail can help; it can trigger awareness of the coccyx and its subtle ability to move in conjunction with the pelvic floor muscles, and this awareness eventually begins to wake up Mūlabandha.

Holding the tail of a serpent is a two-way movement, as if you are pulling a curved sword from its sheath; the movement of two intimately related structures flowing in opposite curves. The two-way action is a function of being able to separate an awareness of the sacrum from an awareness of the coccyx. The sacrum is like the "mother bone" of the coccyx; it is always right there above the coccyx, ready to help. In an extreme, purely apānic movement, the sacrum tends to follow the coccyx's direction of movement, so that as you tuck your tail, you may find that you also contract the abdomen and buttocks muscles and flex the spine. This causes the entire pelvis to tilt or tuck and potentially shuts down the complementary prāṇa pattern throughout the body. In sitting up straight, the sacrum tends to move up and in while the coccyx moves down and in. Separating the movement of the coccyx from that of the sacrum allows the cultivation of Mūlabandha and the refinement of an awareness of the pelvic floor.

The movement of the tail inevitably involves communication with the pubic bone. If we are able to use the tail without too much involvement from the sacrum, we also want to maintain the presence of the prāṇa pattern in the right proportion throughout the body. The pubic bone belongs to the prāṇa family and is reflected as an open heart. When "holding a pose by the tail," we often aim to maintain the complementary openhearted quality of the spine rather than the tuck and flexion associated with the extreme apāna pattern. In these cases, even though we are cultivating a sense of the coccyx dropping down and slightly forward, the sacrum feels as if it is floating up and into the body (moving into the lower abdomen), while the movement of the pubic bone is down and back toward the coccyx. These are all very subtle movements that create a balance of tone in the pelvic floor from front to back and side to side. When done correctly, they can wake up our psoas muscles, alleviate stress in the SI joints, set a base for Mūlabandha to appear, and encourage integrated and full-body movements in the spine and out through the limbs and the entire body.

Feet Reflecting the Pelvic Floor

When working standing poses or even when sitting and articulating our feet and toes into combinations of positions and movements, the pelvic floor comes online to help coordinate the effort. Since it is difficult, especially for beginners, to connect to the pelvic floor, focusing on the different combinations of complementary and opposing muscular and structural tones and forces in the legs and feet—which are far more accessible—can stimulate a spontaneous awakening of the pelvic floor. This is what we refer to as the *feet reflecting the pelvic floor.* It is as if the feet are the embassy of the pelvic floor—an accessible structure through which we can get a message to the homeland of the pelvic floor, which then informs subtle movement and alignment throughout the body.

The various families of muscles around the hip joints flex, extend, abduct, adduct, and rotate inwardly and outwardly through an amazing range and variety of movements. The pelvic floor coordinates all of these movements in a fine balance with each other and with the movements of the spine to produce competent, continuous, and sometimes microscopic adjustments and adaptations. With endless practice, it gradually becomes clear that the feet and pelvic floor are intimately and directly related, so one method for cultivating an ability to articulate the pelvic floor and facilitate integrated movement in all yoga poses is to "wake up" the feet.

In standing poses during which the movement in and out of the poses is almost as important as the "final" form, how the feet respond to the structural needs of the body is essential. Many yoga teachers can diagnose, prevent, or help to heal many structural problems by simply observing how students use their feet. Students sometimes consider standing poses to be basically static warm-up exercises, so they often wander away from fine-tuning the structural lines needed to go in and out of the pose with integrity. Lazy, amorphous, nonradiant feet and legs can cause the entire pose (not to mention the practitioner) to suffer. One way of waking up the feet and legs is to engage the quadriceps without switching off the hamstrings. This can be done by bringing focused attention and a sense of grounding into the sole of the foot; by rooting down through the big toes without abandoning the sense of dropping through the heels. This will bring intelligence into the pelvic floor, and with close observation, you may notice slightly altered patterns of tone in the different quadrants of the pelvic floor.

Each foot has three arches: a powerful medial arch that runs from the first joint of the big toe (near the mound) to the front edge of the heel on the inside of the foot; a smaller but important lateral arch that runs from the first joint of the little toe to the outer edge of the heel; and a transverse arch that runs from side to side across the middle of the foot. These arches give the foot a springlike, bouncing potential. With the feet together in Samasthitiḥ and attention on the feeling of the arches lifting (even if you have flat feet), it is possible to imagine a relationship between the arches of the feet and an awakened pelvic floor. Subjectively, in the practice of Mūlabandha, you can imagine the middle point of the pelvic floor being drawn up in a similar fashion to the arches of the feet, giving it a domelike feeling from side to side as well as from front to back. Of course, distinguishing the pelvic floor from all the nearby muscles is easier said than done, but most of us first get a sense of it by articulating and using the feet intelligently and enthusiastically.

You can use your imagination to tap into this feeling of waking up the feet by imagining in the standing poses that you are putting on a pair of long, high socks in which you have to push each foot and leg out away from the body as you pull the sheath of the sock up toward the hip joint. Imagining the sheath to be your skin as you activate the foot to push out and down can create a radiant, awakened state in the leg and an attentive tone in both the feet and the pelvic floor.

In āsanas in which the legs are up in the air—such as Headstand, Shoulderstand, and arm balances—or even when lying on the back with feet up the wall, the tone and structure of the feet and legs are key to bringing the pose into a full expression. For example, when practicing Piñcha Mayūrāsana (Peacock Feather Pose), it is possible to balance precariously upside down with inactive feet and legs and, almost as if by chance, not fall over. But for a fully inspired pose, one in which the spine feels as if it is being extended up toward the ceiling and the base of the pose feels stable and steady, the feet must be fully articulated with the legs active and awake.

Like so many aspects of the practice, you must work slowly and patiently to feel the immediate and more generalized benefits of connecting the feet to the pelvic floor. Gradually subtle patterns of Prāṇa and connections between muscles and fascia lines will automatically come to life. Outside of your own thought process or your attempts to apply technique to poses, movements will become inspired and integrated on their own.

Palate-Perineum Reflex

During a vinyāsa practice in which the movement in and out of poses is just as important as the poses themselves, we can easily find a simple yet profound relationship between the palate (roof of the mouth) and the perineum (pelvic floor). This *palate-perineum reflex* is an essential element that integrates wavelike patterns of movement between the outer and inner body. In any pose, adjusting even a small corner of the pose—like the shape of the hand, the tone in the tongue, or the movement of the collarbones—can have a ripple effect throughout the entire body. One of the most fundamental of these interpenetrating patterns is along the spine from top to bottom and is associated with the prāṇic inhaling pattern of rising, extending, and spreading and its complementary opposite, the apānic exhaling pattern of descending, flexing, and contracting. In prāṇāyāma practice, keeping the essential pattern of the prāṇa when the apāna is active, and vice versa, is the key to calming and clarifying the mind. So too in āsana, we discover there is a reflexive relationship between these two patterns that inspires a more integrated movement within the practice.

For example, while we are bending forward into Dve position (which is an apānic movement) in Sūrya Namaskāra, we keep the spine relatively straight and the area of the heart open. This is easily accomplished by releasing the upper back of the palate, as if silently saying *ah*. During that phase of the pose, there is a sense of riding the breath as if it were a wave. The palate becomes like a surfboard on a wave, and our attentiveness to the details of movement makes us surfers. When we pay attention to every small, informative shift that arises, it makes the ride smooth and even. As the exhalation comes to an end, the wavelike pattern shifts, and an apānic flexion and slight coiling pattern appears in the body as we detect a toning of the pelvic floor. This happens because the condensed seed of the apānic pattern is in the center of the pelvic floor and can be felt at the end of a full prāṇāyāma-like exhalation. As the breath shifts and the inhalation begins, we refine the emphasis structurally to stay in touch with the seed-point of the exhalation; we do so by cultivating the feeling of "scooping up" in front of the sacrum during the inhalation. At the very top of the in-breath, as the wave of the breath crests, the palate is released and the pelvic floor resets. Then the wave pattern begins again as breathing continues.

This palate-perineum relationship is a whole-body pattern. Focusing the attention on the perineum and palate is never an exclusive focus, but it serves as a gateway within the field of awareness into the entire body. It is extremely pleasant and often relieves strain in a pose when we become too dogmatic and attempt to force the body into some contrived ideal form. Practicing this way—riding the wave of the breath and connecting palate to perineum—leaves a pleasant meditative residue within any form of yoga practice.

Plumb Line

After we get warmed up in our āsana, prāṇāyāma, or meditation practice, it is easy to experience a central axis, a central channel, or a plumb line running top to bottom within the body. The plumb line provides a reference point within the subtle body for feelings, thoughts, sensations, and the movement of Prāṇa to be organized and understood as a reflection of the body's natural intelligence. The plumb, which is easy to sense when the mind is still, gives our structure a clear axis of orientation so that through smooth and even breathing, movements fall spontaneously into place.

A good time to begin feeling and understanding the plumb line is while practicing āsana, particularly while moving in and out of poses. When we twist from side to side or do forward bends followed by backbends, for example, we gradually come to a point where opposite yet interdependent physical patterns become balanced and integrated. As these patterns sync with one another, we no longer fall into habitual patterns that may favor one direction of movement over another. We feel balanced left to right and front to back, with both patterns fully awake so that Prāṇa (and therefore the mind) comes to a natural pause. In that pause, the physiology of the yogic state of nirodha, or suspension of the process of mind, which is the state of pure, unbiased attention, arises. Within this state, it is easy to feel the central line of the body as being the channel for the flow of our attention. When standing or sitting straight, this central channel corresponds to the plumb line; when lying down, we refer to it merely as the middle path or central axis.

Āsana practice can reveal the plumb line, and you can augment an awareness of it through visualization. Imagine, for instance, that you were attempting to balance a pole on your nose like a circus performer might. You would have to make many compensatory movements to the front, to the back, to the left, to the right, and all around. With much practice, you would occasionally get to a point where the pole is balanced; all the minor adjustments would be temporarily suspended, and you would be captured by the process of balancing, finding yourself in a highly attentive, peaceful space. The technique involved is that of appropriate compensation blended with an equalization of present-moment attention and nonattachment to outcome. Finding the plumb line is actually an embodiment practice of the process of effort and letting go, as described in the Yoga Sūtra:

> **abhyāsa-vairāgyābhyāṁ tan nirodhaḥ**
>
> Through practice and releasing, the fluctuations of mind are suspended.
>
> —Yoga Sūtra, Samādhi Pāda, v. 12

Abhyāsa can be translated as "practice" or "effort" and is essential whether you are balancing a pole on your nose, moving into a difficult āsana, or simply dealing with the complexities of life. At the same time, *vairāgyam,* letting go of techniques, theories, and expectations, while staying in the present moment is essential. It simply doesn't work if you put too aggressive an effort into the process, nor does it work if you completely let go. In so many situations in life, and certainly in yoga practice, you must have a full, devoted, and directed effort but, at the same time, an absolute sense of release without a hint of laziness or the abandonment of ideals or form. You must have it all and both ways too.

The same is true when we polish the subtleties of form while standing in Samasthitiḥ. We balance the prāṇa and the apāna, sometimes squeezing them together, sometimes relaxing and letting the alignment of the pose be. The external pose is a conversation between heels and toes, inward and outward rotations, top and bottom, palate and perineum, pubic bone and coccyx, and on and on into infinitely subtle levels of perception, form, and alignment, all of which make us able to access the sense of a plumb line. Wherever the attention falls along that plumb line, a feeling floods the body and mind of an equal opening in all directions arising in conjunction with a joining of prāṇa and apāna. Much like a flower would open to the sun, this spreading of Prāṇa and the intricacies of awareness feed back into our ability to maintain a connection to the central channel through the pelvic floor and the root of the palate.

To tap into this feeling on a more visceral level, the plumb line can be visualized as a straw that extends down into the earth from the middle of the body and between the legs. The straw rises up through the center of the pelvic floor along the midline and continues on and out through the crown of the head. As this image is clarified in the nervous system, we feel that the line corresponds to a conduit through which attention can flow easily. The straw might be perceived as a generalized sensation; a movement of energy, light, or liquid; Prāṇa flowing through a tube; or what we might eventually call the suṣumṇā nāḍī.

LIBERATING AND ILLUMINATING

Visualization practices can be entire paths in and of themselves, enriching the practice as different images and meditations intersect. Different viewpoints reveal a multiplicity of self-reference paradoxes that, when looked at through an open mind, help to refine the intelligence. Watching changes in form, thought, and sensation underscores the liberating insight that, although in a very real sense we are embodied beings, we are not *this* body. Or rather that this body is not a solid and permanent phenomenon. We are reminded again and again to keep the senses fresh and awake—opening the ears, releasing preconceptions along with the palate, tuning in to the breath, and always delving deeper into the experience at hand.

That's why you have to be extremely careful if you try to practice yoga when you're angry, unsettled, or distracted. When the mind is dominated by extreme mental or emotional imbalance, or if there are subtle levels of physical tension and resistance within the body, it is virtually impossible to truly surrender to the entirety of what is occurring and to fully examine (and possibly embrace) an opposing perspective. Misperception, misinterpretation, injury, and unskillful actions are most likely to govern your thoughts and actions when you cling to a single point of view where tension and imbalances dominate. That is not to say you cannot practice when unsettled—in fact, sometimes practice is just the antidote needed to bring balance. But especially when you are off-kilter, you must practice carefully and with a sense of surrender, of not knowing, and of starting over again and again. When approached in this way, the practice will often smooth out imbalances, especially if you practice "all day every day."

And that is the key: we must carefully continue to practice through the ups and downs of life and the practice itself. Visualizations and whole-body patterns of alignment facilitate the visceral experience of connecting, integrating, and unifying opposing patterns. There are thousands of visualizations and many whole-body patterns of sensation through which this integrating experience of letting go of the ego can be found. Any one of them can facilitate a release of your preconceptions so that "you" disappear and a significant and paradoxical understanding is revealed. Once you are fully in your body, it disappears; it becomes open and empty, and the discursive mind, cloaked in all its natural processes of avoidance and grasping, automatically falls back into meditation. There is no one path to this form of insight, you have to get into it from wherever you *really* are—inside, outside, still mind, agitated mind—so that you find a suspension of thought processes and of habitual body patterns.

Just as in meditation, when working with these subtle levels of body, almost anyone who practices long enough may go into what feels like an altered state or a trance. That can be fascinating yet dangerous, because without proper grounding, altered mind states can take us off on tangents. We may not see that a "trance" does not mean we're special. In fact, if we are practicing honestly and openly, everything that arises makes us feel more ordinary, more normal, more like ourselves. The most important insight is not a vision of a deity shining in the center of your heart, but an understanding that you are actually not all that special in terms of standing out from others. Rather you are special because you are inspired and delighted by being nothing special at all.

4

Mechanics

Essential Anatomical Perspectives

CLASSICAL ANATOMY COMPLEMENTS AND GREATLY informs visualization and the idea of vinyāsa in yoga practice. This chapter includes a limited selection of anatomy topics that are of particular relevance to yoga poses and internal forms. Hopefully this basic information will serve as a springboard to deepen your ongoing study of anatomy.

SYSTEMS

With regard to yoga, a good starting point for studying anatomy is seeing how movement patterns within the vinyāsa of a pose relate to the skeletal, respiratory, and muscular systems.

The *skeletal system,* made up of bones and joints, allows movement and provides both a scaffold of form and a protective framework for the soft tissues of the body. The specific shape and size of the bones and their connections at the joints through ligaments (bone-to-bone connections) and tendons (muscle-to-bone connections) contribute to range of motion and affect proper alignment for maximum support within poses. One way of practicing yoga is to visualize a pose from the perspective of either the *axial* (vertebral column, rib cage, and skull) or the *appendicular* (shoulder and pelvic girdles, arms, and legs) skeleton. Focusing on the axial skeleton, we can eventually *feel* the plumb line by imagining the bones of our spine stacked on top of each other in their natural S-shaped curve, providing strength, stability, and mobility to our extended or upright form. Feeling movement in the rib cage, which encases the lungs and is attached to the diaphragm, as we breathe is highly informative for prāṇāyāma and movement. Envisioning our body from the perspective of the appendicular skeleton reveals a solid and intelligent pelvic basin and pelvic floor with connections from the core of the body that both go out into space and are grounded into the earth.

The *muscular system* is perhaps the most tangible system within the body. We can actually see muscles as they move, as when we engage the biceps. Focusing awareness on the character, function, and form of particular muscles and how they relate to bones and the breath can immediately "wake up" a pose. Muscle tissue is composed of elongated cells that vary in size and texture (striated or smooth) according to function. There is a continuous layer of connective tissue called *fascia* that surrounds muscle bundles, individual muscles, and groups of muscles and connects us from head to toe. As we move, envisioning muscles contracting or releasing in line with their fibers, in conjunction with the breath, and in relationship to bones—all facilitated through the fascia—is fascinating.

Visualizing and sensing the *respiratory system* from the gross-body perspective of the organs and structures involved in breathing—the lungs, ribs, diaphragm, and so on—and from a more subtle-body level of nāḍīs and Prāṇa flow is invaluable to our āsana and prāṇāyāma practices. Visualizing the flow of breath within our movements and in harmony with the other systems of the body is central to practicing yoga as a meditative, unifying form.

BASIC TERMS

Active and *passive range of motion:* The range of motion in a joint is active when local muscle groups that impact the joint directly contract to move it to a certain degree of rotation, flexion, or extension. Passive range of motion is when the forces that move the bones at a joint do not come from the muscle groups immediately around the joint. Instead, those "local muscles" remain soft so they do not interfere with or restrict the movement. In a vinyāsa practice, it is common for active and passive movements to complement one another in support of the desired outcome.

Agonist or *antagonist:* A muscle can be described as an agonist—one that is a "prime mover," or causes movement—or an *antagonist*—one that inhibits or counters the movement. The erector spinae and abdominal muscles, for instance, are all involved in extension or flexion of the spine. Working together, they switch roles as agonist and antagonist during a graceful movement of the spine.

Anatomical position: A spatial context for structures is called their anatomical position, described when the body is facing front, arms by the sides, palms forward. Structures closer to the head are *superior,* those closer to the feet are *inferior. Anterior* structures are positioned more toward the front plane of the body, and *posterior* structures are those toward the back. *Medial* refers to structures closer to the midline of the body, and *lateral* refers to structures farther from the midline. The terms *proximal* and *distal* describe structures that are either closer or more distant, respectively, from another reference point—usually the core of the body. *Superficial* and *deep* refer to how far a structure is from the surface of the body, with superficial being closer.

Co-contraction: This is the term for the simultaneous contraction of opposing sets of muscles. In co-contraction the relative forces of the muscles involved are continuously adjusted to achieve the necessary results of movement and stability. For example, co-contraction of the hamstrings and quadriceps is imperative when balancing on one foot, allowing stability and competent reversibility of movements, a basic principle in vinyāsa practice.

Eccentric contraction: When a muscle is contracting and lengthening at the same time, in cases when it is causing resistance to a chosen direction of movement, the action is called eccentric contraction. For example, in Ūrdhvā Dhanurāsana (Upward Bow Pose) one should slightly contract the rectus abdominis muscle and yet allow it to lengthen (eccentric contraction). This keeps the opposing muscles, the psoas and the erector spinae of the back, from contracting, thereby protecting the lower back from compression.

Origin and *insertion:* The origin of a muscle is a point that is more proximal (closer to the center of the body) and is therefore typically more stable. The insertion point is onto a bone that is more mobile—the one that is drawn toward the point of origin when the muscle in question contracts. In complex actions, a muscle may not follow this rule of movement. For example, when you stand up out of Dve during Sūrya Namaskāra, the hamstring muscles pull and make the sitting bones move down toward the floor. This makes the sitting bones the insertion points in this case. Whereas when swinging the leg back, as in walking, the *ischial tuberocity* (sitting bone) attachment is considered the origin because it does not move relative to the leg that is being pulled back.

Reciprocal inhibition: When two muscles (or sets of muscles) create opposite actions, they work with reciprocal inhibition. This happens automatically in the nervous system. For instance, when the quadriceps fire while closing or opening the knee joint, the opposing hamstrings automatically relax. Reciprocal inhibition can be consciously interrupted through co-contraction.

STRUCTURES

Spine

Sensing and understanding movements and form within the practice is greatly informed by a simple overview of the *spinal column.* Composed of thirty-three bones (vertebrae) stacked in a natural S shape running from the coccyx up to the cranium (head), the spine is the main structure that allows us to stand straight, bend, and twist. Sections of the spine are differentiated according to their shape and function as cervical (neck), thoracic (upper back), and lumbar (lower back). Shorthand for various spots on the back, such as L4 (lumbar vertebra 4), is helpful in understanding muscular and skeletal relationships when describing our poses. Between each set of vertebrae is a disk that cushions and contributes to smooth movement within the spine. Due to the natural aging process, accident, or misuse, disks can become damaged or "herniated," oozing out from between the vertebrae. In a yoga practice, this type of injury is one that should be addressed with particular care and caution by both practitioner and teacher.

Palate and Tongue

The *palate* refers to the entire roof of the mouth. It includes the *hard palate,* the bony structure that lies directly behind the front teeth, and the *soft palate,* the soft, movable structure at the top of the back of the mouth, composed of five muscles sheathed in mucous membrane. These muscles are essential to breathing, swallowing, and shutting off or allowing airflow from the mouth to the nasal passages. From an internal forms perspective, the uvula—the teardrop-shaped projection of tissue in the back of the throat—is included as part of the soft palate because it is intimately informed by movements of those five muscles. When we speak of the root of the palate, we are actually moving our awareness back and up behind the soft palate into the hidden yet highly sensitive area near the pituitary gland.

The palate is tied intrinsically to breathing patterns and is also connected to the toning of the pelvic floor and Mūlabandha. Though the tongue is not actually part of the palate, it is an interesting and important muscle to contemplate. It represents the language function, toning even when we think, and activity in the tongue directly affects tone or tension in the palate that is then felt throughout the body.

Pelvic Floor

In an Aṣṭāṅga Vinyāsa practice, the pelvic floor is a place of pilgrimage. It is the seat of Mūlabandha and the trampoline from which movements of Prāṇa rebound to help relate any movement to the rest of the body.

The pelvic floor, or pelvic diaphragm, is composed of the muscles directly attached to the coccyx. The *coccygeus* attaches to the outermost edges of the coccyx and spreads out to attach to the lowest portion of the sacrum. The *iliococcygeus* attaches just in front of the coccygeus and fans out to the left and right to attach to the inner rim of the pelvis. The *pubococcygeaus* (PC) muscle attaches to the sides of the coccyx and travels across the pelvic floor, attaching to the back inner rim of the pubic bone. All of these muscles are found on both the left and the right side, which is relevant to asymmetrical movements and the position of the legs and spine. Any asymmetries in the abdominal wall, spine, pelvis, or hip joints are intimately connected to movements in the pelvic floor. Learning to feel and imagine the pelvic floor in relationship to its peripheral structures is challenging but incredibly helpful to our yoga practice.

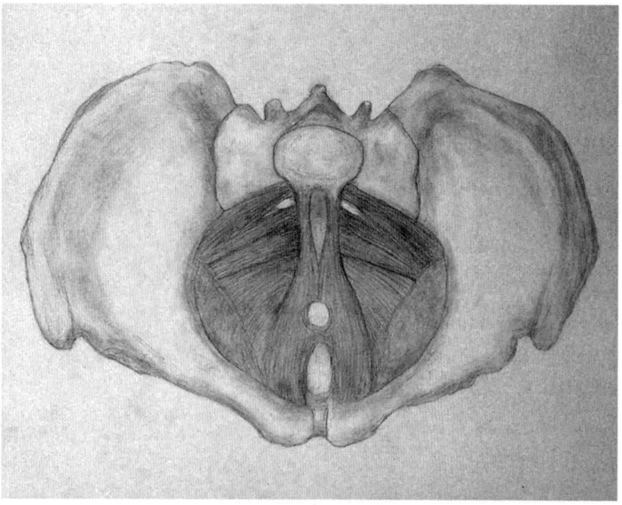

From each side of the coccyx the PC muscle connects across to the pubic bone. The two sides of this muscle along with other closely related muscles affect the functioning and the perception of the anus and the urogenital triangle. Also attached to the coccyx are the illiococcygeus and the coccygeus muscles, which fan out to the sides to help in creating integrated movement through the legs, hip joints, spine, abdominal wall, and the entire body. Balancing the pelvic floor, front to back and side to side, is one of the basic practices of yoga.

SI Joint

Most people are unaware of their *sacroiliac (SI) joints* until the lower back begins to hurt or they feel referred pain in the buttocks or along the outer leg. The SI joint is the juncture of the concave, triangular *sacrum* and the *ilium* (the largest of the three pelvic bones)—hence the name SI joint. The two bones are tightly bound by ligaments that allow the sacrum to tilt slightly in the joint. This tilting is called *nutation* (forward tilt) and *counternutation* (backward tilt). When the two sitting bones are drawn closer together, as when the thighbones are externally rotated, the top of the pelvis broadens and the sacrum counternutates. When the sitting bones are spread apart (as with an internal rotation of the legs), the opposite occurs and the sacrum nutates. In asymmetrical movements, like walking or twisting, there is a small rotation of the two halves of the pelvis—and sacrum—in opposite, complementary directions.

The SI joint, designed for stability rather than mobility, is healthiest when nutations are small. These movements influence and are influenced by pelvic floor muscles and relate directly to the full, rhythmical movement of the spine and completed movements through the legs. Proper activation of the muscles attached to the coccyx—cultivating a sense of the bone dropping down and forward to help the pelvic floor tone—is essential to keeping the SI joint happy.

Isolating movements of the coccyx is difficult. It is important to remember that, although the sacrum and coccyx are actually fused together, on a subtle level we can *imagine* that they move independently, with the coccyx dropping down and forward toward the pubic bone and the sacrum lifting up and into the body. This flow of sacral movement is subtle and illusive, but simply imagining it can stabilize the SI joint.

Abdominal Muscles

The abdominal wall defines the front of the torso and the boundary of the abdominal cavity, containing the abdominal organs. Abdominal muscles integrate patterns of movement from head to toe and impact prāṇāyāma practice profoundly.

Literally front and center is the *rectus abdominis,* a set of paired muscles joined together along the midline by a strong band of connective tissue called the *linea alba.* The fibers of the rectus abdominis follow the vertical line of the muscle along the front of the torso, attached to the *pubic symphysis* and *pubic crest* and running all the way up to the *xiphoid process* (lower end of the sternum) and *costal cartilages* of the fifth through seventh ribs. Three bands of connective tissue traverse the rectus abdominis from side to side, at approximately the levels of the xiphoid process, the navel, and about halfway between the two. This connective tissue reinforces and strengthens the length of the muscle so it can be engaged more efficiently. When highly developed, the rectus abdominis is visible from the outside and may appear to be separate, short muscles running along the front of the body, sometimes referred to as "six- (or eight-) pack abs."

The rectus abdominis tones and stabilizes the trunk and core of the body. When engaged, it contributes to flexion of the lumbar spine if the pelvis is fixed, and it helps in drawing the pelvis toward the upper body when the rib cage is stable. In most movements, the right and left sides of the rectus abdominis are contracted simultaneously; however, in yoga they are sometimes articulated separately, as when practicing nauli (see pages 23–25).

The *internal* and *external oblique* muscles work in conjunction with the rectus abdominis, toning in an oblique crisscross pattern across the abdomen in certain twisting movements. The fibers of the external obliques line up precisely with the fibers of the *external intercostal* muscles on their respective side and with the fibers of the internal obliques on the opposite side to facilitate these movements.

In general the *transversus abdominis* is the deepest muscle of the abdominal wall. From the sides of the rectus abdominis it wraps around the sides of the waist to attach to the lumbar spine behind the *quadratus lumborum* (QL) muscles. Like a girdle, it can give various shapes to the ball-like mass of the abdominal viscera. In the lower belly in front, at about two inches below the navel, is a horizontal seam called the *accuate line*. Here an amazing reversal takes place. The rectus abdominis goes behind the tendon and connective tissue of the other abdominal wall muscles to connect to the back edge of the pubic bone, just above tendons of the pelvic floor's PC muscle. The lower horizontal bands of the transversus then appear as the most superficial. These small strips of transversus act like an elastic belt along the top edge of the pubic bone and allow the shaping of the abdomen into the "floating pot" or the "Gaṇeśa belly" forms.

Diaphragm

The most important muscle impacting our breathing is the *respiratory diaphragm*. It is a unique and elegant muscle that, like other skeletal muscles, can be controlled voluntarily, expanding and contracting along the lines of its fibers from the edges of the diaphragm toward the center as we breathe in and out. It is one large, thin, dome-shaped structure of muscle and fibrous connective tissue that is attached peripherally to the abdomen and ribs. The attachments converge into a central tendon located at the crest of the dome. The diaphragm curves upward like an umbrella when we exhale or are at rest and its central area drops down when we inhale.

At the end of an exhalation, it is possible to feel a toning of the external intercostal and abdominal muscles as well as the muscles of the pelvic floor. When inhaling, we may feel the diaphragm dropping and spreading as the ribs broaden, due to activation of the interior intercostal muscles. During a deep inhalation, the scalene muscles also tone. All of this happens unconsciously to allow room for the lungs to inflate and deflate properly. We can uncover, reveal, and refine unconscious breathing patterns as we cultivate movements that support a more full yogic breath. For example, when inhaling with the mind in its normal, distracted state, the erector spinae muscles that run along the sides of the spine tend to contract to hold the spine straight. However, their involvement can be excessive, activating the hip flexors, overstimulating and stretching the front of the diaphragm, and collapsing the lower back. When exhaling with a distracted mind, the opposite pattern can occur, abdominal muscles contracting to excess and erector spinae muscles releasing, causing the chest to collapse. In yoga, we work to minimize either extreme from manifesting by keeping the opposite form awake while the dominant pattern is at work.

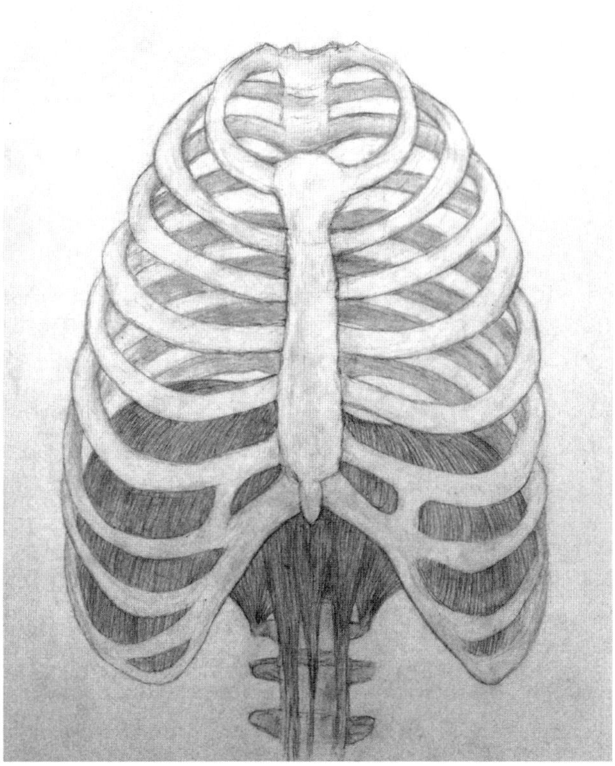

The respiratory diaphragm attaches all around the lower edge of the rib cage and then down onto the fronts of the lumbar vertebra. Its movement profoundly affects the shape of and the tensions in and around the rib cage, which in turn affect the entire spine, pelvic floor, throat, and head.

Scalene Muscles

The *scalenes* are a set of three pairs of muscles that run along the sides of the neck (anterior, middle, and posterior scalenes). They originate along the cervical spine (from C4 to C6) and attach to the first, second, and occasionally third ribs. The scalenes are engaged when tilting the head, but, along with the *sternocleidomastoid* muscles on the front of the neck that look like straps, the scalenes are also the primary muscles involved at the crest of an inhalation, lifting the first two ribs and the collarbones so the top lobes of the lungs can fully inflate.

In an integrated practice, scalenes release and lengthen while remaining toned to facilitate full extension of the lower cervical spine, an action integral to every Upward Facing Dog Pose, among many other poses. As they are the primary actors in maximizing the crest of the inhalation, sensing the toning of the scalenes is central to finding the plumb line, lifting the heart, and connecting to the kidney wings when we reach the arms overhead.

Legs and Arms

The arms and legs have interesting similarities in terms of our yoga practice. Each is attached to the trunk of the body through a single large bone (the humerus of the arm and the femur of the leg) at a ball-and-socket joint that allows for a wide range of motion. The knee and elbow—both hinge joints—connect to the lower portions of the leg and arm to two smaller bones (the tibia and fibula in the leg and the radius and ulna in the arm). The wrist and hand also have obvious similarities as do the ankle and foot. It is through the legs, feet, arms, and hands that we express the feeling of luminous extension, groundedness, and "reaching to infinity."

Articulation of the hands and feet has a direct influence on the healthy functioning of the knees, elbows, shoulders, and hips, and ultimately on the entire spine and every pose. Using the hands and feet correctly is often challenging due to semiconscious habits and how we interact with the world. For example, the inner edge of the hand, from the heel of the thumb out through the tips of the index and middle fingers, is the area that should bear weight because the radius of the forearm is thicker than the ulna (on the outside of the forearm) and strong as it comes into the inner wrist. Yet often when we're doing arm balances or even Downward Facing Dog the index finger uproots, and our weight shifts to the outer edge of the hand unconsciously. The feet are structured so that they too should ground evenly so the arches come to life and the legs engage correctly. In both hands and feet, if the weight is distributed poorly, it will eventually cause injury somewhere along the line—whether it's the wrist, elbow, shoulder, ankle, knee, or hip. These are basically rotational problems that proper alignment can resolve.

There are muscular similarities between arms and legs too. The *biceps* and *quadriceps* work in similar ways to wake up the legs and arms, respectively, and the *hamstrings* and *triceps* working to stabilize and strengthen. Of course, there are also numerous differences between the arms and legs. For instance, the *greater trochanters* of the femur, a vital point of postural assessment and adjustment for teachers in the legs and pelvis, are not paralleled in the arm. Nonetheless, considering similarities in an overview of anatomy provides insight into many movements and poses.

Hips

The pelvis consists of two curved flat bones, together called the *ilium*, that join in the front of the body at the pubic symphysis and are fused to form the pubic bone. In the back of the pelvis the sacrum connects to the ilium to form the SI joint. The coccyx, which is fused to the sacrum, curls down and forward like a tiny tail. Two protrusions at the bottom of the pelvic bowl, one on each half of the ilium, are called the ischial tuberosities, or sitting bones.

The hip joint, or *acetabulofemoral joint,* where the femur and pelvis meet is a ball-and-socket joint. The femur is secured by a thick ligament (the *foveal ligament*) that extends out from the center of the top of the head of the femur, attaching to either side of the *acetabular notch,* a rough-edged depression on the sides of the socket. This ligament and the shape of the socket make the hip stable.

Four groups of muscles facilitate hip movement, flexibility, strength, and stability. Those primarily responsible for flexing the hip and drawing the top of the femur toward the torso are the *iliopsoas, rectus femoris,* and *sartorius* muscles, commonly referred to as the *hip flexors.* Those primarily responsible for extending the thigh from the hip are the *gluteus maximus* and the hamstrings. The muscles responsible for drawing the leg toward the midline of the body, adducting the leg, are located along the inner thigh. When these muscles are weak, the hamstrings may become compromised, particularly in forward bends. The abductor muscles (all of the gluteus muscles and the tensor fasciae latae muscle) are located on the outer thigh and hip and draw the leg away from the body's midline. Another important group of muscles associated with the hips are the "deep six" (the pieriformis, gemellus superior, obturator internus, gemellus inferior, quadratus femoris, and obturator externus). These muscles are responsible for helping to rotate the leg out; they stabilize and protect the hip joint and have an intimate relationship to the pelvic floor muscles.

Psoas

The psoas (*psoas major*) is a long, smooth-fiber muscle that connects the torso and the legs, functioning to link, move, and stabilize the body. On a subtle-body level, the psoas helps to link earth, which is our embodied situation, with our emotions and our concepts about our predicament. So similarly, it links and stabilizes our mental and emotional states to our actual embodied circumstances. The psoas attaches along the lateral border of the spine from T12 down to L2, where it joins the *iliacus* muscle (which lines the inner surface of the upper bowl of the pelvis) to form the *iliopsoas* muscle. After passing through the pelvic bowl, the iliopsoas attaches to the posterior surface of the femur at the *lesser trochanter.* Some

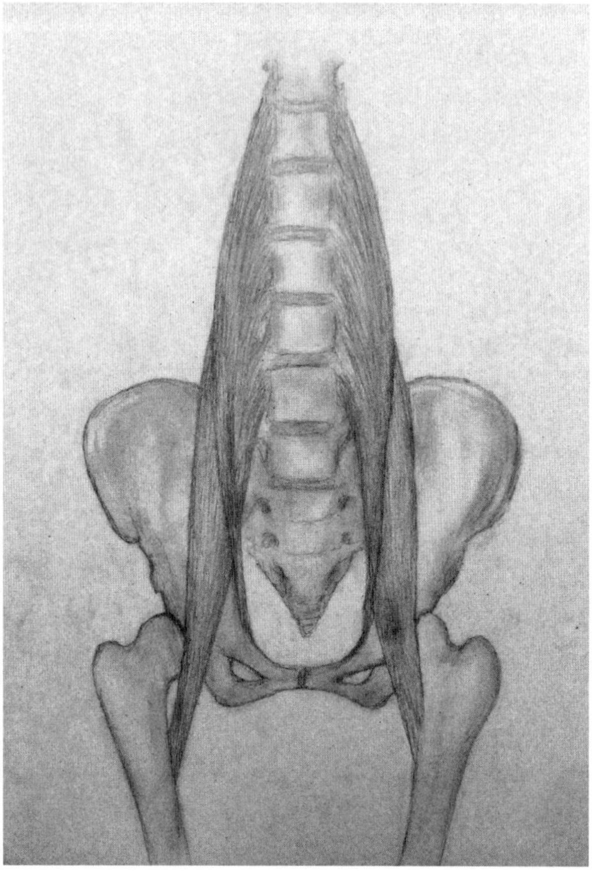

Imbalance and unconscious tensions in the psoas muscles affect the pelvic floor and the respiratory diaphragm. Learning to release them and then to balance them side to side allows a deeper meditative awareness of the body.

people also have a psoas minor muscle that lies anterior to and follows the line of the psoas major, usually attaching to the spine at T12 at one end and below the ilium at the other.

The primary function of the psoas (major and minor) is as a hip flexor—responsible for the first 30 percent of lift in the leg. When we are walking, it is mostly the psoas that swings the leg forward to take a step. When contracted unilaterally, the psoas also contributes to lateral flexion of the spine. When we are lying down and engage the psoas laterally with the pelvis stable, the psoas functions to help raise the torso off the floor.

Hamstrings

Many yoga practitioners learn to love and respect their hamstrings, usually after a few years of fearing and cursing them for being so tight that forward bends are next to impossible. The three hamstring muscles—the *semitendinosus*, the *semimembranosus,* and the *biceps femoris*—lie along the back of the femur. The biceps femoris has both a long and a short head: the short head attaches to a small ridge of bone just below the posterior side of the sitting bone, and the long head and other hamstrings attach to the pelvis just beneath the gluteus maximus at the ischial tuberosity (sitting bones). All of the hamstrings cross the knee joint and attach to the lower leg: the semitendinosus attaches to the medial surface of the tibia, the semimembranosus attaches to the medial tibial condyle, and the biceps femoris attaches to the lateral side of the head of the fibula.

Together the hamstrings function in knee flexion, hip joint extension, and stabilization of the knee joint. They are stubborn muscles; the more you tug and pull on them to demand length so that poses are accessible, the more resistant, stiff, and short they become. Pushing to overcome hamstring limitation usually results in injury. In fact, one of the most common yoga injuries is strain, or tearing, of the hamstring attachment at the sitting bones. Less common is strain at the lower attachment (insertion) points. Working with hamstring injuries takes patience and should be addressed with intelligence and the guidance of a good teacher.

Knees

The knee is one of the strongest and most complex joints in the body. Its function is intimately related to the hip and ankle joints and articulation of the feet. The knee connects and facilitates movement between the lower and upper leg, and it supports and distributes body weight. It is a synovial hinge joint whose primary function is to bend the leg into flexion. When the joint is closed, it also allows for a small amount of lateral "swing" in the lower leg, a movement that is key as we work safely toward poses such as Vīrāsana (Hero Pose) and Padmāsana (Lotus Pose).

The knee joint connects the tibia, *patella* (kneecap), and femur through a complicated design of muscles, tendons, ligaments, and bones that fit together for maximum stability and ease of movement. Two concave processes, or *condyles,* on the distal end of the femur fit exactly into corresponding concave condyles at the proximal end of the tibia. They are separated by a shock-absorbing, figure-eight-shaped piece of cartilage (the *meniscus*) that lies between them. The meniscus can become compromised or injured through misuse of the knee joint or accidents in life that torque the knee. Folding the leg into a strained Padmāsana without allowing for proper rotation of the upper and lower legs is one common way yoga practitioners injure their knees.

The patella lies on the front surface of the knee joint and attaches to the femur and tibia via the *patellar ligament,* the distal portion of the quadriceps femoris. To "wake up the legs" in standing poses, we are instructed to lift the kneecap, which is partially a function of engaging the quadriceps.

Four primary ligaments serve to reinforce the knee joint. The *medial collateral ligament* (MCL) connects to the medial side of the femur, then crosses the knee joint and attaches to the medial side of the tibia. The MCL stabilizes the joint when force is applied to the lateral side of the knee. The meniscus is attached directly to the MCL, so it is not uncommon for the meniscus to be torn when the MCL is injured. The *lateral collateral ligament* (LCL) runs laterally along the outer seam of the leg from femur to fibula. It inhibits forces applied to the medial side of the knee when the knee moves laterally. Two cruciform ligaments cross within the joint to stabilize it front to back. The *anterior cruciate ligament* (ACL) extends obliquely from the inner surface of the lateral condyle of the femur to the upper medial front of the tibia. The ACL is helpful in maintaining stability and preventing hyperextension of the joint. Immediately behind the ACL is the *posterior cruciate ligament* (PCL), which extends obliquely from the inner medial condyle of the femur to the posterior intercondylar space of the tibia.

Shoulder

In one sense, the shoulders are extremely familiar territory—we shrug them when we're uncertain, slide them in and out of clothing without a thought, and bear the weight of the world on them day in and day out. The shoulder area of the body is complicated, so understanding and controlling shoulder movement and mechanics can be confounding, but a basic understanding of shoulder anatomy can demystify the actions we attempt in yoga.

In common usage, the term *shoulder* usually refers to the *shoulder girdle*—the entire part of the upper body that connects the arms to the torso. It includes three bones: the *clavicle* (collarbone), *scapula* (shoulder blade), and *humerus* (upper arm bone), which are all supported and stabilized by a number of associated muscles, tendons, and ligaments. The shoulder comprises two joints—the *glenohumeral* and the *acromioclavicular* (AC)—but strictly speaking, when we talk about the shoulder joint, we're referring to the former. It is a ball-and-socket joint formed where the *glenoid fossa* (a concave hollow on the lateral end of the scapula) interfaces with the convex head of the humerus. This joint has more mobility than any other joint in the human body and is also more vulnerable to injury than most due to the shallowness of the fossa and the available range of motion. The AC joint is a synovial joint at the juncture of the uppermost part of the scapula (the *acromion*) and the clavicle. This is the only place the scapula actually attaches directly to another bone. The *sternoclavicular* joint, also considered part of the shoulder, is at the center of the chest where the clavicle interfaces with the upper part of the sternum to provide stability.

The shoulder joint is also stabilized and protected by the *labrum,* a strong, cup-shaped cuff of cartilage within the joint that cups the head of the humerus. There is also a small sac of synovial fluid, the bursa of the shoulder, that cushions the tendons of the rotator cuff and protects the joint.

Four of the seven muscles that stabilize the connection of the upper arm to the torso are grouped and called the *rotator cuff* because their tendons form a "cuff" over the end of the humerus at the joint. They are the *supraspinatus,* the *infraspinatus,* the *teres minor,* and the *subscapularis.* The supraspinatus helps to abduct the arm at the shoulder. It lies in the fossa (trough) of the top section of the scapula, between the spine of the scapula and its uppermost edge, and the muscle attaches laterally to the greater tubercle of the humerus. The infraspinatus is a relatively thick, triangular muscle that lies on the back portion of the scapula, attaching the upper arm to the shoulder blade. The teres minor connects the humerus directly to the scapula with fibers running obliquely upward and laterally to a point on the upper arm. The subscapularis lines the inner surface of the scapula and shares the same tendon as the serratus anterior. It inserts on the humerus and the front of the glenohumeral joint capsule. The subscapularis works in conjunction with the serratus anterior to stabilize the shoulder and is key to many yoga poses that involve the arms, as it rotates the humerus inward and cues the inner edge of the hand to bear weight, even when the shoulder blade is protracted.

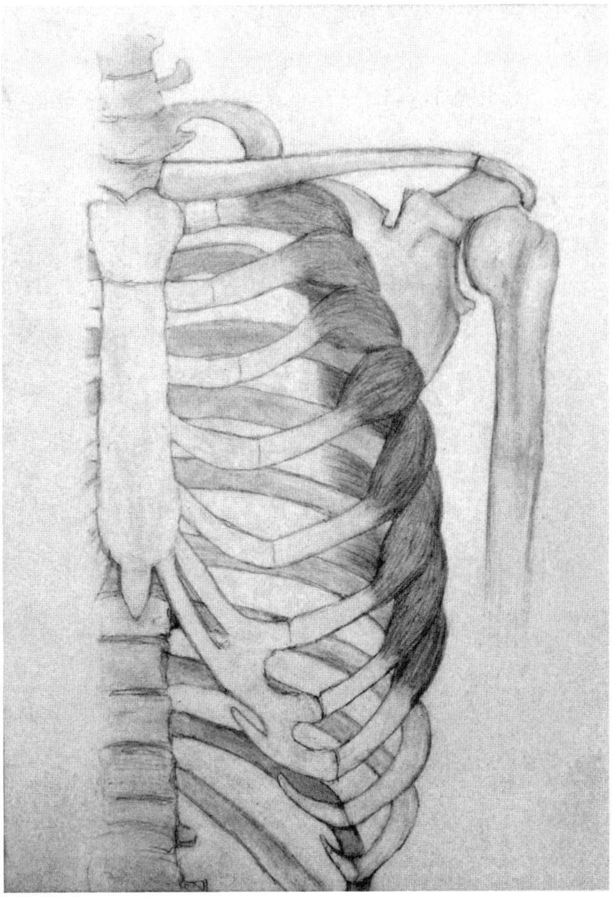

The serratus anterior protracts (spreads and outwardly rotates) the shoulder blades, fixing them firmly onto the ribs. With such a solid connection, force can be transferred through the arms without strain in the neck or danger to the shoulder joints.

Serratus Anterior

Within an āsana practice, the *serratus anterior* muscle is critical to many patterns of movement in poses from backbends and arm balances to twists and headstands. It attaches to the ribs (from the first through the ninth) and along the anterior medial border of the scapula; it holds the scapula flat on the rib cage, which stabilizes the shoulder girdle. It also helps to protract the shoulder blade and is the primary path of structural strength between the back of the diaphragm and the arm. It opposes the *rhomboid muscle,* which also attaches along the medial border of the scapula and along the sides of the spine. The rhomboids retract and lift the shoulder blades, while the serratus anteriors protract to stabilize—they work together in well-aligned, full-shoulder action.

PART TWO

ĀSANA

Movements and Poses Strung Together Like Jewels on the Thread of the Breath

For Aṣṭāṅga Vinyāsa practitioners, the simplest and possibly the "only" way to consider the poses is from the perspective of the order in which they appear in the traditional sequences: Sūrya Namaskāras, the standing poses, the specific series, and the finishing sequence. This is good. But we can also gain understanding by examining the postures in terms of some of their common features, regarding them as twists or backbends or balancing poses. Looking at postures in terms of the overall category into which they fall is informative in terms of alignment for any practitioner, and for Aṣṭāṅga practitioners, pulling poses out of the usual sequence can be a good practice for shifting perspective.

This book presents the poses first in detail within "families" to show the underlying patterns of breath and movement that tie them together. It also gives the traditional sequences as a quick reference. All poses found in the Primary and Intermediate Series and a small number of other poses that demonstrate a particular form or idea are included. Some can belong to more than one family. Yoga is a fluid, flowing, evolving system of breath, movement, and form, forever resisting our need to categorize it yet benefiting from our attempts to do so.

5

Building Sūrya Namaskāra

Sūrya Namaskāra (Sun Salutation) serves as the foundation of an Aṣṭāṅga Vinyāsa practice. It contains all of the subtle alignment as well as the cues for and process of joining together complementary opposites from which the internal forms of the practice unfold. When Sūrya Namaskāra is practiced carefully, with vitality and enthusiasm, it sets a tone for our entire practice and informs the movements in every other posture. Many of the traditions of yoga believe that the sun is not only far away in space, but also simultaneously in the center of our hearts. Practice Sūrya Namaskāra as if you were the radiant sun to fully feel and express internal forms and alignment.

There are two forms of Sūrya Namaskāra: form A and form B. Both begin and end standing in Samasthitiḥ. There are nine poses, or subforms, within form A and seventeen within form B. The quality of the movement in and out of each pose is a key to the effectiveness of both sequences. It is important to work slowly and patiently when first learning Sūrya Namaskāra so you can refine the movements, cultivating a strong, integrated, and meditative flow.

In this section, Sūrya Namaskāra is broken down into constituent parts. Working on them individually can help encode the coordination of breath and gaze within each form into the body, making Sūrya Namaskāra—and the entire practice—fluid and meditative. Many of these foundational movements are also beneficial for therapeutic purposes. If Sūrya Namaskāra is not appropriate for someone, the foundational movements with modifications, such as the Puppy Pose, can be explored in a way that might still be beneficial.

Once the transitions within Sūrya Namaskāra are smooth and integrated, you can use the traditional method of "counting out" the forms, using Sanskrit numbers assigned to each position as a kind of shorthand to flow continuously on the thread of the breath. Moving in a smooth and fluid manner helps to give the entire practice a truly meditative quality.

During a traditional Aṣṭāṅga Vinyāsa practice, Sūrya Namaskāra A and B are each practiced a minimum of five times before moving into the standing sequence and then on to the body of the specific series or sequence to be practiced.

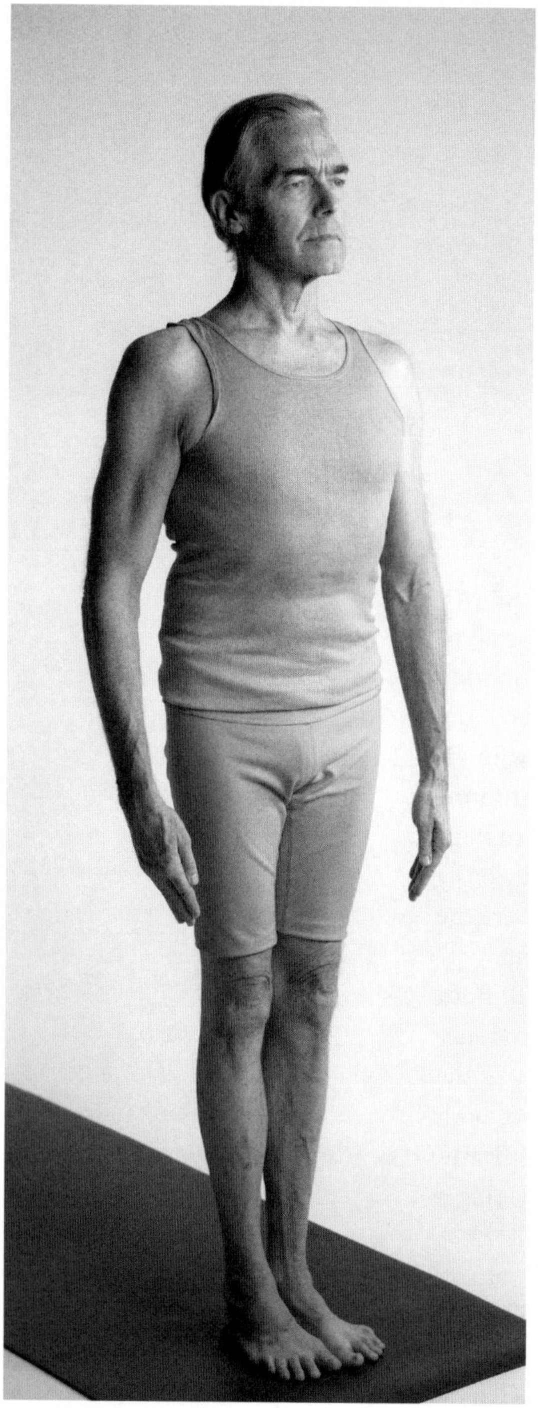

SETTING UP FOR SŪRYA NAMASKĀRA

Samasthitiḥ

Equal Standing

1. Stand straight and tall with the feet together, sides of the big toes touching, and the arms down at your sides. Linger for a moment in Samasthitiḥ. At this point, the eyes become steady in dṛṣṭi, which releases the palate and allows you to begin ujjāyī breathing. The simple waves of the breath initiate the process of natural alignment. This is merely the intelligence waking up in the central channel.
2. It is easy to feel a sense of floating at the center of the upper chest on the inhalation. Staying with the sensations as they arise, the middle of the pelvic floor will begin to feel like it is becoming centered on the plumb line. The back of the diaphragm—along the kidney wings—lifts and floats, as does the heart. The sitting bones, pubic bone, and coccyx all drop down, while the pelvic floor tones. As you soften into the breath you may experience a constant sense of tuning and retuning—even microtuning—on the current of the breath. Everything is there if you remember to continue to inhale and exhale into the pose. This is similar

to the process that manifests in sitting meditation, except here you're standing.

3. The radiant seed-point of the inhaling pattern is in the heart. Its extended pattern all through the body is experienced as a feeling of upward expanding and floating. The seed-point of the exhaling pattern is the center of the pelvic floor, and that pattern gives the feeling of downward contracting and grounding throughout the body. When you inhale, you pull your attention like a thread up through the seed of the exhalation at the middle of the pelvic floor. When you exhale, you release the upper back of the palate to keep the heart open. Every time you inhale, you concentrate on the residue of the exhalation and with each exhalation your mind rests in the feelings and sensations of the inhalation.

   Hold this position for five to ten rounds of the breath, with the hands folded in *Añjali Mudrā* (prayer position) in front of the heart. At this point, you may chant invocations to center the mind and begin the practice. (See Appendix 2.)
4. Standing like this in Samasthitiḥ is prāṇāyāma practice, and essentially that's what you do in all of the poses. Yoga āsana, when practiced in a contemplative manner with the poses strung together like jewels on the thread of the breath, is nothing less than prāṇāyāma in motion. The technique of relishing the essence of the inhalation as you exhale and delighting in the essence of the exhalation as you draw breath in is the root of all your practices.

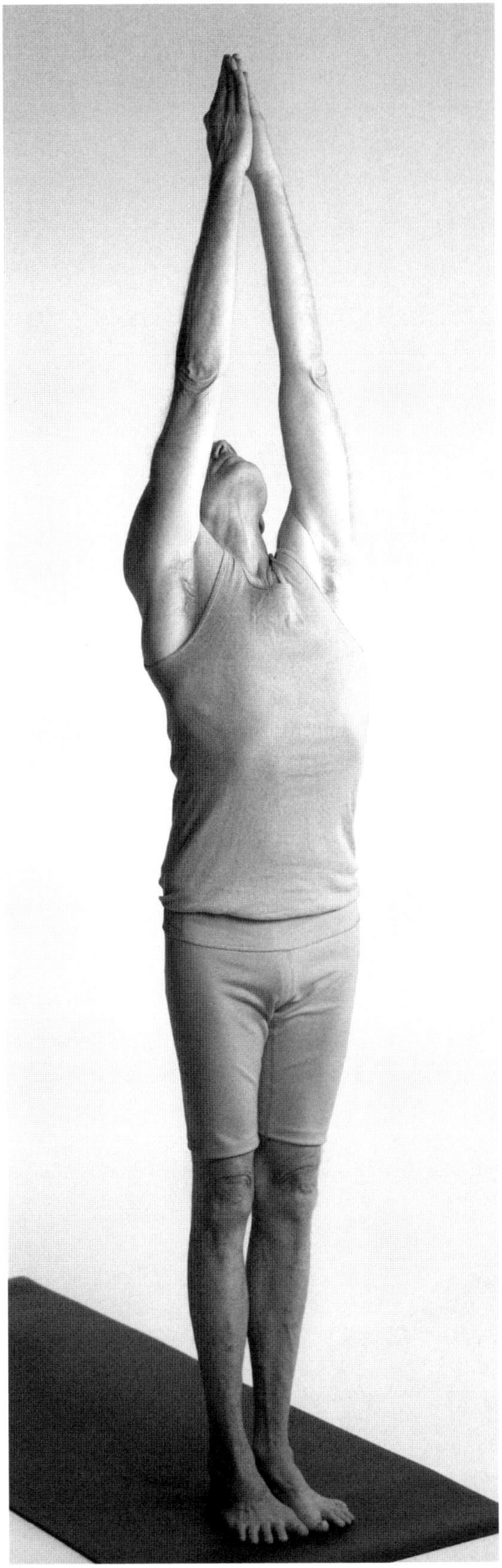

Ekam

Ekam, or "one," is the first position of Sūrya Namaskāra, and it begins the vinyāsa process of moving in sync with the breath and the gaze.

1. Standing in Samasthitiḥ, inhale as you lift the arms up and out slightly in front of the body. Spin the arms by reaching up toward the ceiling and placing the palms together.
2. As you reach up through the arms, they should feel as though they are extensions of a spreading in the back of the diaphragm, the kidney wings, and by keeping awareness

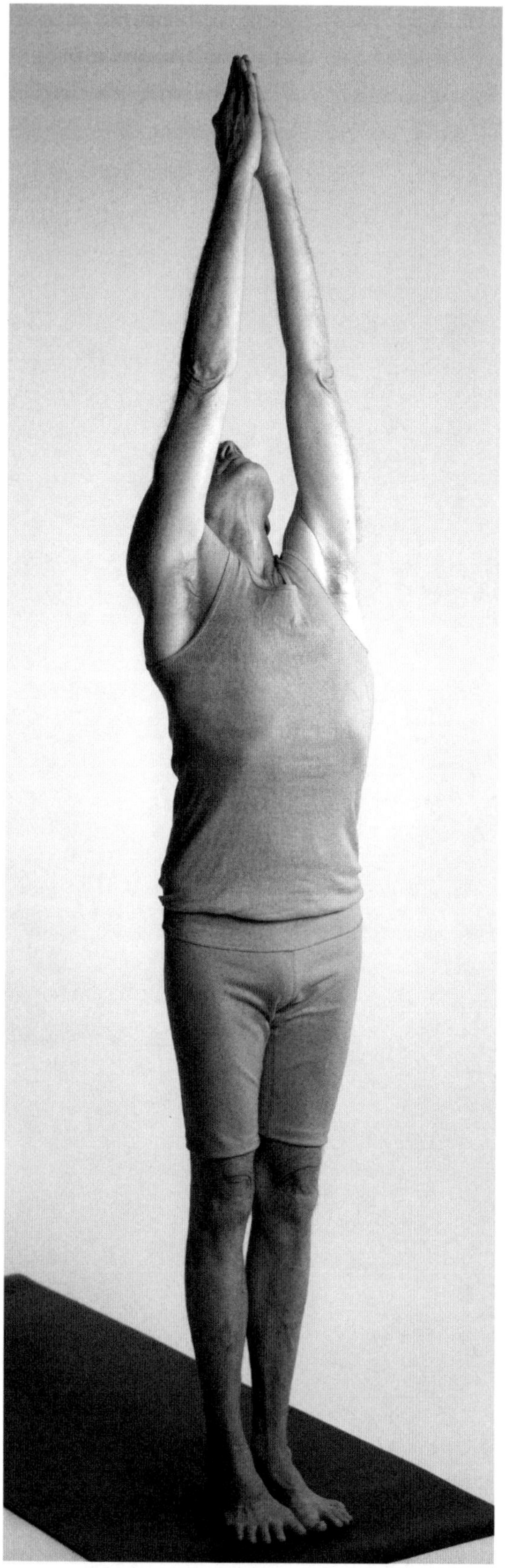

in the coccyx and pelvic floor you can sense into a full stretch of the psoas line. Firm up the legs—quads and hamstrings—so that as the inhalation fills the body, the edges of the diaphragm open like an umbrella.

3. The shoulder blades spread wide (protract) as the palms turn toward each other, so you can really lift the arms as you reach the peak of the inhalation.
4. Finally, tilt the head back, keeping it behind the arms and gazing to the thumbs, along the line of the nose; there should be no strain in the neck. This stretches the throat, and you get a broad, comfortable backbend in your lower neck without your head falling back on the atlas (the first vertebra in the neck). The entire head, including the chin (even if you have a beard!) should be *completely* behind the arms.
5. In the gap at the top of the inhalation, lift the arms even more, as if you are trying to reach the ceiling. Really lifting in this way protracts the shoulder blades and stimulates the edges of the diaphragm so those edges start to sparkle.
6. The residue from those diaphragmatic sensations percolates as you exhale and allows the arms to float back down to the sides. Keep your arms toned as they descend, and work the legs to stand taller than ever right up through the crown of the head. This helps create a sense of stability and allows the unfolding of proper geometry within the body.
7. Remember, all the movements are based in the sound of the ujjāyī breath. If you get the sound, everything is easy. As you move, keep the legs engaged and reach up on the inhalation, like you're a swimmer. Then exhale with the soft, aspirate ujjāyī sound, and push on up through the crown of the head to glide back down into Samasthitiḥ.
8. Repeat these movements from Samasthitiḥ to Ekam and back to Samasthitiḥ with feeling at least three more times.

Ekam, Dve, Trīṇi

Numbers One, Two, and Three

Next we add the second and third movements of Sūrya Namaskāra. This begins to work the whole body rhythmically in time with the gaze and the breath.

1. As you inhale, tone the quads and pull down on the sitting bones with the hamstrings. Open the wings of the kidneys extra wide as you lift and spin the arms to reach up into Ekam.
2. Keep the heads of the femurs back slightly in the hip sockets, so the groins are hollow. This keeps the center of the pelvic floor on the plumb line, which makes the center point float.
3. The shoulder blades wrap out wide and lift while the pot of the belly is lifted up and out of the pelvic basin. This will subtly awaken Mūlabandha, like a little flame in the middle of the pelvic floor, which will maintain reversibility and core awareness through the coming movements.
4. Gaze at the thumbs, using the image of cobra hoods rising and spreading in the back of the head. This keeps your head behind the arms and the lower neck gently curved into a backbend.
5. Exhale and "swan-dive" up and over. As you begin to fold forward, keep the spine straight, the arms full of breath, and the legs toned. From the sun in your heart extend through the crown of the head. This will keep the pelvic floor online and ready for counteractions.

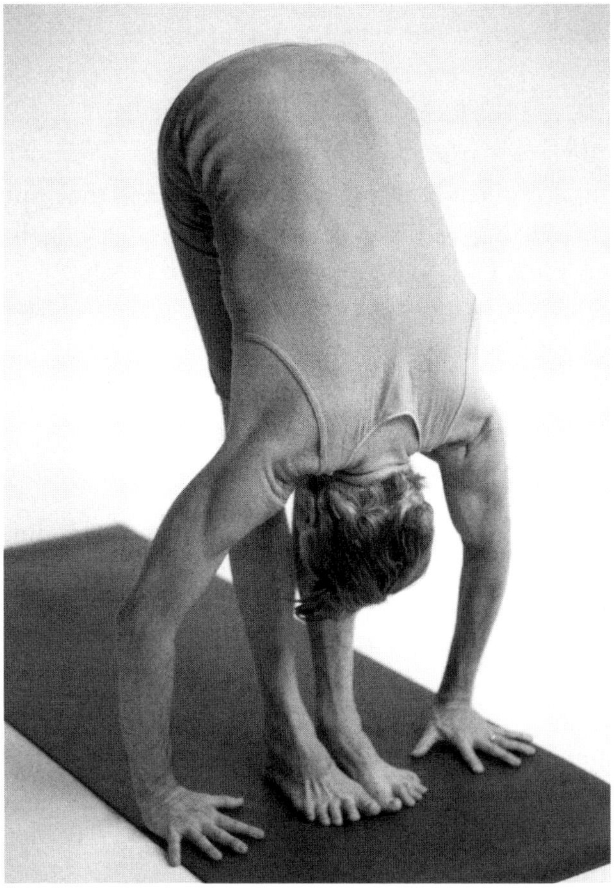

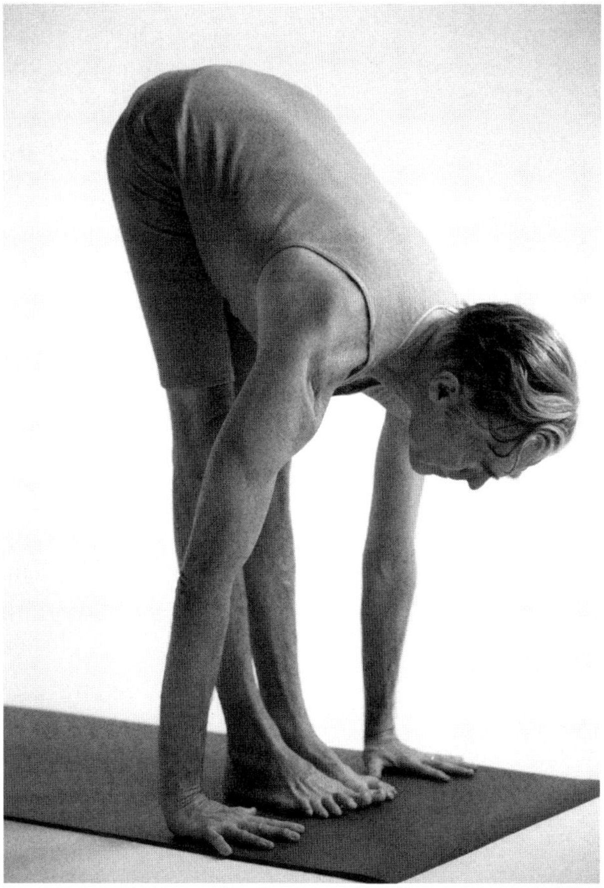

6. Keep the chin slightly out for the first 90 percent of the fold, then just as you run out of air, look toward your nose so the spine begins to flex. At the very end of the exhalation, contract the abdomen and the PC muscle, creating a coiled feeling at the very end of the breath to complete Dve position.
7. If you are unable to touch the floor beside your feet with your hands, bend the knees as you fold. Even with the knees bent, keep the legs toned by grounding down evenly through the mound of each big toe and the other corners of the feet. Lift the kneecaps. Keeping your legs engaged, work the edge of sensation in your forward bend, taking care not to overengage or overextend and not losing integrity in the muscular patterns awakened by these movements.
8. Inhale as you lift your head and elongate the spine through the crown, moving into Trīṇi. To keep your PC muscle toned during this inhalation, spoon up under the belly and create a vacuum under the belly right above the pelvic floor, as if drawing breath in through a straw that comes up the midline of your body between your legs. Again, you'll use the end of the exhalation to set this particular intensity of the apāna, then inhale and pull the seed-point of the exhalation up inside.
9. On the next exhale, lengthen your spine and return rhythmically to full Dve position.
10. On the next inhale, feel the form of the legs, feet, and coccyx as you reach back up with vibrant arms into Ekam.
11. As you exhale, your arms float back down to your sides and the heart floats up as you return to Samasthitiḥ. Keep the gaze steady along the line of your nose to a point out in front of you.
12. Repeat this sequence of movements—Ekam, Dve, Trīṇi—at least three more times.

Ekam, Dve, Trīṇi Variation

If you're stiff, that's good. Who wants to hit their face on their shins anyway? You can still look toward your navel at the end of the exhalation to get that apānic coil after you fold forward. Rather than being concerned about how flexible you are, you can base the action in the pelvic floor and be happy.

1. With the feet hip-width apart, inhale and open the arms as if they were extensions of the kidney wings. Grip the legs with your awareness and keep them parallel as you inhale and reach up to a modified Ekam.

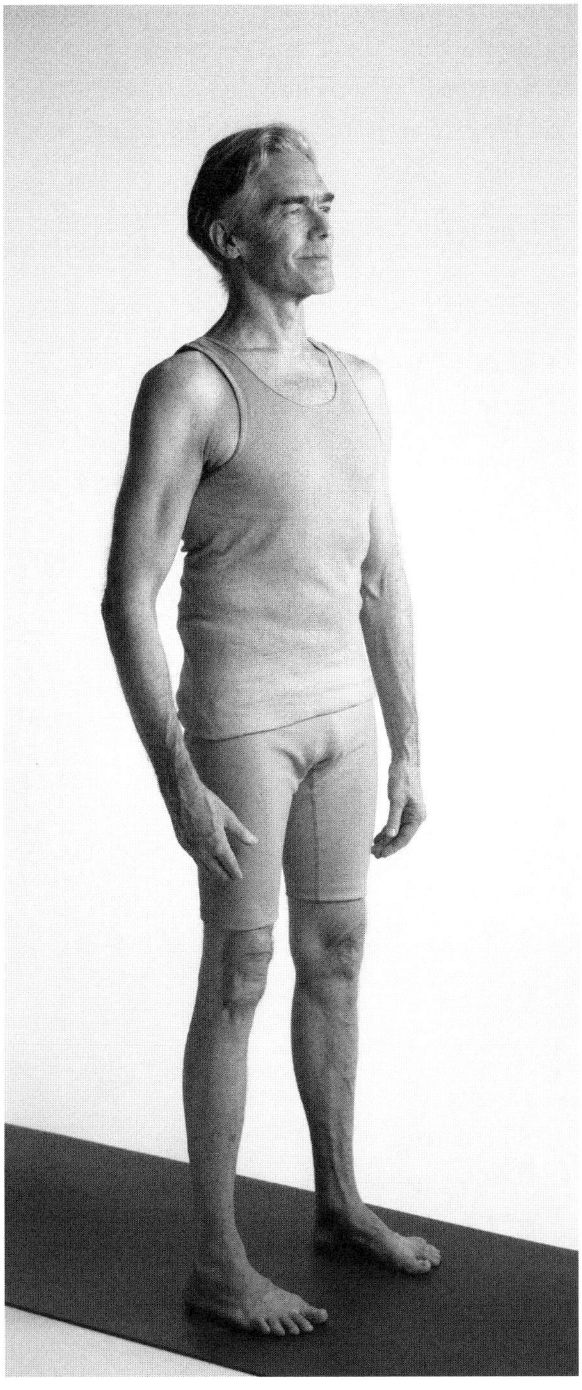

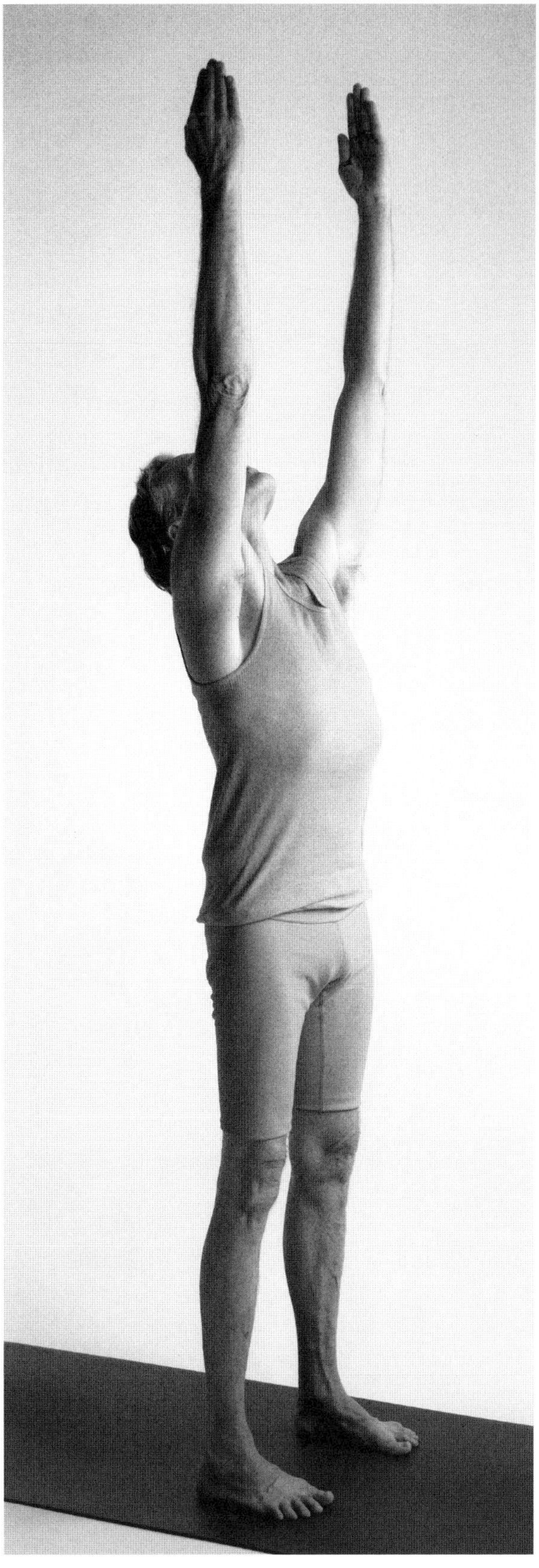

2. Swan-dive up and over, looking up and out as you fold forward. Gradually bend the knees and place your elbows on your thighs just above the knees.
3. Having folded forward as far as is appropriate for you, at the very end of the exhalation tone the abdominal muscles and drop the head. This is a modified Dve.
4. As you inhale, find the line of the PC muscle and abdomen, and lift the head to Trīṇi . Extend through the crown so the spine straightens, and imagine that the pubic bone and coccyx are moving back and then together. Relax your palate. Have a good time.
5. Exhale and fold forward again to Dve, keeping the legs toned and the spine straightening, as before.
6. Lift your head and, inhaling, reach back up to the ceiling as you straighten your legs. As you exhale, allow the arms to float back down to your sides as you return to Samasthitiḥ.

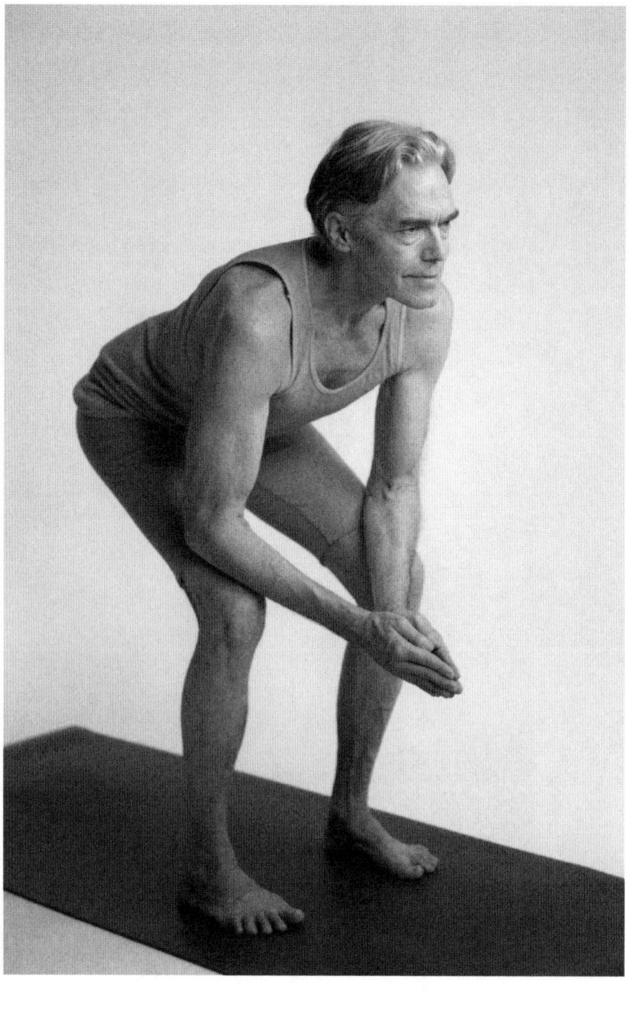

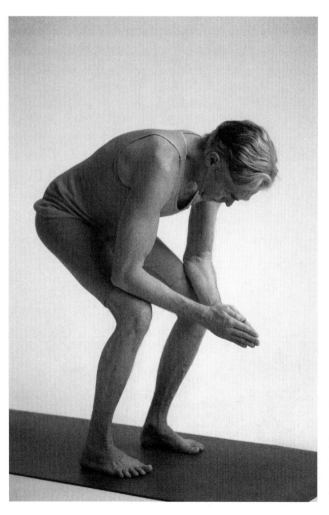

ESTABLISHING A BASE FOR SŪRYA NAMASKĀRA A

For the first Sun Salutation of the day, while learning Sūrya Namaskāra, or if you have injuries that prevent you from doing the full form, it is helpful to break the sequence down into component parts. (See the full sequence of Sūrya Namaskāra A in Appendix 5.) But remember, even when separating the movements, you must still move in sync with the breath and the gaze. When you slow down movements and concentrate on particular subtleties of form or precise points of alignment, the mind may take it as an invitation to wander or to co-opt the practice and turn it into a theoretical mind game rather than an internal physical experience. So stick with the breath, the gaze, and the internal forms, flowing mindfully with whatever full body patterns you have.

By exploring modified forms, some of the restrictive or distracting external factors—such as tight hamstrings, theories of alignment, or SI joint pain—can be removed from the equation so the internal forms are easier to observe. Slowing down the movements within Sūrya Namaskāra provides an opportunity to "relearn" how to move; this can help you to recover from an injury and to avoid creating unbalanced habitual patterns of movement that may be limiting or eventually *cause* injury.

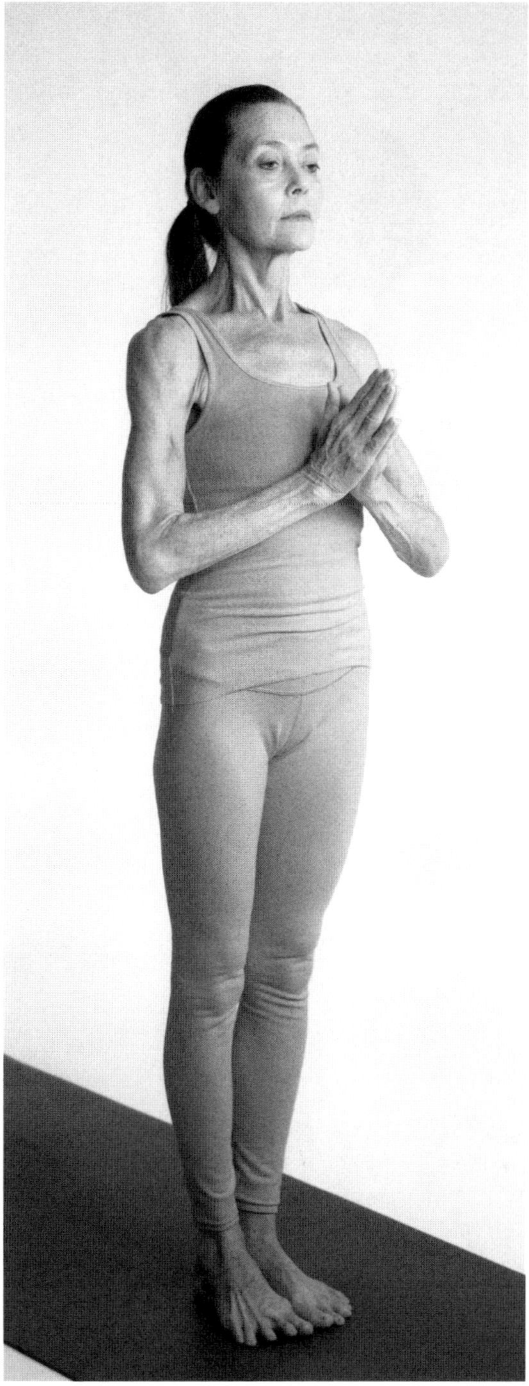

Samasthitiḥ

1. Establishing the plumb line, steadying the gaze, softening the tongue, and releasing the palate you can enter Samasthitiḥ. Bring your awareness to the sound of the ujjāyī breath, and notice the ends of the breath as they join together deep in the belly behind the navel.

Ekam, Dve, and Trīṇi

1. As you inhale, create a vacuum under the belly right above the pelvic floor, as if drawing breath in through a straw that comes up the midline of the body between the legs. Fill the arms with breath, as you lift and spin them reaching to the sky and looking at the thumbs in Ekam.

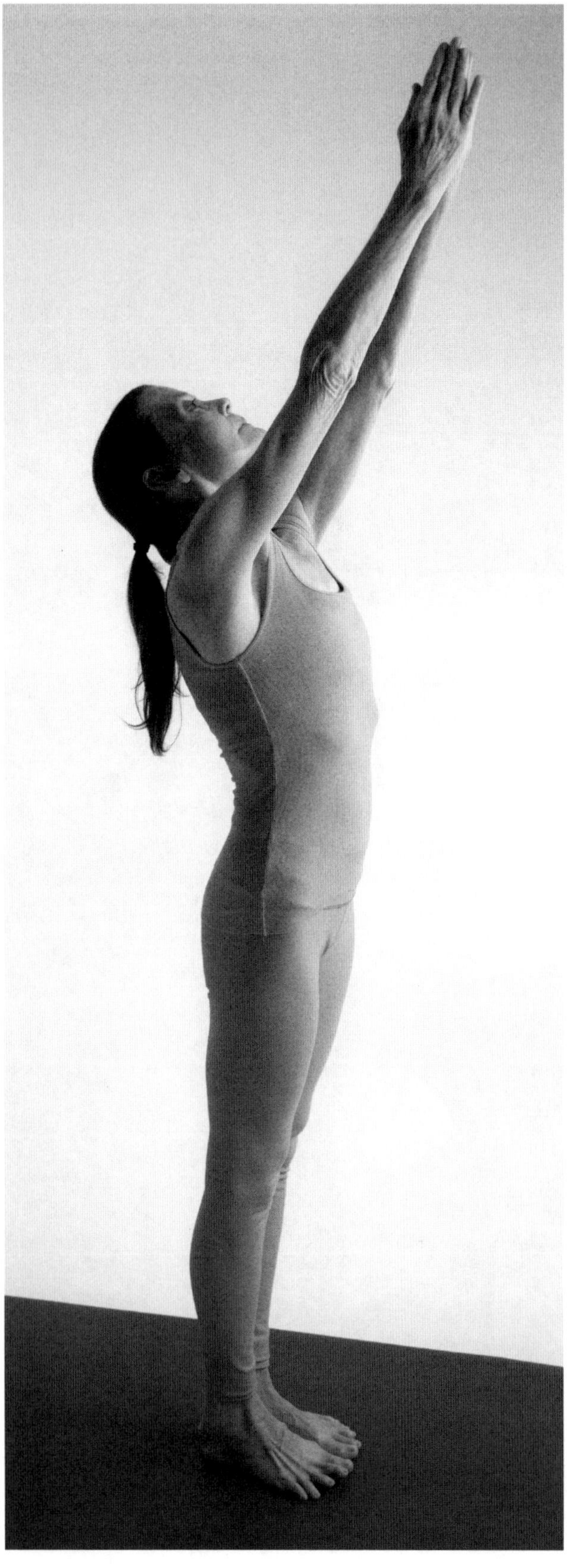

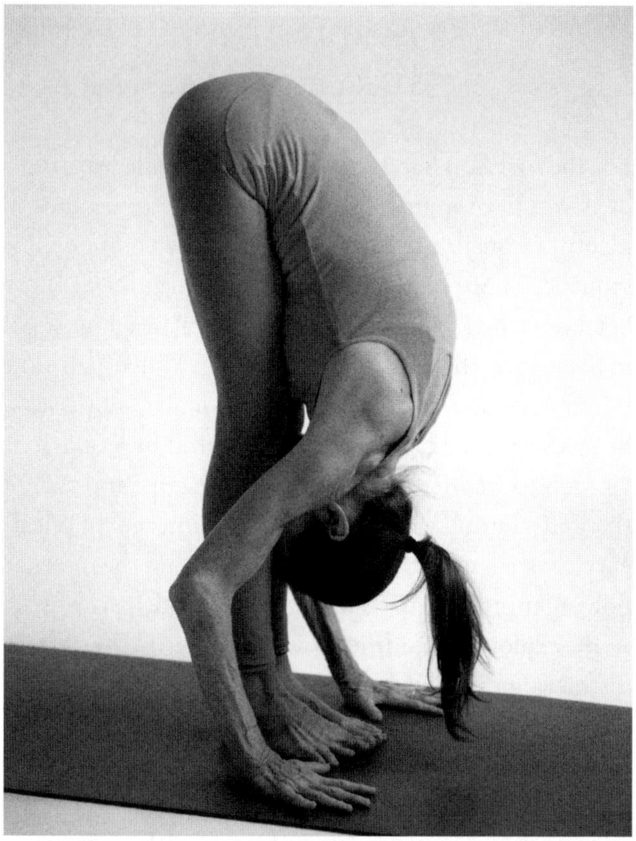

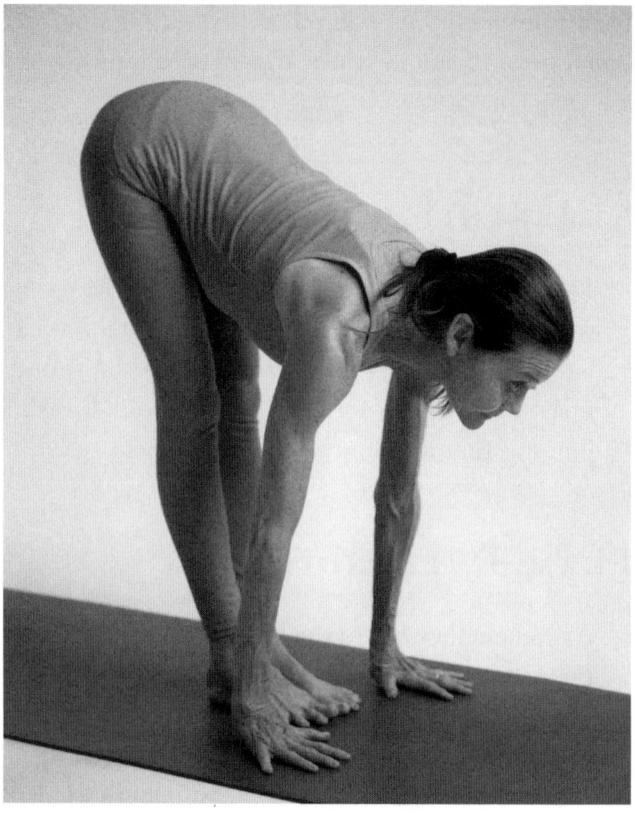

2. On the exhalation, release the palate up and back to do a swan dive—moving up, over, and around to fold forward into Dve. Keep the toes and fingers open for guidance.
3. At the end of the exhalation, curl the spine, contract the abdominal muscles, tone your PC muscle, and look toward the nose.
4. Lift the head as you inhale and extend the spine long, out through the crown of the head, placing your hands next to the feet for Trīṇi.

Catvāri and Variations

Number Four

1. Exhale, step back, and lie down on your belly. This is an introductory form of Catvāri, the fourth movement within Sūrya Namaskāra. You will expand on this initial form as your practice evolves. The full form of Catvāri is like a well-aligned push-up position, but in the beginning as you build strength, or for educational purposes anytime, lying on the belly can be very effective.
2. Alternatively, when learning Catvāri, you may step back into a high plank position. In this form, the arms are vertical with the elbows slightly bent to about five degrees. Push the shoulders down, away from your ears, and ground your thumbs. Keep the abdomen toned

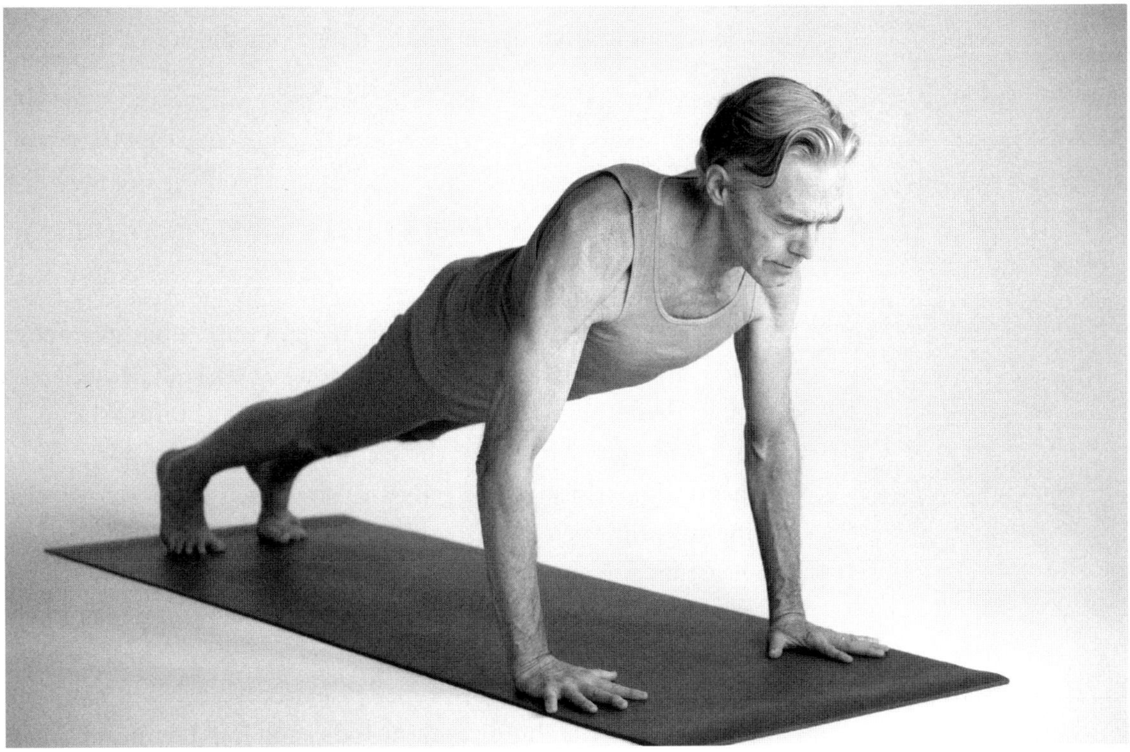

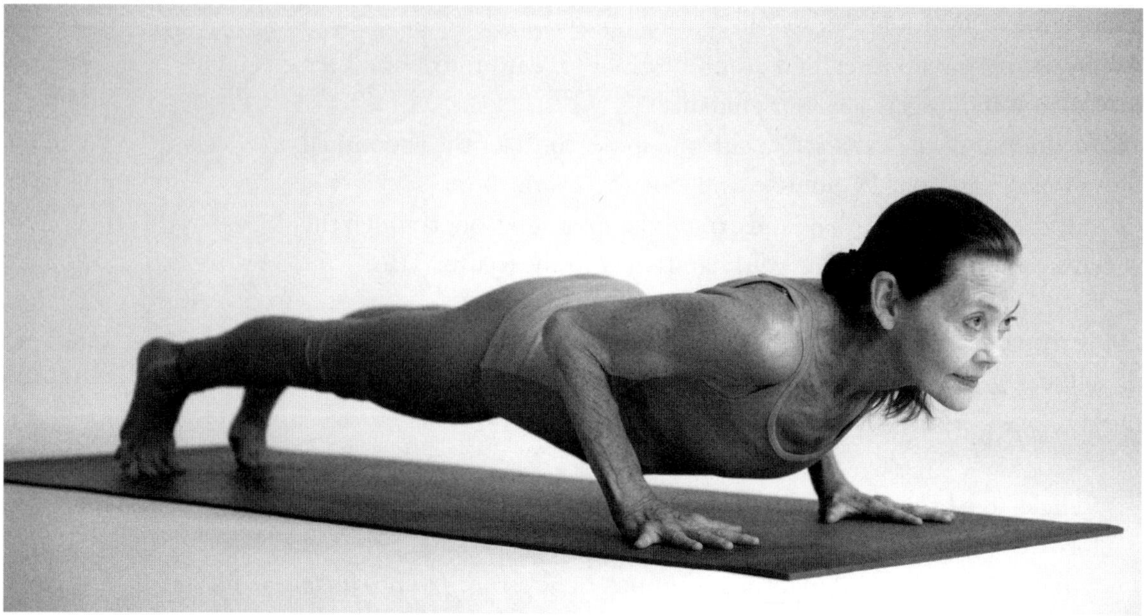

and the legs fully extended and engaged so that your body is in a straight line. Direct the gaze out in front along the line of the nose.

3. For the final form of Catvāri, come into a low plank position with the sternum about four inches from the floor. Align the top edge of the shoulders just over the tips of the fingers. Position the feet about hip-width apart, strengthen the abdominal muscles, and pull back the groins. Keep the shoulders squared and elbows fairly close to your sides. Gaze out in front of you on the floor along the line of the nose.

Pañca

In Sūrya Namaskāra, the fifth full form is Ūrdhvā Mukha Śvānāsana (Upward Facing Dog Pose).

1. From the end of the exhalation in Catvāri, pull your pubic bone about one inch farther back from the floor. As you begin to inhale, allow the coccyx to dive straight down into the pelvic floor. Pulling the spine forward, roll onto the tops of the feet as you unroll the spine into a backbend. Press through the hands to straighten the arms without locking your elbows.
2. The heart area floats up high in front of the arms. The pelvic floor will feel as if it's being pulled way up into the body, as you maintain a slight inward rotation so the "eyes" of the elbows do not look straight ahead. This keeps the weight properly distributed on each hand between the heel of the thumb and the index and middle fingers.

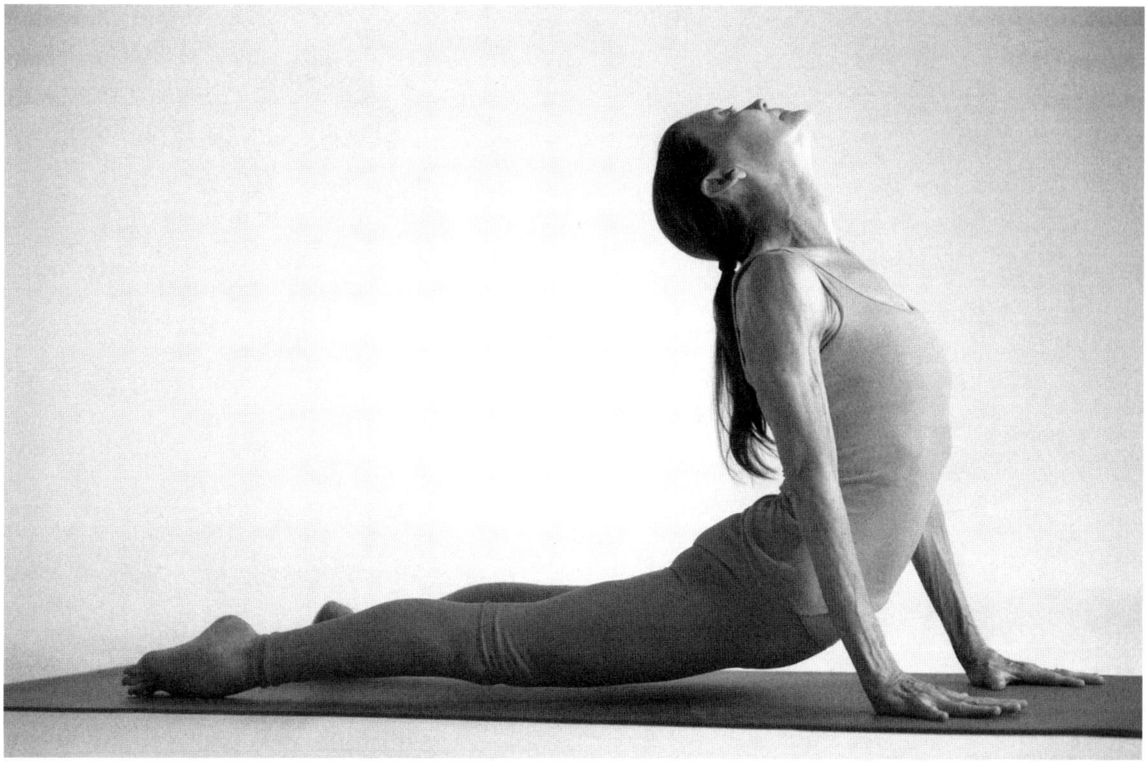

3. When you unroll your spine, it's as if the spine were uncoiling from bottom to top, the head being the very last component to roll back as you gaze down the nose. This is Pañca, the fifth position in the Sun Salutation.

Pañca Variation

Sphinx Pose

Two important poses that can help us train for Upward Facing Dog Pose are Sphinx Pose and Bhujaṅgāsana.

1. Lie on your belly and crawl up onto the elbows, placing them approximately under your shoulders. Position the forearms and lower arms parallel to each other, with palms facing down.
2. As you inhale, pull isometrically through the forearms back along the sides of your body. Draw the sternum forward and up to gently encourage the spine to elongate into a subtle backbend. It will feel as if the collarbones are spinning backward and being drawn up and back over the shoulders. Keep the pubic bone on the mat.
3. Meanwhile, imagine the coccyx is heavy, like gold, so that it drops easily down. Keep the eyes steady, gazing at a point out in front

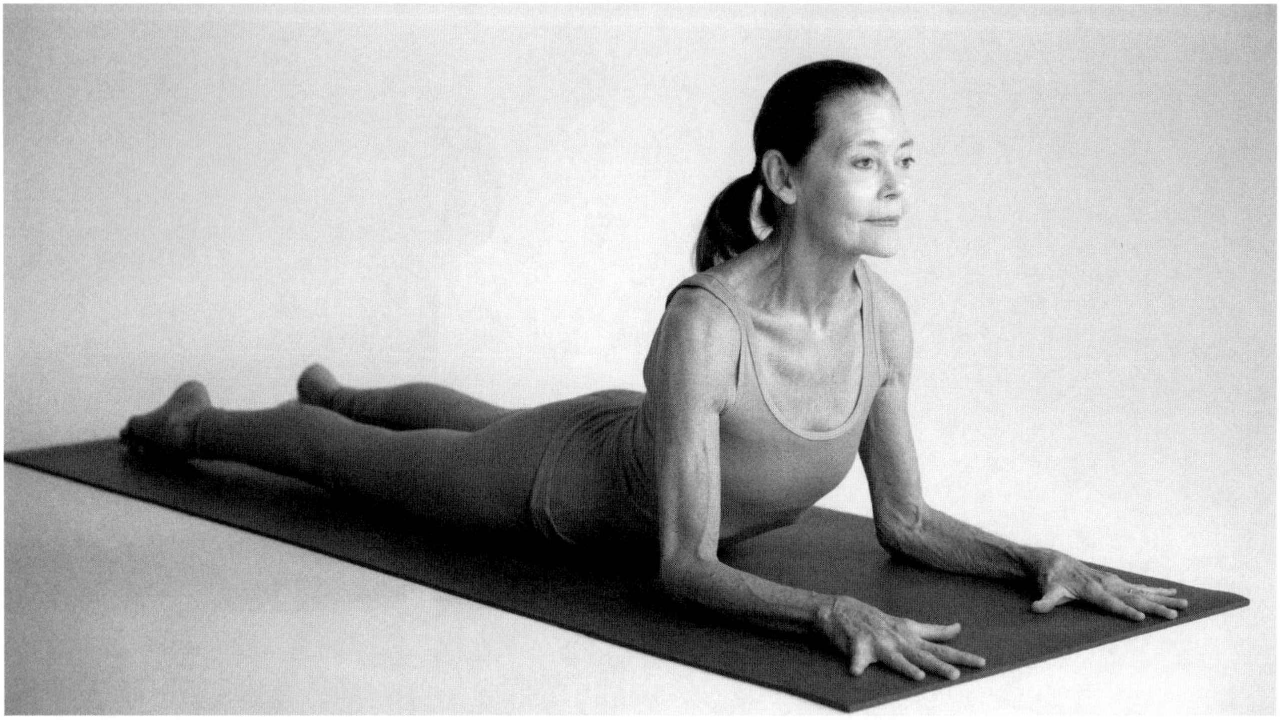

of you on the floor along the line of the nose. Roll the tops of the arms up, back, and down to cue the shoulder blades to slide down the back, the collarbones to spread, and the heart to float. Keep the head steady, kidney wings wide, palate released, and the crown of the head light.

4. When you inhale, you should feel the weight of the coccyx as if it were a slightly heavy tail flowing into the PC muscle. As you exhale, release the pull through your forearms and soften into the pose. On the next inhalation, again pull the spine forward and feel the breath as it spreads the kidney wings. Drop the coccyx but keep the buttocks soft.
5. If you experience compression or pain in the low back or SI joint, experiment with small shifts in form to alleviate the discomfort. Slightly changing elbow position—moving them forward or back, a little bit wider or somewhat closer together—can help. Also, focus fully on rolling the tops of your arms back and dropping your coccyx down while softening your belly—maybe sinking a little lower down through the upper body—as you pull with the forearms. Tone and reach back through the legs so there is a sense of the spine being pulled forward as the sitting bones are held back evenly in the opposite direction.
6. On the inhalation, lengthen the psoas muscle behind the belly, almost like you're breathing *through* the muscle itself. Eventually the

inhalation will pull the middle point of the pelvic floor up into the midline. On the exhalation, maintain, observe, and keep the tone that is building in the pelvic floor and throughout the body.

Pañca Variation

Bhujaṅgāsana (Cobra Pose)

1. After five rounds of ujjāyī breath in Sphinx Pose, take a big breath in. At the top of inhalation, lift and spread the elbows out to the sides. Use the pressure of the palms of your hands to pull yourself forward into Bhujaṅgāsana. You may also enter Bhujaṅgāsana directly from any variation of Catvāri.
2. Roll the tops of the arms back in space. The shoulder blades will automatically slide down the back, broadening and supporting a gentle lift to the heart from behind. Keep the coccyx dropped, the pubic bone and thighs on the floor, and the legs gently toned. Stay in Bhujaṅgāsana for several rounds of the breath or move immediately into Ṣaṭ, the sixth form.

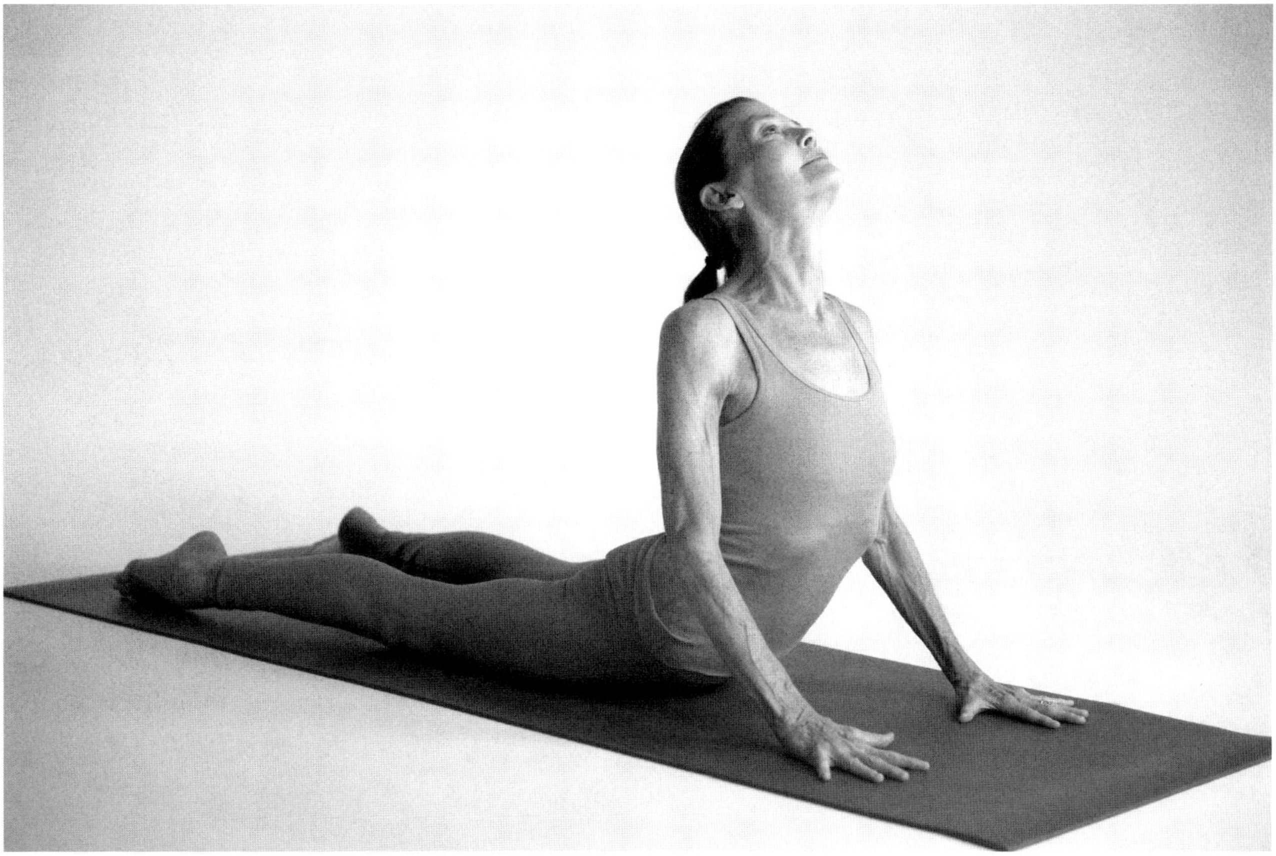

Ṣaṭ

The sixth form in Sūrya Namaskāra is Adho Mukha Śvānāsana (Downward Facing Dog Pose). In an Aṣṭāṅga Vinyāsa practice, practitioners spend more time in Downward Facing Dog Pose than in any other single pose. It is one to work on and refine endlessly.

1. At the crest of an inhalation in Upward Facing Dog Pose, release the palate to stimulate a wavelike, rolling movement that, on the exhalation, triggers the feet to pull back and flip over. This closes the hip joints and creates the perfect counterpose to Upward Facing Dog Pose.
2. Entering the pose, the shoulder blades must be fully protracted. As your weight shifts forward from the heels of thumbs to the roots of the index and middle fingers, the shoulder blades rotate back. Focusing on the collarbones, you may experience a sense of them rolling back and spreading.
3. The head gradually falls through the arms to complete the form. Keep the legs and arms activated and the fingers and toes spreading.

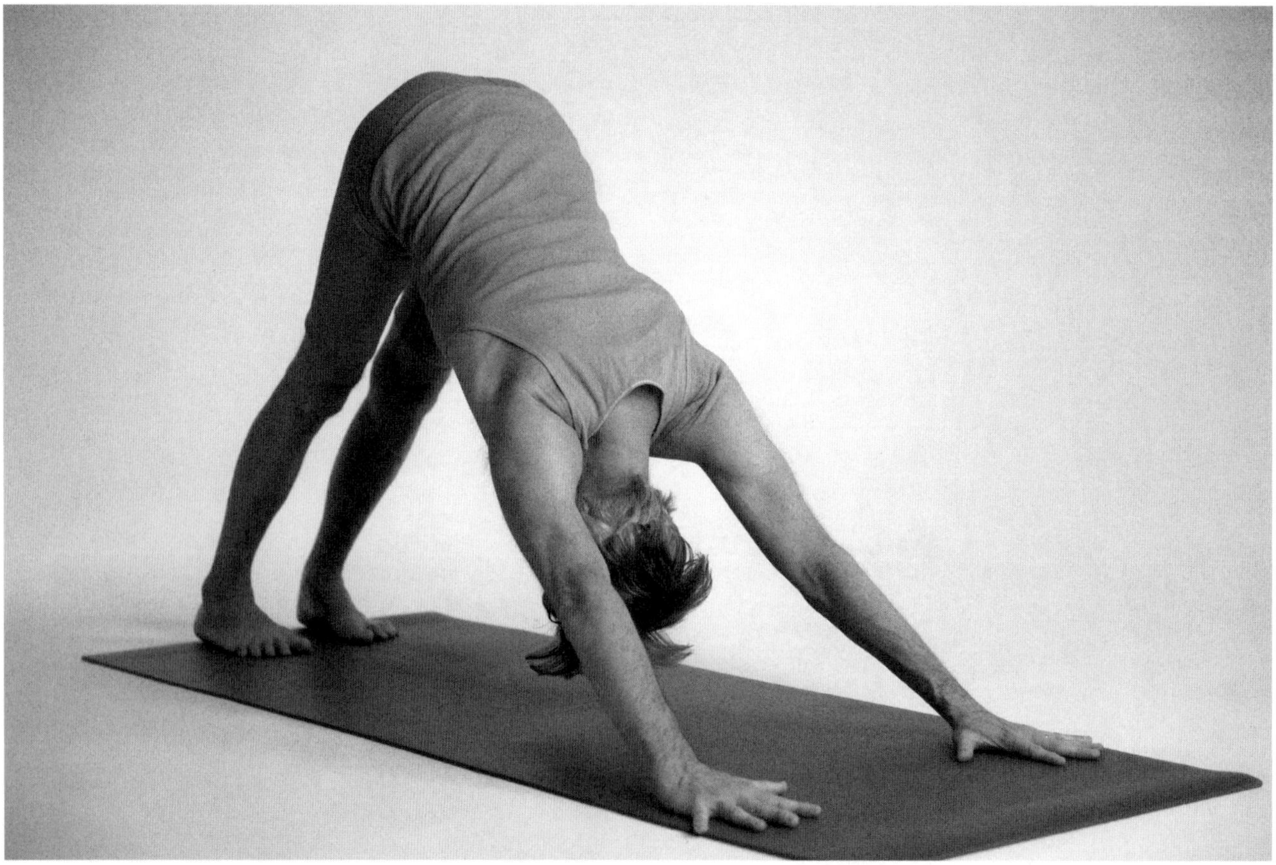

4. Hold the pose for at least five full rounds of the breath, gazing at a point on the floor between your feet or, eventually, at your navel. Gradually lengthen the arms to move the sitting bones farther back and to release and lengthen the psoas muscles; this allows you to find Mūlabandha and the central channel.

Ṣaṭ Variation

Puppy Pose

1. From Pañca or one of its variations, exhale and push up onto the knees with the toes turned under.
2. Position the thighs vertical to the floor, walk the hands as far forward as possible, and place the forehead on the floor. (If your forehead doesn't reach the floor, put a block under the forehead as support.)
3. Come up onto the fingertips as you reach through the arms, cupping the palms away from the floor and protracting the shoulder blades. Pushing your fingertips down moves the middle of the armpit back and up, away from the floor. This is one way of learning the illusive shoulder form in full Downward Facing Dog Pose.

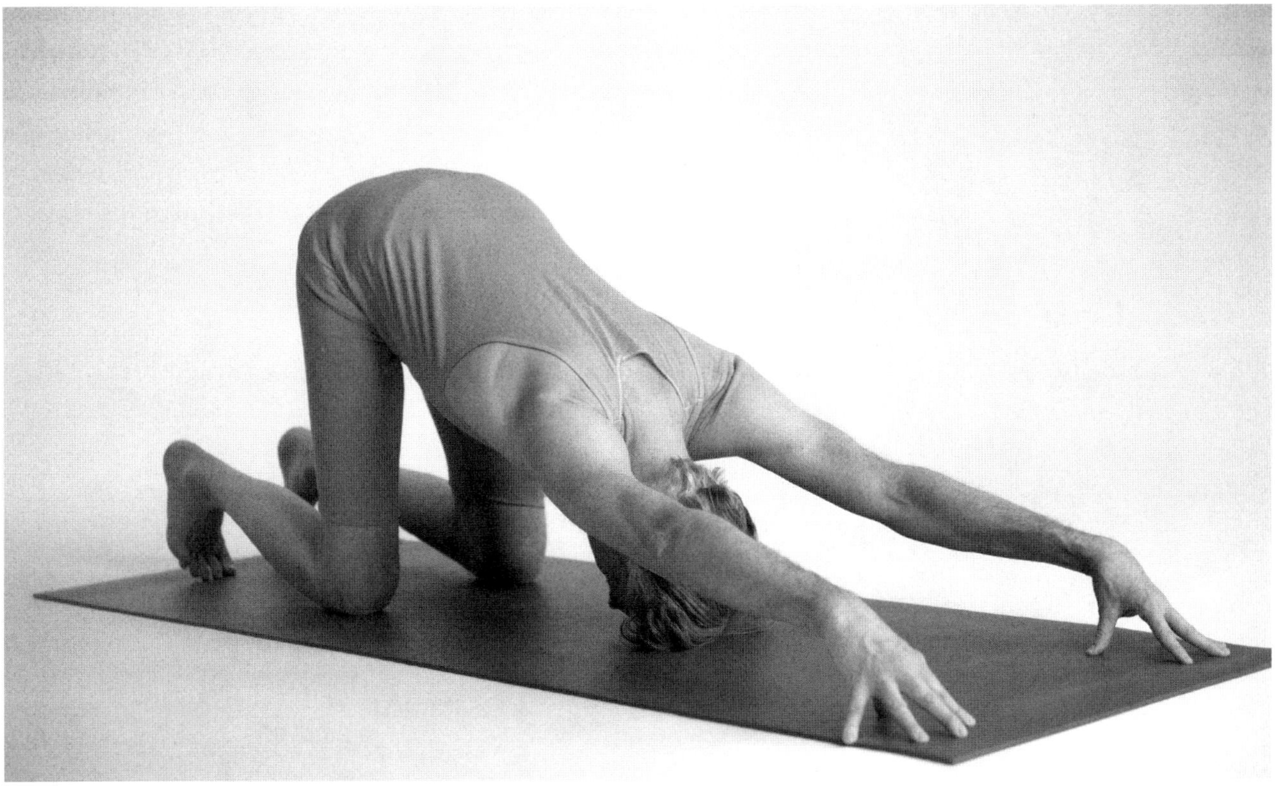

Ṣaṭ Variation

Old Dog Pose

1. You may come directly into this variation by pushing up onto the knees when transitioning out of Pañca. Alternatively, you may practice the Puppy Pose first and work into the Old Dog.
2. Begin on all fours, with the arms and thighs vertical and the toes turned under. Move the hips back in space until the knees automatically begin to lift off the floor. You will experience a sensation of the buttocks expanding just before the knees automatically lift away from the floor. This is good because it makes the pelvic floor shrink.
3. Leave the knees bent deeply, and notice that your thumbs naturally ground to the floor. Keep the knees bent until you've moved the coccyx, pubic bone, and sitting bones as far back as possible.
4. This variation is particularly good if you have tight hamstrings that prevent you from deeply folding the groins closed in Downward Facing Dog Pose. Tight hamstrings may also inhibit the primary prāṇic action of the pubic bone moving up and back in the full form. Because the hamstrings are such strong muscles, when tight they pull down on the sitting bones, which prevents the pelvis from rotating

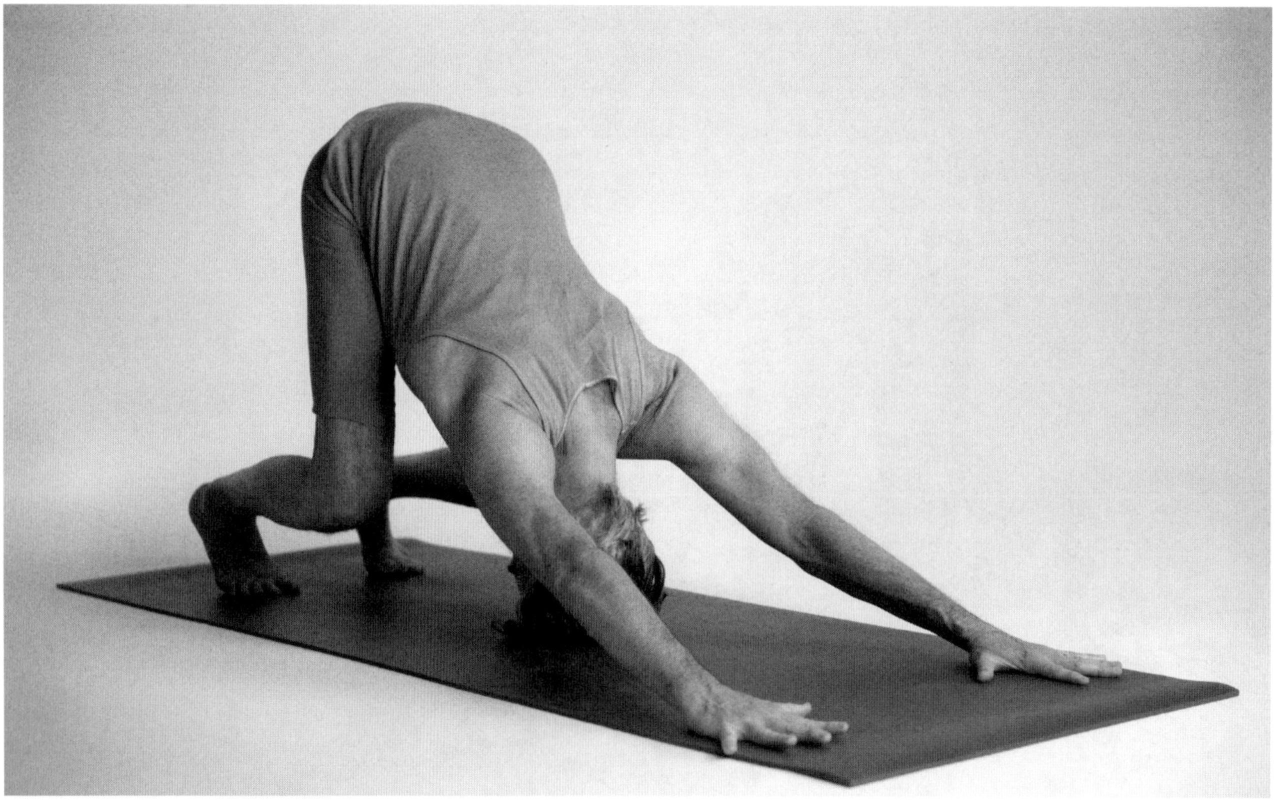

around the femurs and keeps the coccyx tucked. All this can prevent the primary action of the pubic bone. In the final form of the pose, both actions are present: the pubic bone moves back and up, while the coccyx moves back and down. Too much action from the coccyx at the beginning of the pose may move the sacrum in the same direction as the coccyx, which will overpower the desired up and back motion of the pubic bone.

5. Stay in the pose for five breaths. Then, if appropriate, gradually straighten the legs into the full Downward Facing Dog Pose form and hold for five more rounds of breath.

Transitioning

1. When practicing Puppy Pose, transition to the front of the mat and the next movement of Sūrya Namaskāra by lifting the hips and walking the feet forward until they are between the hands.
2. For Old Dog or the full form of Ṣaṭ, at the end of the fifth exhalation, bend the knees to prepare to jump forward. The end of the exhalation pulls down on the coccyx by toning and setting the PC muscle. That stability gives you the control to get your feet back to the front of the mat.

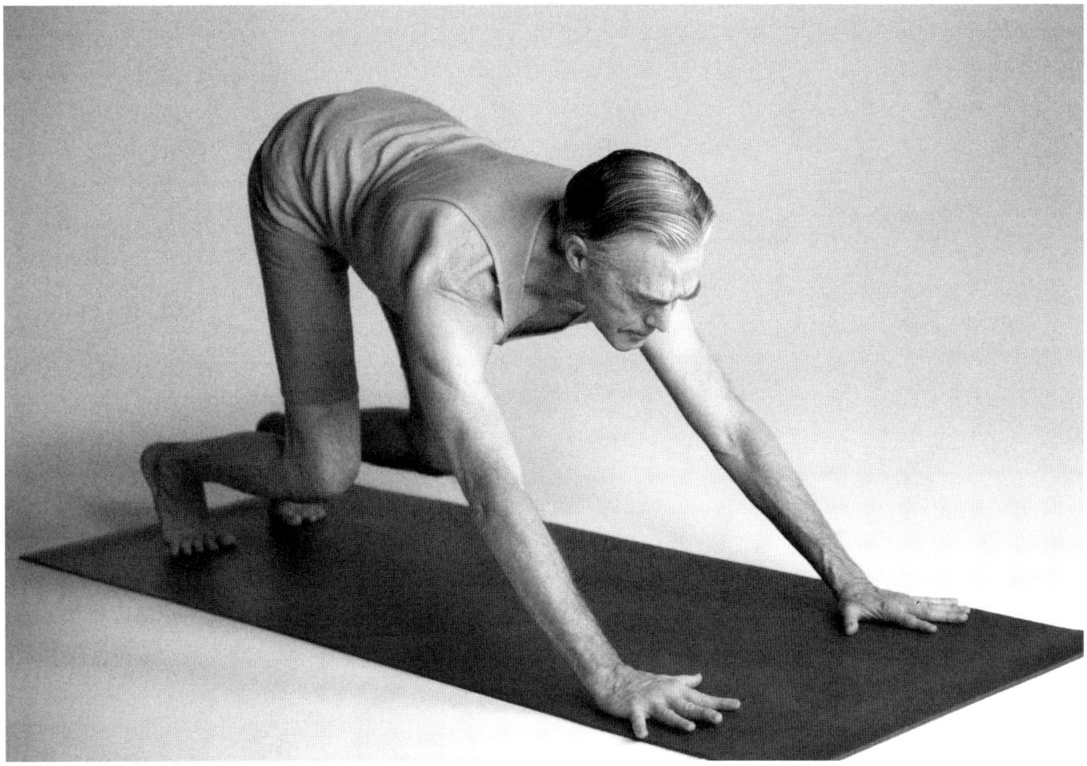

3. As you bend the knees, lift the head to look at the floor between the hands. Keeping the head away from the floor and behind the arms, walk, step, hop, or float forward, landing with the feet approximately between the hands at the front of the mat. However you get there is fine. Over time and as your strength and trust in your own movement increase, you will eventually be able to hop easily and land lightly.

Sapta, Aṣṭa, Nava, and Samasthitiḥ

Seven, Eight, Nine, and Samasthitiḥ

1. Just as the feet land, extend the spine and inhale, looking up and lifting into Sapta (the seventh position, which is the same as Trīṇi).
2. Exhale and fold forward, engaging the legs and abdomen. Gaze down the line of the nose. This is Aṣṭa (the eighth position, which is the same as Dve).
3. Lifting the head, inhale as you stand up. Reach up and place the palms of your hands together above and in front of the head, gazing down the line of the nose at your thumbs. This is Nava (the ninth position, which is the same as Ekam).

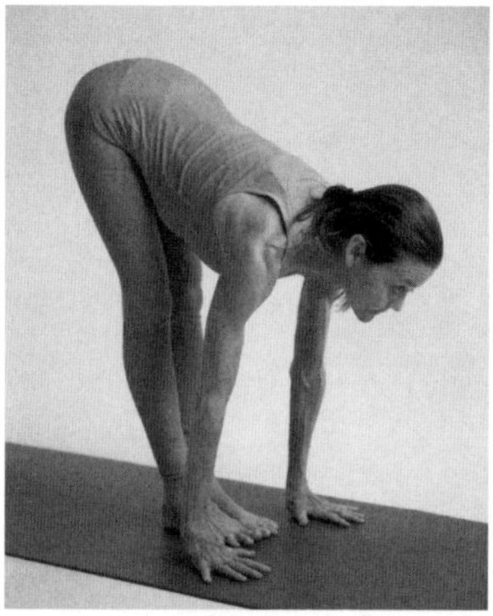

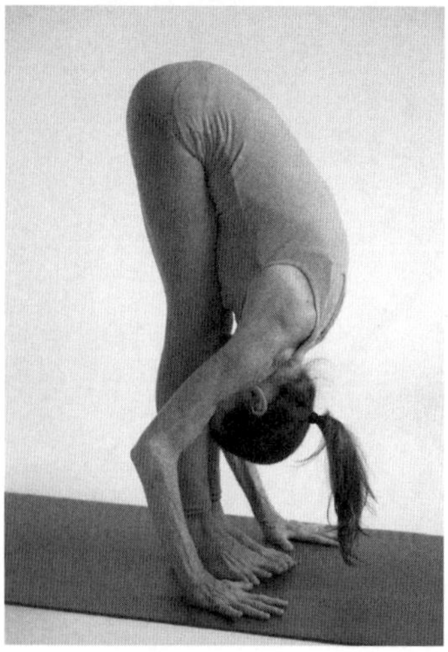

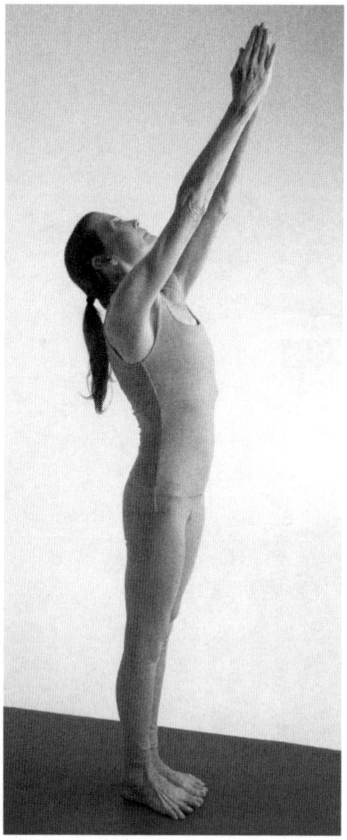

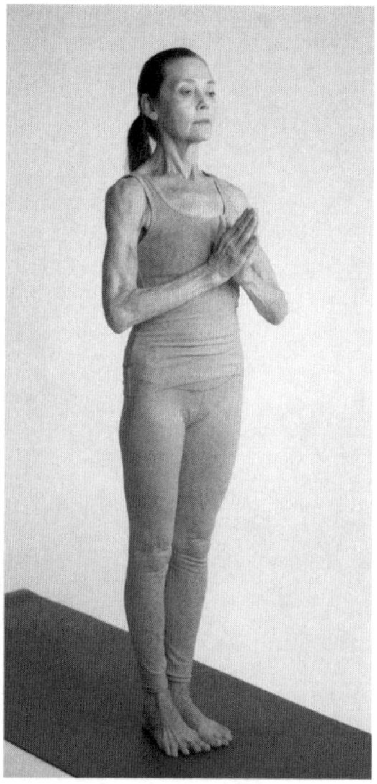

4. Exhale, lengthen up through the midline, and return to Samasthitiḥ, allowing the arms to float back down to the sides.
5. Once you have become familiar with the movements and underlying structure within Sūrya Namaskāra A, you should practice it as a rhythmic, moving form, synchronizing the breath, gaze, and movement into a smooth and continuous pattern. All of the movements except Ṣaṭ (Downward Facing Dog Pose), from Ekam back to Samasthitiḥ, are held for only one breath, inhaling to enter the movement and exhaling to transition out of it. Ṣaṭ is held for five rounds of breath before transitioning forward into Sapta.

Sūrya Namaskāra B

Sūrya Namaskāra B has seventeen forms and builds the heat before the full practice. Refer to the earlier descriptions of Sūrya Namaskāra A for more detail on some of these movements. (See full sequence of Sūrya Namaskāra A in Appendix 5.)

1. Stand in Samasthitiḥ with the hands together in prayer position.
2. Inhale into Ekam. As you inhale, bend the knees 90 degrees into a half squat and lift the arms over the head. Place the palms together and look along the nose at the thumbs. Keep the lower belly hollowed just above the pubic bone, inner knees touching, and the arms reaching up but in front of the head. This is Utkaṭāsana.
3. Exhale into Dve by straightening the legs, then coming up and folding over on the wave of the breath.
4. Inhale into Trīṇi, straightening the spine as you lift the head.
5. Exhale into Catvāri. Jump or step back into a high or low plank position (whichever is appropriate for you) with the corresponding gaze.
6. Inhale into Pañca. Pull yourself forward and roll the feet over into Upward Facing Dog Pose.
7. Exhale into Ṣaṭ, pushing back into Downward Facing Dog Pose.
8. As you complete the exhalation, bring the left heel onto the centerline of the mat, toes pointing out, and the right foot forward between the hands into a lunge position. Inhale into Sapta by lifting the arms and placing the palms together, keeping both feet well grounded. Bend the right knee until it is over the right ankle. Keep the left leg firm and straight and the left foot entirely grounded. Draw down the coccyx, pubic bone, and sitting bones, while opening the left groin. Gaze at the thumbs with the head behind the arms. This is Vīrabhadrāsana A (Warrior Pose A).

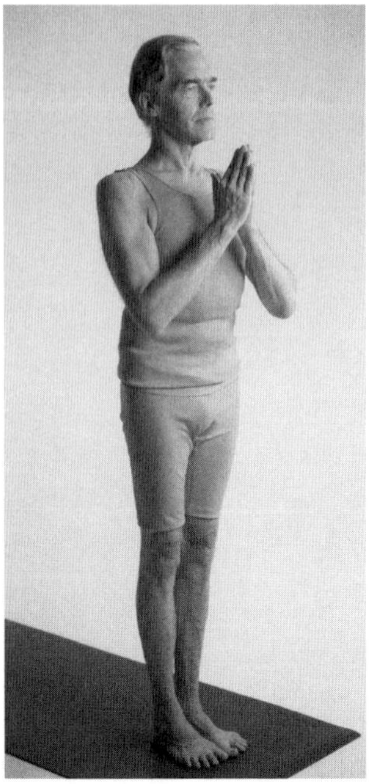
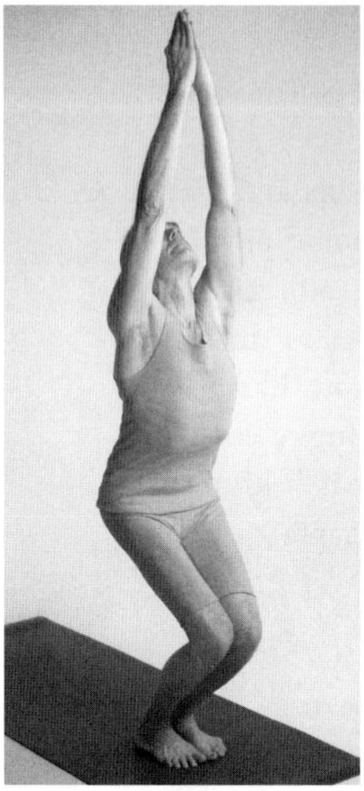
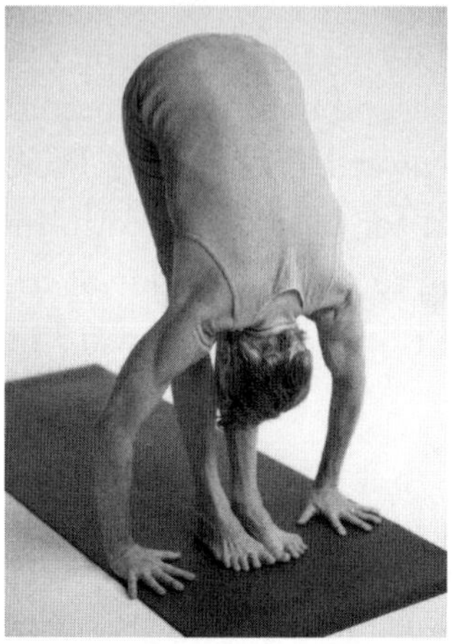
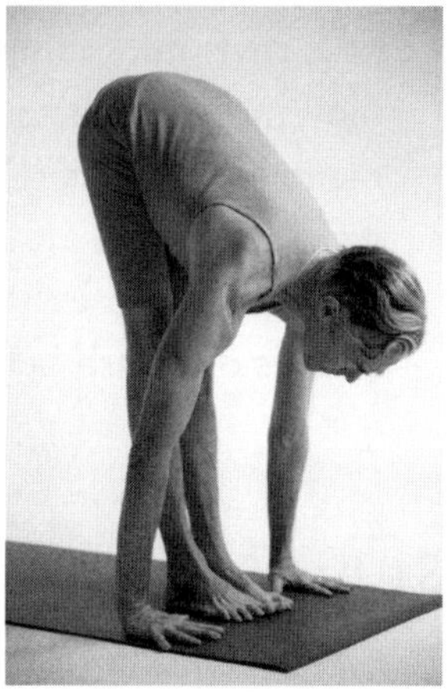
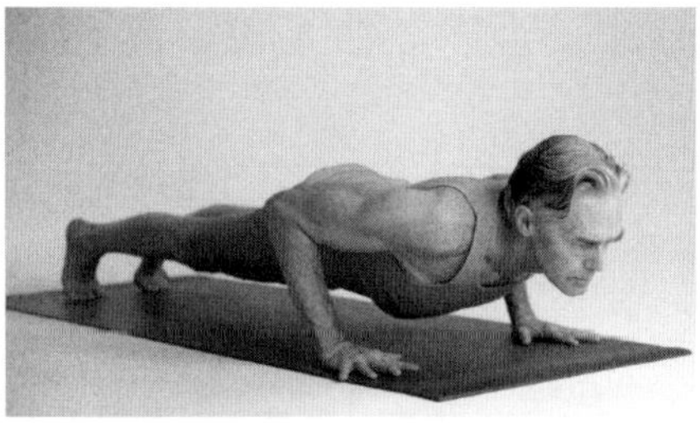
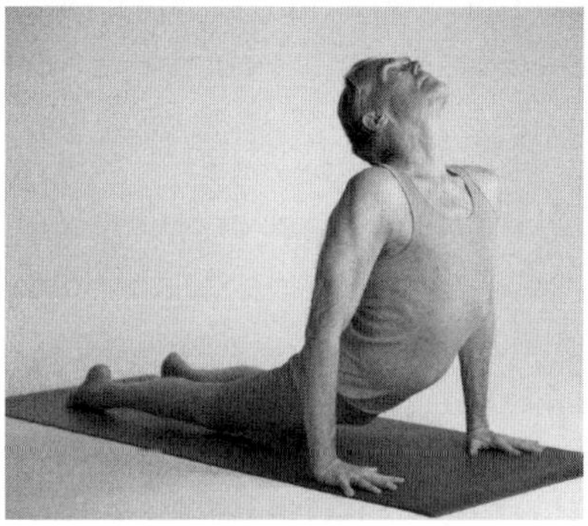
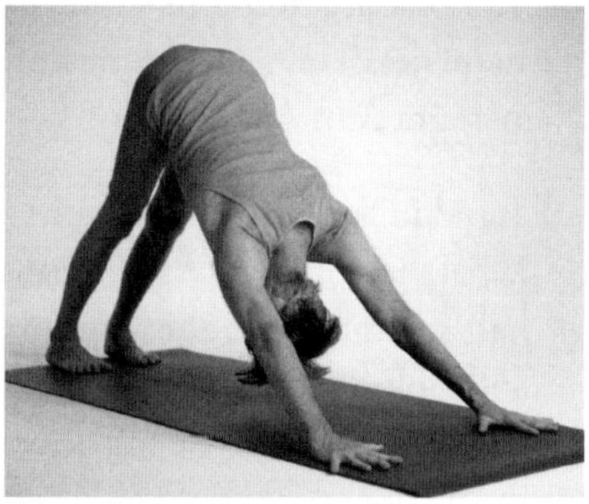
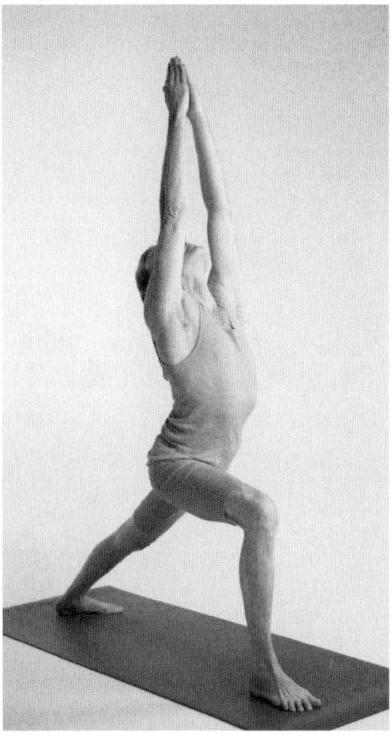

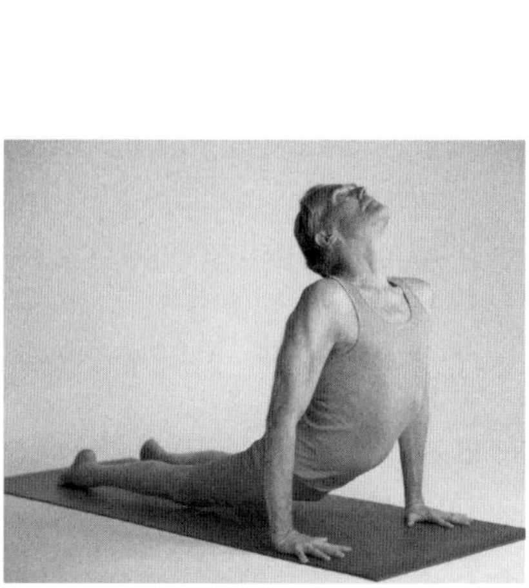

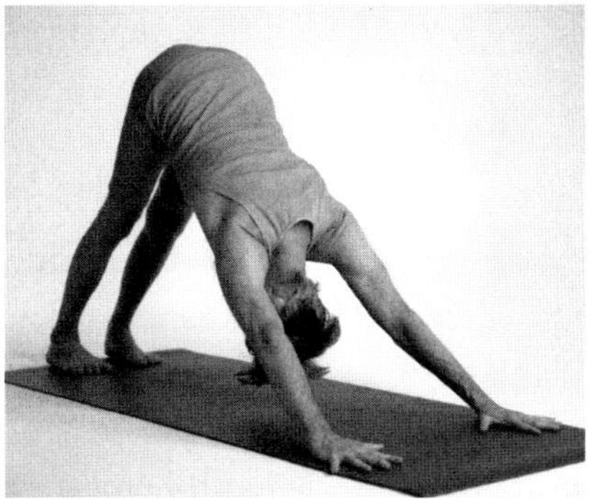
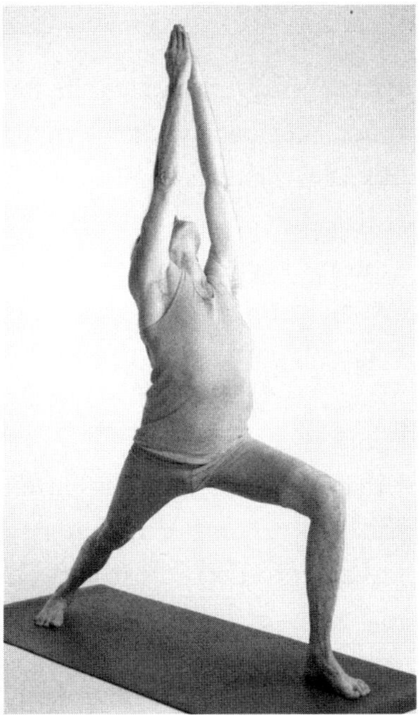
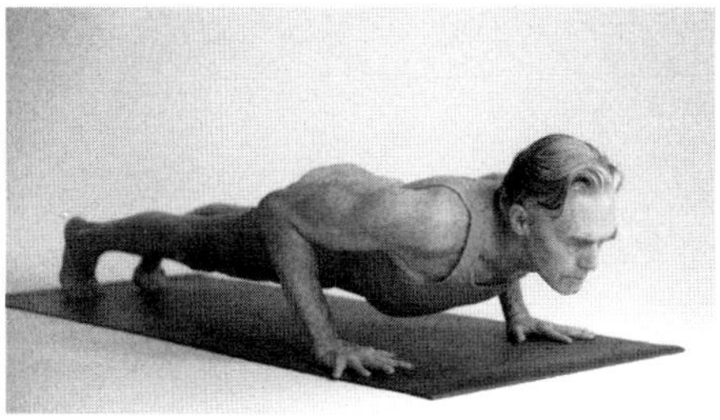
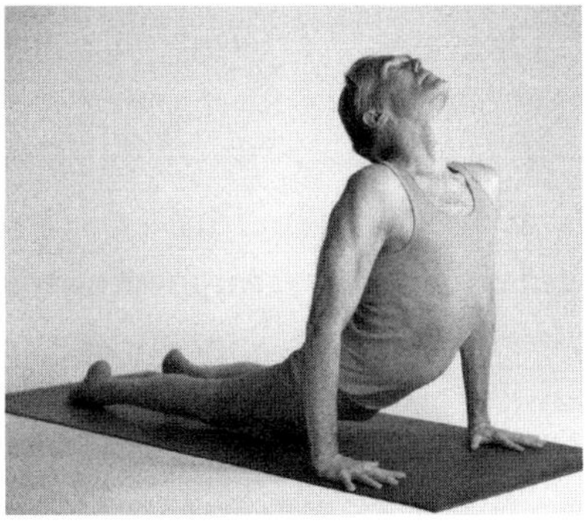
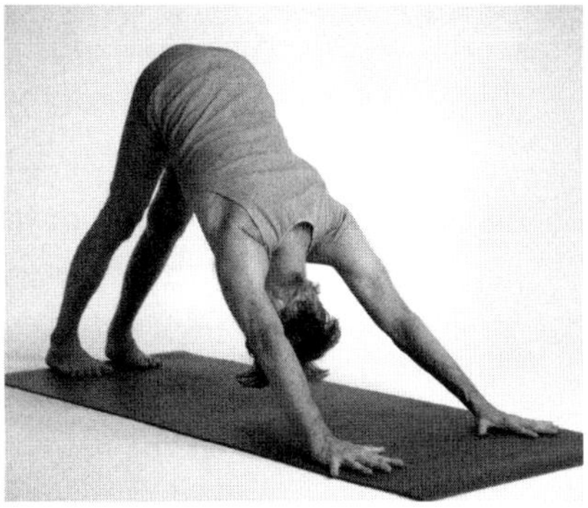
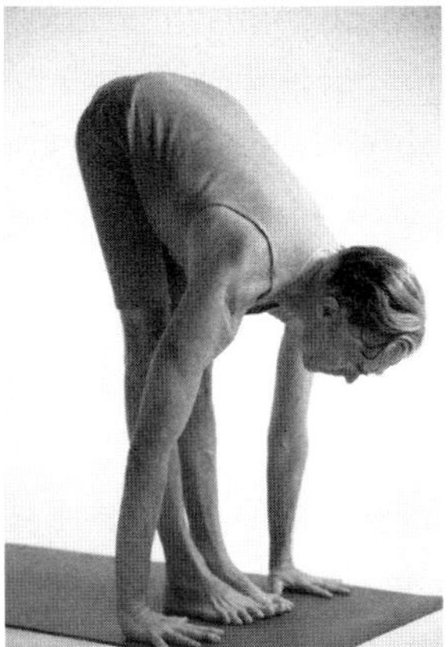
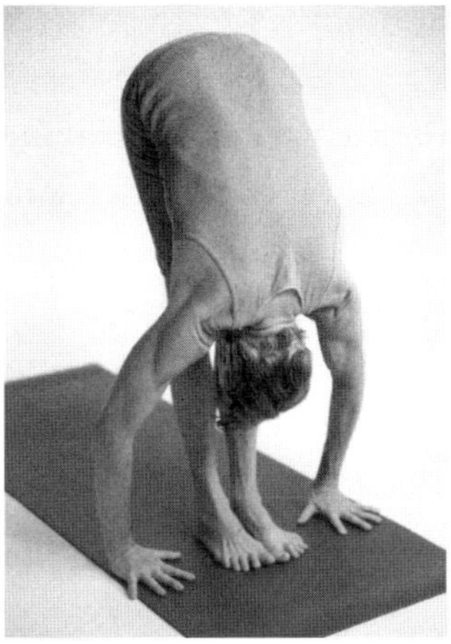
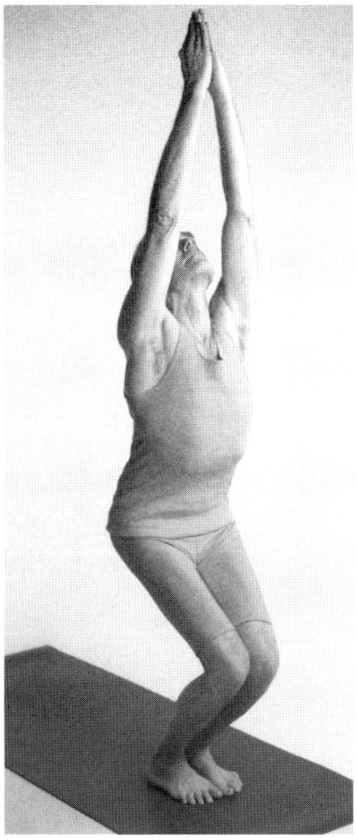
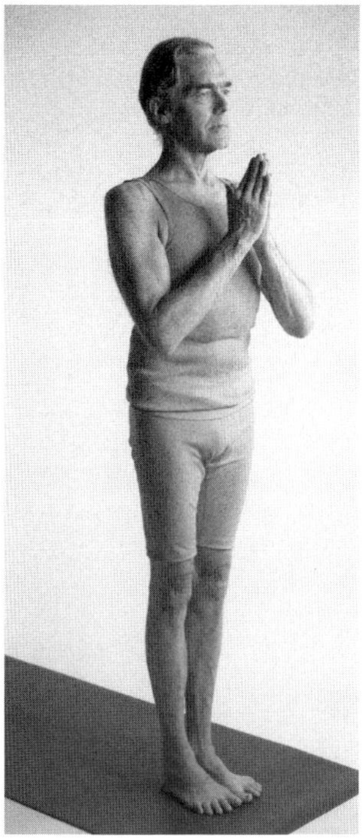

9. Exhale into Aṣṭa. Place the hands on the mat at shoulder-width distance. Step back with the right foot and lower the body into the form of Catvāri that is appropriate for you.
10. Inhale into Nava. Lift the heart, point the toes, and come up into Upward Facing Dog Pose.
11. Exhale into Daśa (the tenth movement). Pull back into Downward Facing Dog Pose on the out-breath, and at the end of the exhalation, bring the right heel in and step forward with the left foot between the hands in a lunge position.
12. Inhale into Ekādaśa (the eleventh movement). Lift the arms and bend the left knee into Vīrabhadrāsana A, the mirror image of step eight.
13. Exhale into Dvādaśa (the twelfth movement). Place the hands on the mat and step back into whichever plank position you did for Catvāri, with the elbows bent and drawn in toward your sides.
14. Inhale into Trayodaśa (the thirteenth movement) by pulling forward into Upward Facing Dog Pose.
15. Exhale into Caturdaśa (the fourteenth movement). Draw the hips back and wrap your shoulders out, engaging the serratus muscles so they protract easily as you move into Downward Facing Dog Pose. Remain in this position for five breaths.
16. Inhale into Pañcadaśa (the fifteenth movement). At the end of the fifth exhalation, bend the knees, look up, and hop forward, placing the feet in Samasthitiḥ position. Just as your feet land, inhale and lift the head.
17. Exhale into Ṣodaśa (the sixteenth movement) by folding forward and looking at the tip of the nose.
18. Inhale into Saptadaśa (the seventeenth movement). Bend the knees deeply and raise the arms into Utkaṭāsana.
19. Exhale as you press back up to standing tall in Samasthitiḥ.

Sūrya Namaskāra A and B should each be practiced a minimum of five times at the beginning of each practice. It's best to do them until a feeling of stability arises, and the breath seems to pervade your whole body. Sūrya Namaskāra is the great elixir among yoga practices; beginners and those who feel weak or emotionally distraught should do many repetitions! Sūrya Namaskāra builds the foundation for the rest of the series by creating coordination, endurance, and strength. Its importance cannot be overemphasized. Sūrya Namaskāra B helps to open the *granthis* (energy blockages) around the sacrum. Remember to keep the shoulders away from the ears and the heart open throughout all the movements.

In a vinyāsa practice, poses are not done in isolation from one another. Instead, one unfolds into the next as a moving meditation, linked together by the breath and the gaze. They flow naturally, like waves within patterns of breath, movement, alignment, form, and mind. Ujjāyī breathing and a steady, nongrasping gaze, combined with a sense of bandha and mudrā, construct the foundation on which this integration of body and mind is built. To maintain this sense of a pattern of movement and form rather than independent poses, the entrance and exit to any pose are considered as important as the pose itself. Keeping the internal, meditative connection alive, we move between poses with Full or Half Vinyāsas or by returning for a full breath cycle to Samasthitiḥ.

FULL VINYĀSA AND HALF VINYĀSA

A Full Vinyāsa may be practiced between any and all poses, if time and energy permit. Typically, however, it is practiced during the second half of the standing sequence, and Half Vinyāsa is practiced between every pose (and eventually between the sides of most poses) after the standing sequence. Both forms increase strength and stability and serve to keep the practice moving as an interconnected series of movements while helping to reset the mind and nervous system to neutral between poses. Upward and Downward Facing Dog Poses and the rhythmic movements in and out of them are full, symmetrical expressions of the interlinking prāṇa-apāna patterns that help to process the residue of a pose and take you back into the middle path of breathing, bandha, mudrā, and dṛṣṭi.

A Full Vinyāsa follows the pattern of Sūrya Namaskāra A, returning to standing through the two Dog Poses and then starting again the Sūrya Namaskāra A pattern, and from Downward Facing Dog Pose moving into the next pose on the following inhalation. Half Vinyāsa is when you jump back into Catvāri between poses; move into Upward Facing Dog Pose on the next inhalation followed by Downward Facing Dog Pose on the exhalation; then glide into the next pose on the following inhalation.

TWO EXTRAORDINARY LINKING MOVEMENTS

To accommodate the cyclical return to the two Dog Poses, there are two other wonderful movements that defy easy categorization: Jumping Back and Cakrāsana (Wheel Pose). While you are learning the movements, or if you have physical limitations, these poses may feel (and be) out of reach; however, there are alternatives so that everyone can work on the same patterns of strength, counteraction, and movement and perhaps move into the full form one day. Remember, it is the patterns of Prāṇa and the thoughts that ride upon them that are of interest. The mindful, meditative step-by-counterstep process of intelligent vinyāsa is the actual practice. The achievement games that the mind constructs are to be observed by an unbiased intelligence.

Jumping Back

1. From a sitting position on the floor, begin by crossing the legs, drawing the thighs and knees in toward the chest, and placing the hands down at the sides while finishing a firm exhalation. This helps the apāna pattern bring the rectus abdominis muscle into its most contracted and toned form.

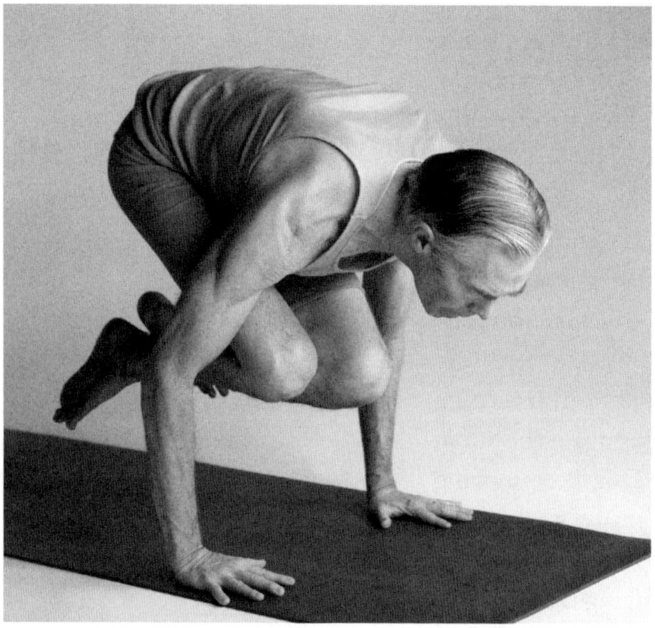

2. Lift the hips off the floor and inhale into the higher portion of the lift. As you lift and swing the legs back between the arms, move your chest and face forward and down.
3. Extend the legs to land in Catvāri once the chest and shoulders are down in correct Catvāri position.
4. If you can't perform this entire movement, merely lift the hips and feet off the floor as you balance for a breath resting on the hands. Then lower back down, place the hands in front of the knees, and step or hop back into Catvāri. Practicing the lift alone initiates the desired pattern in your body. Whether lifting up to jump back or simply lifting and stepping back, the movements should be done elegantly and on

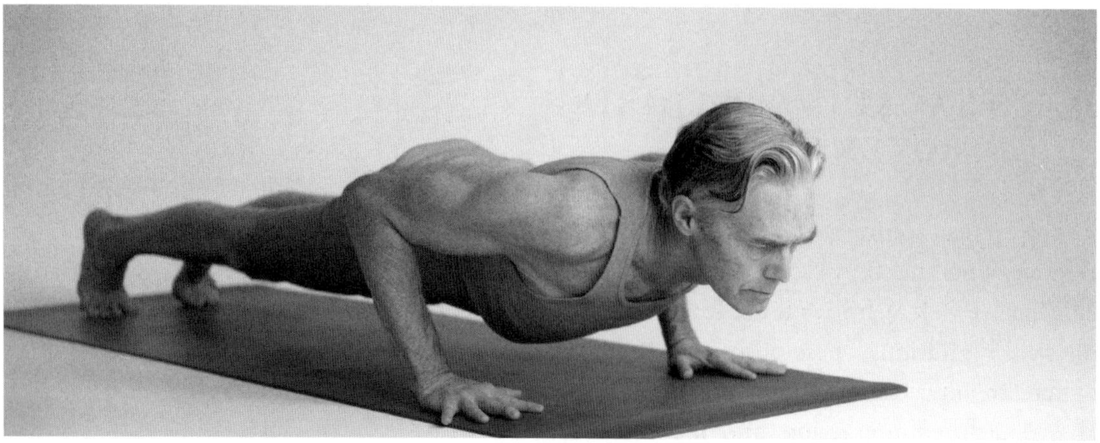

the wave of the breath. Straining and using yoga as a competitive ego sport is usually counterproductive in the long run.

Cakrāsana

Wheel Pose

Another useful and potentially wonderful vinyāsa linking movement is Cakrāsana, a backward roll. This pose can cause fear or trepidation because it's disorienting to roll backward, and it may seem that your neck is in danger. Actually with practice and some trust in the breath, Cakrāsana is accessible to most people.

1. Lie on your back in Tāḍāgī Mudrā (see page 27). Exhale deeply and firm the rectus abdominis muscles.
2. Before inhaling, begin lifting the legs. When they are about halfway up (at about 40 degrees from the floor), begin to inhale.
3. Lifting the pelvis off the floor, place the hands on the floor next to your ears. As your feet travel over the head, turn the eyes slightly upward in dṛṣṭi.
4. As the center of gravity moves between the hands, begin to push with them, almost as if you were pushing up into a backbend. Keep the legs straight, reaching them back toward the wall behind you as you move into a backward roll and wind up in Catvāri. The heart will approach the chin at the point of greatest flexion in the lower neck.

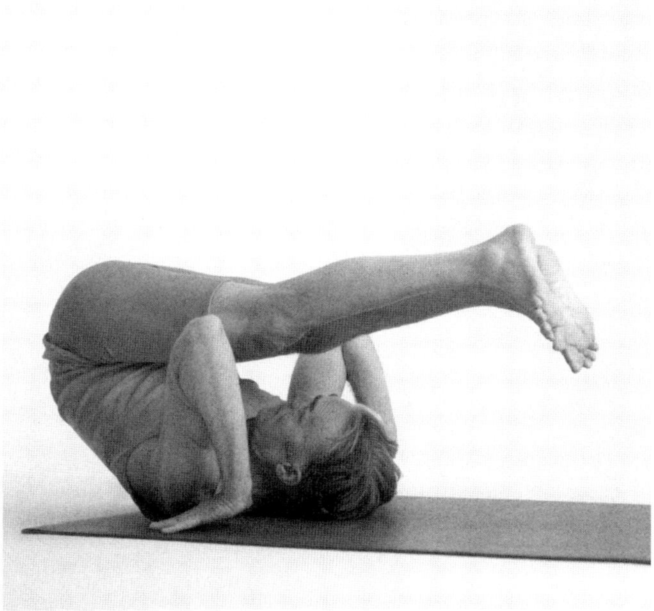

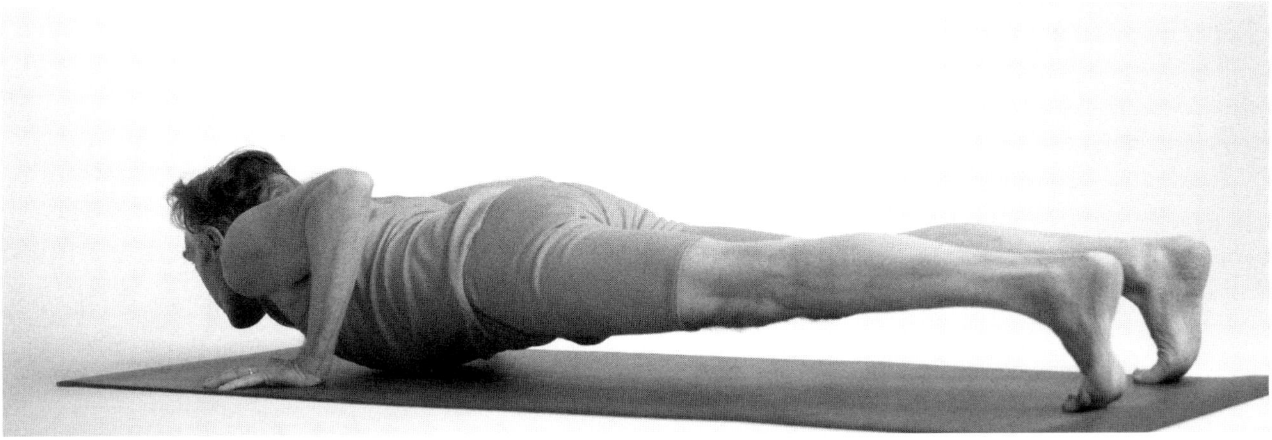

5. In the final stage of the roll, gaze down the line of the nose and roll symmetrically. Never pull the chin into the throat, and do not turn the head to either side.
6. Finish the pose in Catvāri, and then proceed through Half Vinyāsa to the next pose.
7. A qualified and patient teacher can be of tremendous help in learning this movement. It is important to resist doing the cheating method of rolling over one ear or the other. This is mechanically unsound and does not produce the symmetrical stretch that serves as a vinyāsa meditation.

6

Standing Poses

Even if you don't do much yoga, a considerable amount of your time is spent in standing poses: at the sink in the morning brushing your teeth, waiting in line for the bus, or strolling along the beach at sunset. When we begin practicing āsana, we discover that there are many "official" standing poses too, each with specific benefits and identifiable form. Those are the poses we will explore in this chapter.

As we begin to understand the underlying principles of form and alignment required to practice the āsanas as vinyāsa, we see how extraordinarily valuable standing poses are; they are titillating, grounding, and integrating. Most standing poses, such as Samasthitiḥ or Trikoṇāsana, are less dramatic than many other forms within our practice, and we may take them for granted or overlook their importance. For that very reason they are a practical and intelligent place to begin experiencing the internal forms that connect us from palate to perineum, allowing us to feel fully rooted to the earth through the practice. Well-executed standing poses, more than any other āsana form, make it possible for us to wake up and connect to what's happening before our eyes, even when we find ourselves in everyday "standing poses" like walking the dog.

The category of āsanas referred to as standing poses have many virtues. First, most can be done with little or no warm-up, so they may be practiced wherever you happen to be and whenever you feel like tapping into the benefits of the practice. Unlike most seated and balancing poses, backbends, or inversions, standing poses usually do not require a formal vinyāsa of poses to prepare and stretch the body beforehand or to get into them easily and safely.

Second, these poses connect us top to bottom, earth to sky. All standing poses naturally emphasize the feet and legs, and consequently they must involve the hips in a competent and integrated way; otherwise, the practitioner would fall over. With our feet fully awakened and intelligently rooting down, we build standing poses from the ground up. Bringing awareness to the arches, we then focus on the feeling of the leg muscles being drawn up from the feet (as if we were putting on a pair of stockings) as we experience a sense of connection to the earth and grounding down through the feet. This makes it easy to see that waking up the feet is immediately reflected in the pelvic floor. On a more subtle level, standing poses are stabilizing, not only in the literal sense of connecting us to the earth, but because the mechanical requirements they teach underscore the correct use of the pelvic floor, co-contractions of opposing muscle groups, and the obvious value of simultaneously working primary rotations and counterrotations. This deepens the impact of standing poses so we can experience and get the most benefit from the healthy and competent movements in and out of the forms.

All standing poses also require balance and thereby demand that we hone the skill of constantly adapting the forces and movements in the body to different structural plumb lines. On a subtle-body level, this is the function of Prāṇa (intelligence), and it quickly offers a visceral lesson on the wisdom of following the middle path. As such, standing poses, like deity visualization, can be a simple doorway into this internalized experience of the middle way.

Another good thing about standing poses is that, because there are so many of them, we can get a complete and balanced yoga practice using these poses alone. So if you ever find yourself in a tiny space for a long time—say, you get stuck in an elevator one day—you can do a full practice using very little floor space. Such a practice would include poses that fully express extension, flexion, and twisting as well as balancing and meditative form. Even the asymmetrical standing poses such as Parivṛtta Trikoṇāsana, because they are done on both sides, are conducive to meditation, bringing you back to a powerful feeling of symmetry and the invitation to drop into the midline of the body.

For the most part, standing poses are safer for many people than other poses. This is partly due to the fact that standing itself is a familiar form to anyone who ambulates through the world. Usually standing requires that we be awake and relate to the physical necessities of our environment. For this reason, during standing poses, we are less likely to obsess on and strain in any particular movement or position while ignoring the rest of the body (which is not uncommon when doing some other types of poses). Standing forms are simple, and beneath them all messages from the subtle body are constantly bringing our focus back to balancing, the familiar territory of not falling over. This is true even in more difficult standing poses, like Utthita Hasta Pādāṅguṣṭhāsana, where little opportunity is left for strain or distraction even though full expression of the pose may be beyond the practitioner's current reach. Because we are connecting lines of movement and Prāṇa rigorously and intelligently—and in most cases, more simply than in other forms—it is easy to recognize the necessary patterns of moving in sync with the breath in standing poses. They simply and directly invite us to feel and dissolve into integrative, full-body lines of movement and awareness.

This chapter groups together the poses traditionally practiced as the "standing sequence" in the Aṣṭāṅga Vinyāsa form, defining this family as poses that ground us into our legs and the earth. They connect us from top to bottom, from fingertips to toes, so when we wake up through the standing poses the mind no longer tends to separate out āsana and yoga practice as different from every other moment of our day. Standing poses bring with them the clarity, maturity, and competence required to be grounded physically and emotionally in the real world; as such, they are an antidote to neurotic patterns that may arise from attempting meditation, prāṇāyāma, or extreme yoga āsansas in an incorrect manner. Standing poses are of particular importance to practitioners who have difficulty focusing on what is arising in front of them and for those who are dull, distracted, distraught, or dysfunctional, as the benefits of well-executed standing poses can be a remedy to these sorts of problems.

An interesting point of controversy is the question of how far apart to place the feet in standing poses such as the Trikoṇāsana family or Pārśvottānāsana. A general rule is that you should place your feet apart approximately the length of one of your legs (measured from the top of the femur to the ankle). More important is that the feet should be placed at a distance that invites the pose to be "turned on" and that requires the feet and legs to wake up so you can experience the "juice" of the pose. You must discover the most healthy and beneficial distance for your specific circumstances. When your feet are at the optimal distance, a pose works your entire body—including the spine, head, neck, and shoulders—to make the pose a beautiful expression of integrated form.

Ultimately a yoga pose should not damage the joints, ligaments, tendons, or cartilage (or any other body system, for that matter). For example, you can create beneficial poses with the feet fairly close to each other (less than one leg length apart) in Trikoṇāsana or Vīrabhadrāsana, and this may be valuable or absolutely necessary if you have an infirmity, are older, or lack flexibility or strength. But if you are stronger, younger, more flexible, or more athletic, you can move the feet farther apart. Equally, a number of injuries can result from placing the feet *too* far apart and exceeding the structural limits of the hip joints and the many groups of muscles that cross over these joints.

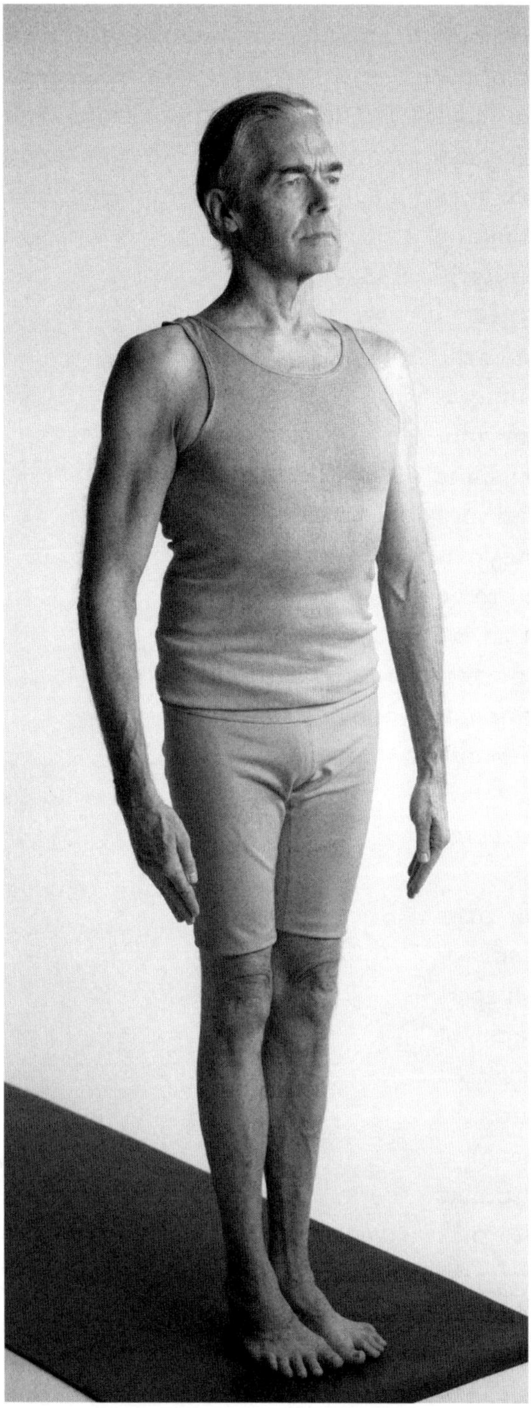

In the end, we must each understand the structural requirements of the poses and the breathing patterns necessary to integrate the form. We then practice with the intention of waking up both the body and the mind through each movement and micromovement as we transition in and out of poses and take on the full forms.

Samasthitiḥ

Equal Standing

Standing in Samasthitiḥ may seem relatively unchallenging, perhaps not even much of a yoga pose, since we stand around all the time anyway. Yet it is actually a very *advanced* and important āsana. It is translated as "equal standing" because we stand rooted deeply into the earth while finding that point in time and space that falls directly along the plumb line and drops us into the present moment. Everything is equal in all directions: perfect efficiency in relation to gravity; a complete lack of bias from left to right, front to back, up to down; and when it's really tapped in, past to future. Samasthitiḥ is a strong yet meditative pose characterized by a clear, soft, open heart.

More than anything, it places the details and difficulties of other poses in the perspective of the present moment. Establishing a solid Samasthitiḥ sets the tenor for the entire practice, and as we return again and again to the form, the seed of connection to our present circumstances arises, inviting us to wake up!

1. Stand with the sides of the big toes touching. The heels can be together or slightly separated, depending on individual preference or limitations. Take a moment to breathe into the pose and settle the attention along the plumb line

of the body, connecting the pose from the crown of the head through the core of the body and evenly down through the feet.

2. The weight drops immediately in front of the heels as the toes spread opening evenly and rooting down through the mounds of each toe into the earth. Draw the kneecaps up, to facilitate a feeling along the whole front surface of the body that it too is being drawn up. The back surface of the body is drawn down.
3. The heart area is lifted and spreads evenly. The front edges of the armpits lift and widen as the back edges drop down and broaden. Behind the kidneys, the floating ribs, the kidney wings, lift up with as much buoyancy as the heart.
4. The centers of the ears are over the centers of the shoulders, which are over the centers of the hip joints. The center of the perineum—the mūla point—ascends, which facilitates lifting the core of the body and making the crown of the head ascend.
5. Draw the lower belly, just above the pubic bone, slightly back to give you an awareness of Mūlabandha. The eyes remain steady, either slightly downcast or at the level of the horizon, resting on a point straight ahead.
6. Tune in to the body's central vertical axis, which runs from the center of the crown through the center of the perineum falling just in front of the heels. If you wish, fold the hands in Añjali Mudrā (prayer position) in front of the heart.

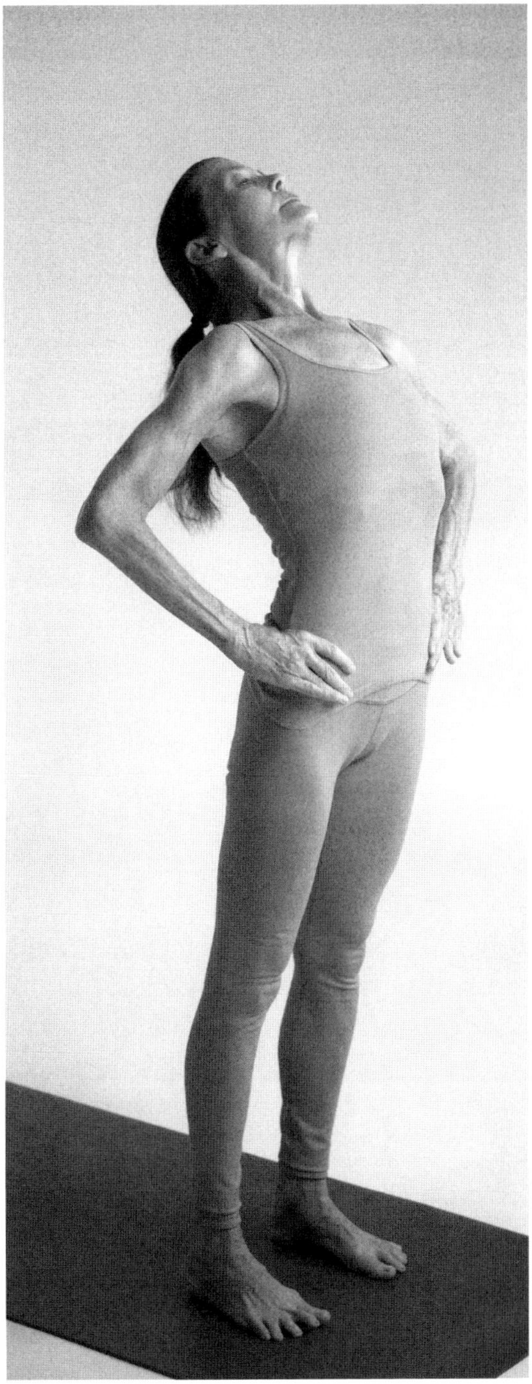

Pādāṅguṣṭhāsana

Big Toe Pose

Pādāṅguṣṭhāsana and Pādahastāsana (the pose that follows it) are usually practiced together, one immediately after the other, without a Half Vinyāsa between them. Of course, they may be practiced separately as well, but they complement and inform one another, both presenting an excellent opportunity for learning to passively rotate the pelvis around the tops of the femurs in a simple forward bend without straining either the lower back or hamstrings.

1. Stand with the feet hip-width apart and exhale to fully ground through the legs and feet. The distance between the legs should be just wide enough so that eventually,

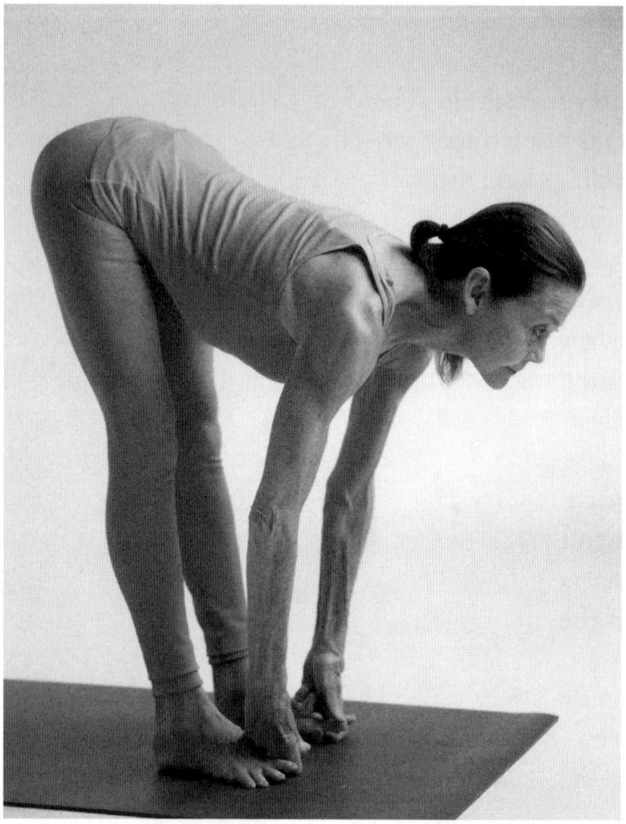

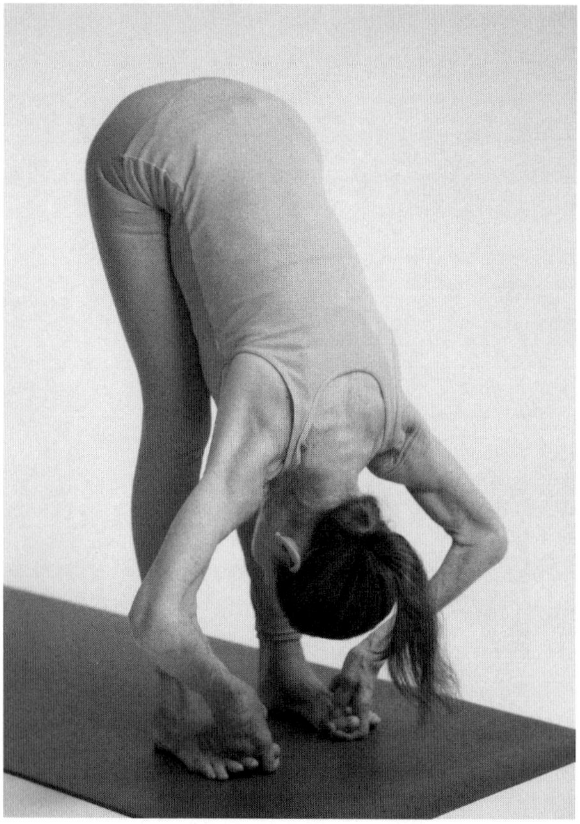

when the forward bend is quite deep, the head can fit between the upper shins.

2. Place hands on waist and on the inhalation, lift the front of the body without strain but with strength to feel an even upward pull through the core of the body, as if you were preparing to do a subtle backbend. Bring awareness to the pelvic floor, toning and dropping the coccyx down and forward as the pubic bone drops down and back.
3. On the exhalation, begin to fold forward keeping the spine straight and the legs active and awake so that the pelvis rotates around the top of the femurs. If your hamstrings are tight or injured, bend the knees slightly, but even while bent, your legs should remain vibrant and engaged, pushing down into the earth through the feet, especially the mounds of your big toes.
4. At the end of the exhalation, wrap the first two fingers of each hand around the big toes. Then inhale and lift the head to reset the pose, elongating the spine as if reaching through the crown of the head. (Remember you may bend your knees.)
5. On the exhalation, fold forward completely, pulling straight out (not up) along the line of the floor on the toes, bending your arms, and spreading your collarbones by reaching the elbows out to the sides. Allow the head, neck, and spine to hang as you fold forward, so there is a feeling of depth in the groins and the weight of the head encourages the spine to elongate. Pull with the arms, but do not put any strain on the neck, throat, or palate. Straighten the legs, if possible, and gaze at the tip of the nose.
6. After five breaths, at the end of an exhalation, tone the abdominal muscles and pelvic floor, bringing awareness to the sense of a heavy coccyx. On the inhalation, keep the awareness in the pelvic floor and coccyx as you straighten the arms. Still holding the toes, lift the head and reach out through the crown, straightening the spine and coming halfway up.

7. Place hands under feet, palms up, and move immediately into Pādahastāsana. Or, to exit the pose, follow step 4 in Pādahastāsana below.

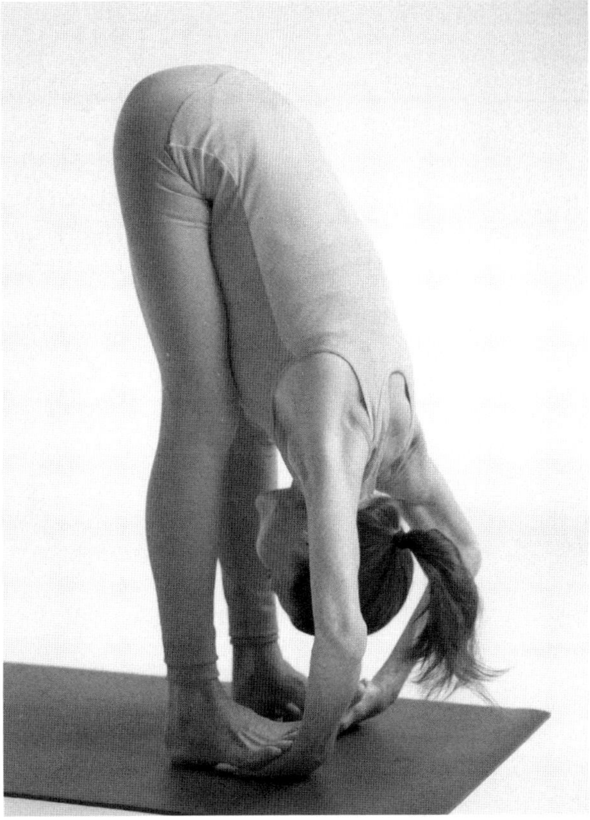

Pādahastāsana

Hand and Foot Pose

Pādahastāsana requires more flexibility in the hamstrings and wrists than does Pādāṅguṣṭhāsana. It is acceptable to bend the knees in order to place the hands under the feet, but remember to keep the legs active and awake, which allows for a "micro-bend" (slight bend) that encourages the kneecaps to lift as the feet remain fully grounded.

1. After lifting the head in the last step of Pādāṅguṣṭhāsana, slide the hands, palms up, under the front of the feet until the toes touch your wrists. Bend the knees, if necessary, but keep the legs engaged. (To enter the pose without doing Pādāṅguṣṭhāsana beforehand, follow steps 1 through 3 for Pādāṅguṣṭhāsana.)
2. Spread the toes and fold the hip joints closed as you exhale. Pull the hands forward toward the front of the mat, as if trying to pull them out from under the feet. Bend the arms and work the elbows out to the sides.
3. Gaze at the tip of the nose with an empty palate and smooth, complete breathing. Hold the pose for five breaths.
4. To exit, as you exhale, tone the abdominal muscles and PC muscle. At the end of the exhalation, keep the coccyx heavy (PC muscle engaged). Lift the head as you inhale and straighten the arms and spine, lifting halfway up. As you complete the inhalation, place the hands on the hips and push the skin there back as you exhale. On the following inhalation, return to standing with the spine straight and the palate released.
5. Hop the feet back together and take one round of breath in Samasthitiḥ before entering the next pose.

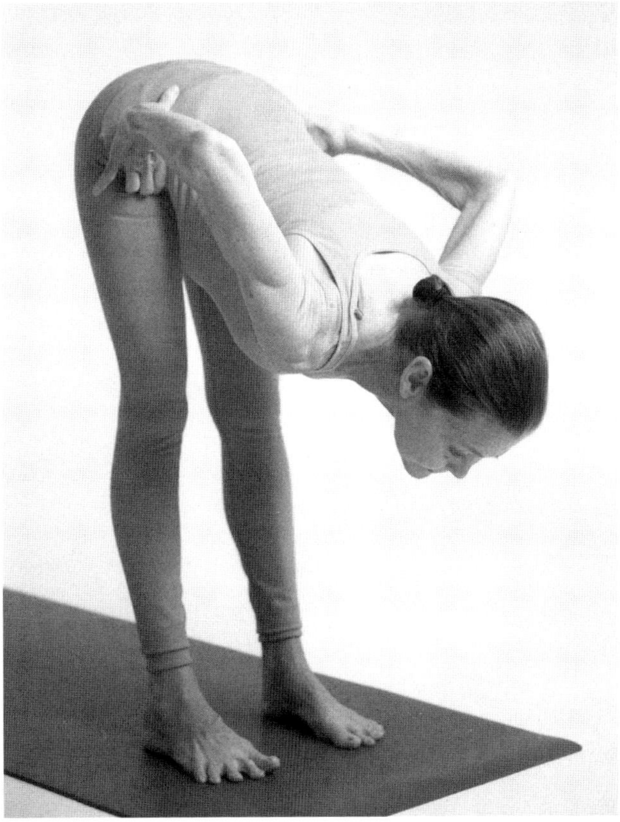

Trikoṇāsana

Triangle Pose

Trikoṇāsana and its counterpose, Parivṛtta Trikoṇāsana, are usually practiced together, one immediately after the other, without returning to the front of the mat. Of course, they may be practiced separately as well, but they complement one another on many levels. For Trikoṇāsana, maintaining a straight spine while entering and exiting the pose is very

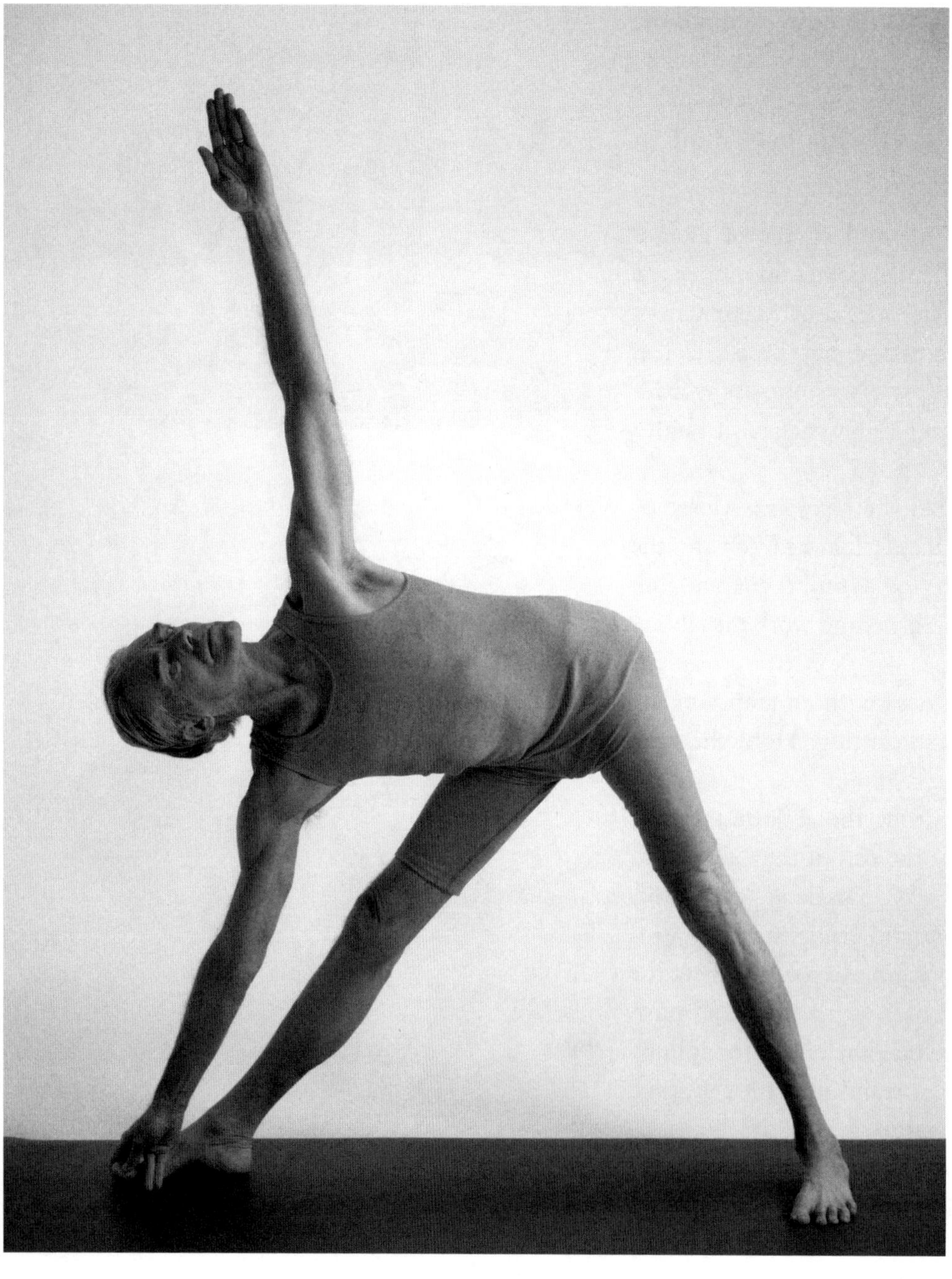

important and is instrumental in cuing the legs to rotate and counter-rotate properly. This allows the pelvis to rotate passively around the tops of the femurs so the full benefits of the pose can be felt.

1. From Samasthitiḥ, on an exhalation, hop open to the right side, placing the feet about one leg length apart. Line the heel of the right foot up with the back of the left arch. Turn the right toes out toward the end of the mat, and turn the left foot in about 20 to 40 degrees. Make sure the right kneecap points in the same direction as the right foot, and engage both legs.
2. With the arms stretched out parallel to the floor, shoulder blades down, and torso facing the side of the mat, inhale and lift the quadriceps, kidney wings, and the center of the pelvic floor, as you scoop up in the cave of the sacrum. On an exhalation, keeping the PC muscle toned and the spine straight, tilt the pelvis to the right for the setup of the initial position.
3. The right leg will rotate slightly outward, and the left leg will rotate slightly inward—the primary rotations of this pose. Keep the spine straight as you reach out through the right arm.
4. Place the right hand in the appropriate position for your physical circumstances. The official placement is to hold the big toe of the right foot with the first two fingers of the right hand. If you are too stiff to manage this, placing the hand on the right ankle or shin, or a block positioned next to the outer edge of the foot can provide a starting point for working toward the full form. At this stage do not sacrifice the straightness in the spine in leaning over to take the big toe if you cannot reach it. Instead, rely on the rotations in the legs and the straightening spine to inform the pose and facilitate the rotation of the pelvis around the tops of the femurs to bring you naturally into the pose.
5. Once in the basic pose, introduce the counteractions in the legs, hips, and torso with the next in-breath. This inhalation wakes up the coccyx to bring it closer to your pubic bone. Ground the outer edge of your left foot while simultaneously reaching down into the earth through the mound of the right big toe. Keep the arches of both feet awake, and as you reach up to the ceiling through the left arm, imagine both arms extending evenly in opposite directions so there is space for the spine to continue to elongate.
6. Turn the head to gaze at the fingers of the left hand as you draw up the kneecaps and thighs on both legs. Make the buttocks firm and draw the shoulder blades down the back. Keep a micro-bend in the right knee and draw the back of your body toward the front of the body, starting with the sacrum; keep the PC muscle toned.

7. Hold the pose for five breaths. At the end of an exhale, keeping the legs engaged, the spine straight, and the pelvic floor toned, take a smooth inhale and reach up and out through the fingertips of the left hand to guide you back up to standing.
8. On the next exhalation, turn the feet to the other side; on the inhalation, repeat the pose to your left. Again, after five breaths, exit the pose on an inhalation. As you exhale, move into the counterpose (Parivṛtta Trikoṇāsana) or come back to Samasthitiḥ.

Parivṛtta Trikoṇāsana

Revolving Triangle Pose

This is the counterpose to Trikoṇāsana and is an example of a pose that is difficult to categorize: it is both a significant standing sequence pose and an important twist. To fully enter the pose, the spine should be elongated while reaching forward into the twist. This facilitates the proper actions and relationships of rotations and muscle tones in pelvis and hips. Once in the pose, watch and play with the interpenetration of actions within the pose; never locking the pelvis or hips helps to refine these relationships.

1. Standing in Samasthitiḥ, exhale, and hop out to the right side. As a counterpose, simply move into this pose after completing Trikoṇāsana on the second side. With the feet about one leg length apart, turn the right toes out toward the end of the mat and turn the left foot in 40 to 60 degrees. Turn the pelvis toward the right foot and draw up the fronts of the legs. Wake up the arches of both feet, and make sure not to lock or hyperextend the knees.
2. Angle the left foot forward enough to accommodate the rotation of the pelvis, which should be squaring (but not locked) toward the wall in front of your right foot. Be sure to keep the outer edge of the left heel and the inner edge of the right foot grounded. For extra stability, the feet can be positioned slightly wider apart—toward the sides of the mat—than they would fall if you were simply to turn directly from Trikoṇāsana. This added width can be helpful if you are very stiff, have hamstring injuries, or have difficulty maintaining balance.
3. On an inhalation, place the right hand on the right hip and reach up toward the ceiling through the left arm, protracting the left shoulder blade and reaching through the fingertips of the left hand.
4. On an exhalation, begin to fold forward at the hip joints. Elongate through the spine, as you reach forward and down through the left arm, allowing the left hand to come flat on the floor outside the right

foot. If you cannot place your hand on the floor without curling your spine too much, position a block on the floor along the outer edge of the right foot and place your hand on the block.

5. On the next inhalation, reach up toward the ceiling through the right arm as you move the right hip back slightly and extend long through the crown of the head. Draw both shoulder blades down the back, opening the fronts of the armpits. Pay attention to your left shoulder so that the top of the humerus does not rotate forward, collapsing the heart. Spread the kidney wings and reach through the fingertips of

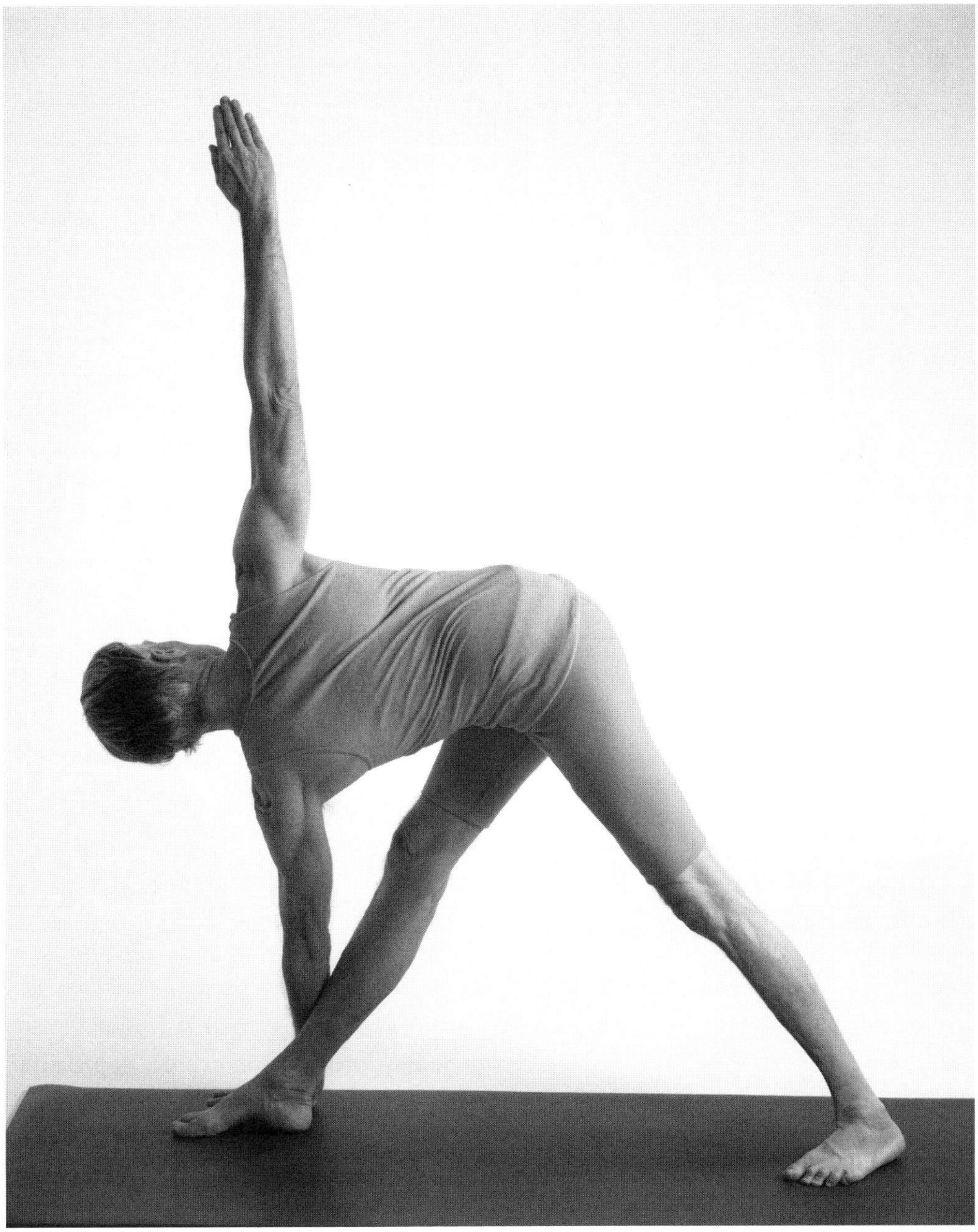

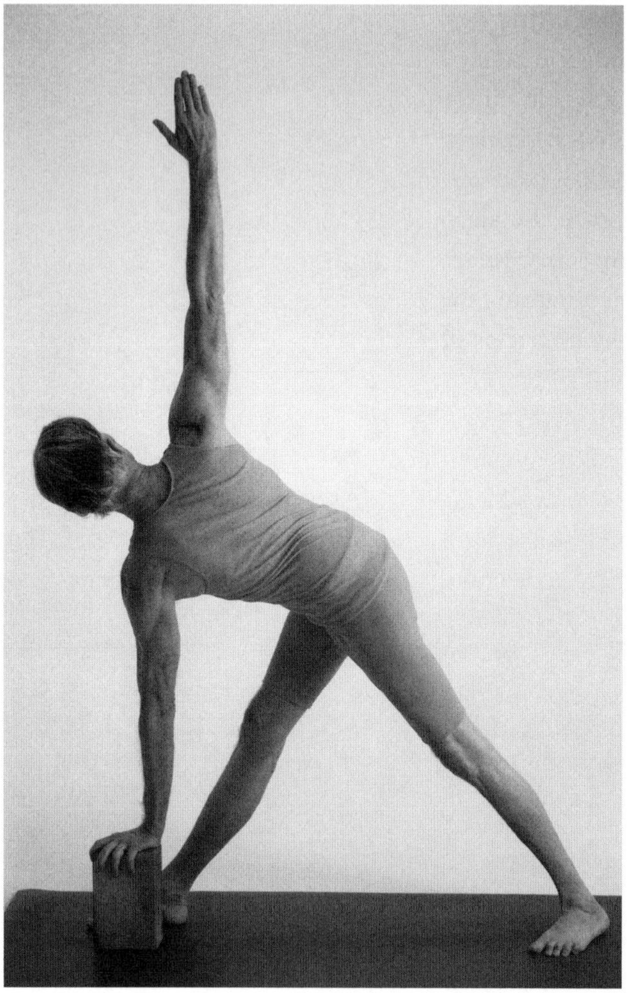

the right hand to facilitate the twist and extension in the spine. Gaze softly at the thumb of the right hand. There should be no strain in the neck, jaw, or palate. Check to be sure the feet remain fully grounded, especially the outer edge of the left foot.

6. Hold the pose for five breaths, breathing smoothly and adjusting the pose with subtle actions and counteractions that will automatically bring you into the final form.
7. To exit, look down at the left hand at the end of an exhalation. With strong legs and a long spine, inhale and spin like a windmill to come up and out of the pose. Turn to the left and on the next exhalation enter the pose on the other side. Move smoothly and rhythmically into and out of this pose to receive maximum benefit from the form. Do not overanalyze the form or microadjustments you "think" you should make. Instead tune in to the feelings and sensations as they are arising and respond so that the pose comes to life with an open heart, strong legs, and a soft palate.
8. Hold the pose for five breaths. Exit smoothly by looking down on an exhalation and, with strong legs, spinning back up to standing. Hop or step back to Samasthitiḥ.

Pārśvakoṇāsana

Side-Angle Pose

This is an important pose for establishing a sense of strength in the legs and learning Uḍḍīyāna Bandha, which helps to lift the lower belly out of the pelvic basin. It is important, especially for those with knee injuries or who have had knee surgery, to drop the weight of the bent leg directly down through the heel so the force is not jammed forward in the knee joint.

1. From Samasthitiḥ, as you exhale, hop the feet out to the right with feet about one leg length apart. With the torso facing the side of the mat and arms reaching out to the sides at shoulder height, begin to lower into the pose. Ground evenly through the right heel as you spread the foot, and bend the knee until the right thigh is parallel to

the ground. Keep the left leg long and firm and the outer edge of the left foot grounded.

2. Be certain to bring the right knee over the center of the right ankle. Keep the knee over the line connecting the two heels when entering and exiting the pose, and keep the upper body lifting toward the ceiling, with heavy sitting bones, as you first enter the pose.
3. Inhale and reach through the right arm to extend the right waist. On the exhalation, keeping the spine straight, tilt the pelvis to the right and place the fingertips (and eventually the flattened palm) of the right hand on the floor outside the right foot.
4. Keep both legs strong, grounding through the outer edge of the left foot, lifting the left thigh away from the floor while keeping the right knee precisely over the ankle.
5. On the inhale and from the hollow in front of the sacrum, generate a spiral extension up the front of the spine as you sweep the left arm up to point fingers toward the wall near your head. Turn the palm down, reaching through the fingertips and keeping the arm at the same angle as the left leg. Firm the buttocks to move your sacrum into

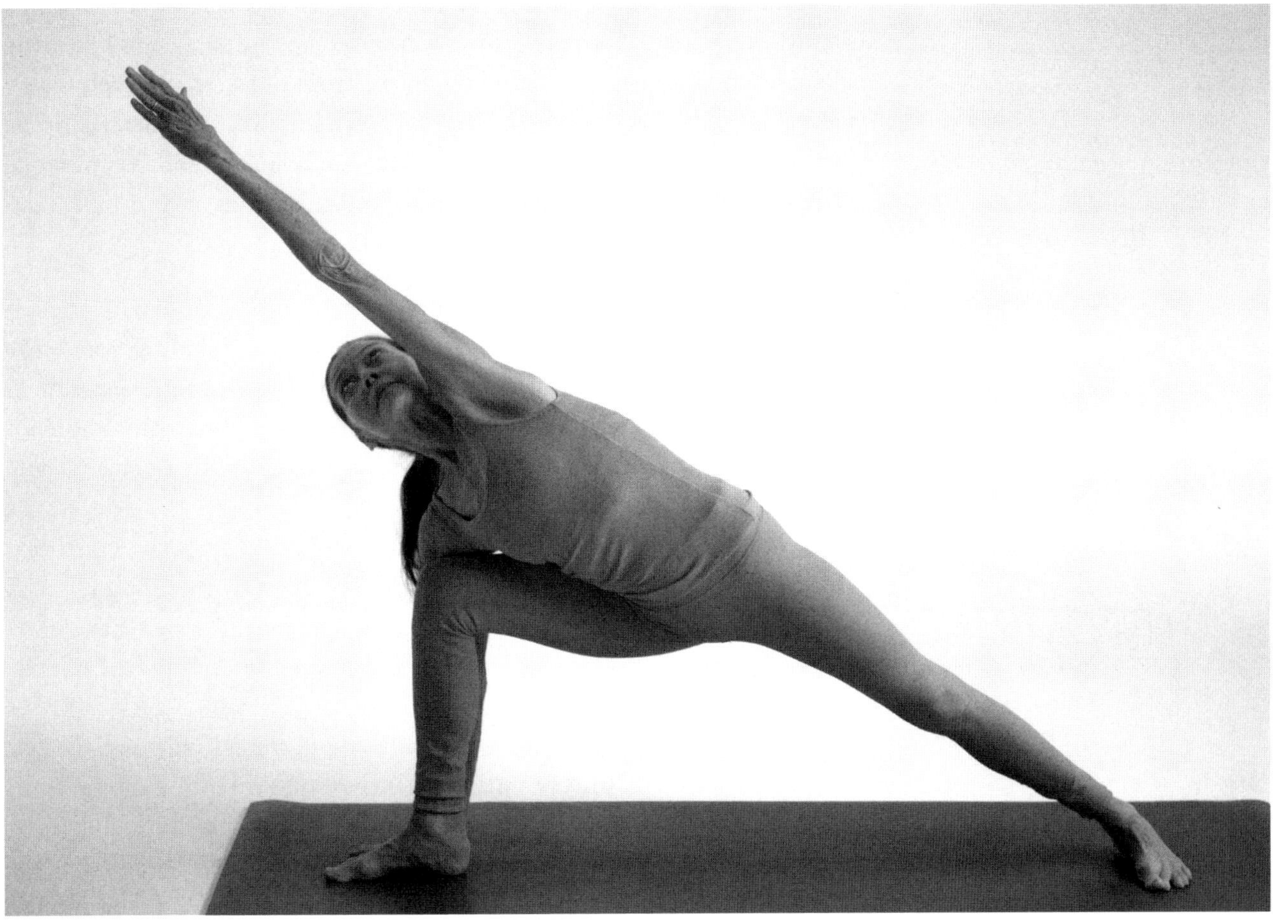

your body. Curl the coccyx closer to the pubic bone and gaze at the palm of the left hand to stretch the psoas line.

6. Do not hunch the shoulders. Externally spiral and lift the left shoulder blade so that the flesh on the back of the neck moves down the back. Be sure that you have spiraled enough so there is no tension when you tilt your head back to look at the center of your palm. Reach as far as you can through the left fingertips, as if trying to touch infinity.
7. At the end of five breaths, root firmly into the floor through the legs and, maintaining strong legs, come back up to standing on the inhale. Immediately turn around to the second side and exhale as you bend the left leg to enter the pose on the other side. Gaze at the palm of the right hand and keep the inner right thigh lifting away from the floor.

Parivṛtta Pārśvakoṇāsana

Twisted Side-Angle Pose

As with Parivṛtta Trikoṇāsana, it is helpful to study this pose as both a standing pose and an important twist. In the traditional Aṣṭāṅga Vinyāsa practice, it is practiced as a counterpose immediately following Pārśvakoṇāsana without returning to the front of the mat, which is why it has been placed in this chapter. It is very important to flex the spine while entering Parivṛtta Pārśvakoṇāsana so as not to collapse into the front hip joint, which can eventually damage the hip and possibly contribute to femoroacetabular impingement.

1. If you are starting from Pārśvottānāsana, exit the pose with the left knee bent, come up to center on an inhale and, exhaling, rotate the right toes out, bending the right knee, and angling the left foot in about 45 to 60 degrees. If you are starting from Samasthitiḥ, hop out to the right so the feet are about one leg length apart. Rotate the feet and legs as already described.
2. With strong emphasis on the legs, on an inhale draw the spine long from deep in the low belly, reaching up. Then, fully exhaling reach forward with the left arm. Curling the spine, as if drawing the navel back to touch the spine, wrap the left upper arm around the outside of the right thigh and knee.
3. Place the fingertips, and eventually the flattened palm, of the left hand, with the fingers pointing in the same direction as the right toes, on the floor outside the right foot. Do not lose the engagement in the left leg. Keep reaching back and down through the outer edge of the left foot without letting the left thigh collapse down toward

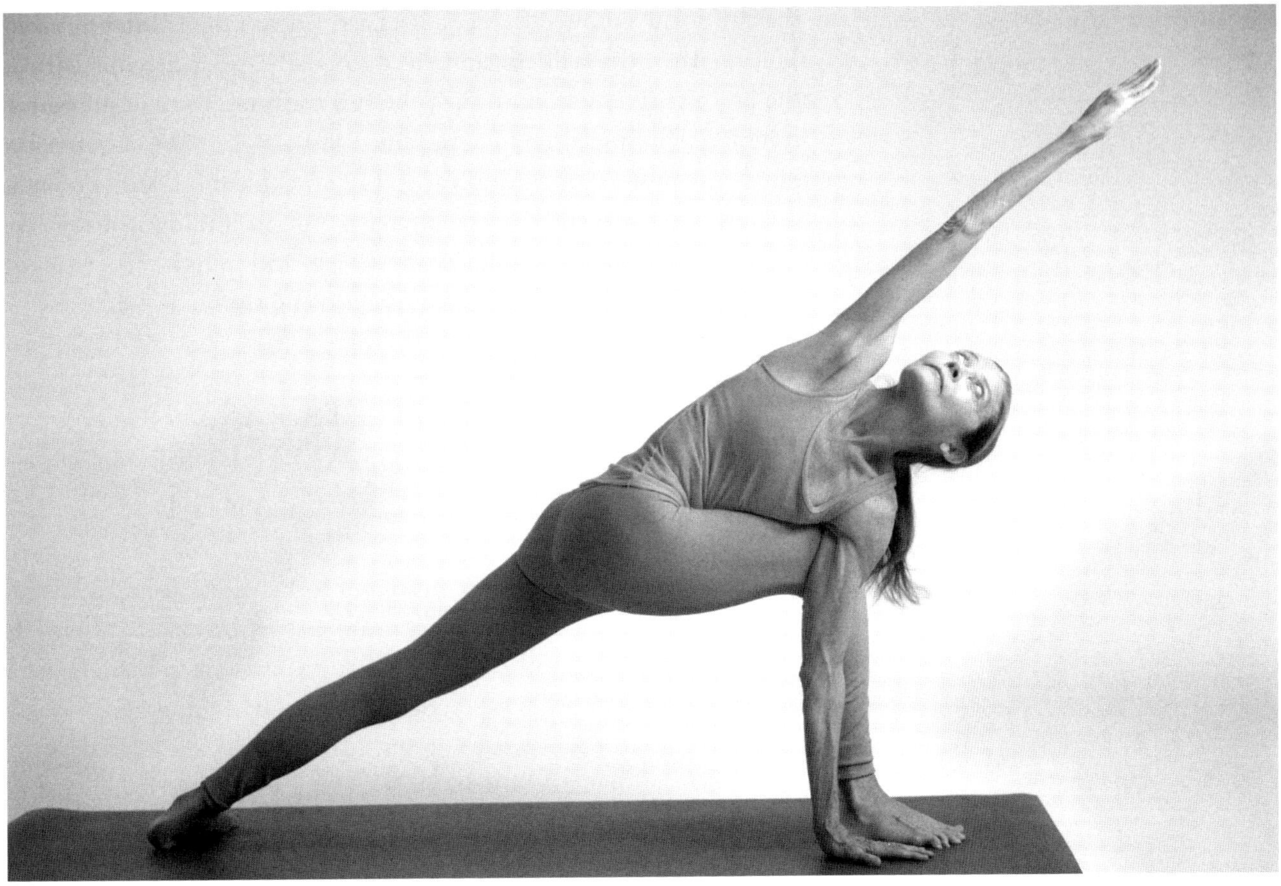

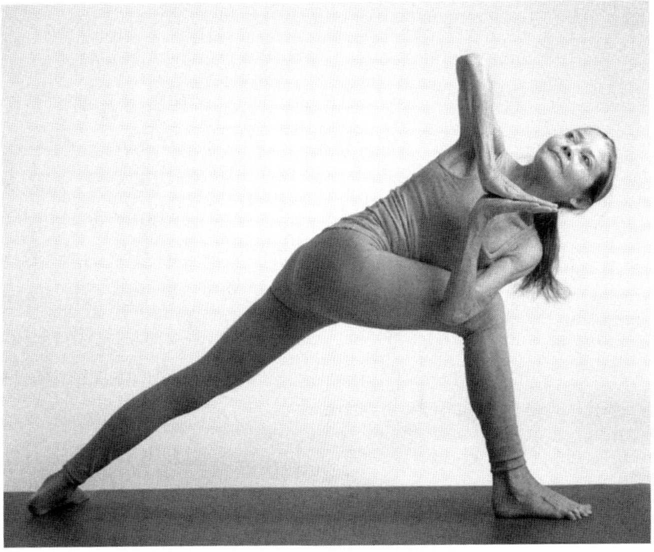

the mat. The foot may not fully ground at first, but that is not a major problem if the intention to keep it grounded is there.

4. Once the legs are firmly established, add the right arm into the pose. As you inhale, straighten the arm and sweep it around in an arc so it is stretched out above your head in the same line as the back leg. The palm should face down toward the floor. Keep the arm connected by using the serratus anterior muscle to protract the shoulder blade out and the humerus away from the ear as you reach in one long extended line from the outer edge of the left foot all the way out through the fingertips of the right hand.
5. If the top of the left humerus does not reach past the right knee as you rotate to enter the pose, you may substitute a modified version of the pose with hands together in Añjali Mudrā until you are flexible enough to do the full form. Do not abandon the aim to shift into

the full form simply because it is easier to keep the hands in Añjali Mudrā. The pose will continue to deepen and offer new insights to the practice if you work toward the full form rather than becoming complacent and settling for a modified form.

6. Hold this position for five breaths. On an exhalation, look down at the left hand. Reestablish the strength and grounding in both legs and the pelvic floor. Inhaling, work the legs and spin the arm to come up, then rotate around to practice the pose on the second side.

PRASĀRITA PĀDOTTĀNĀSANA (FORWARD BEND WITH FEET SPREAD POSE) A, B, C, AND D

Within the Aṣṭāṅga Vinyāsa system, all four forms of Prasārita Pādottānāsana are practiced together, flowing seamlessly from one to the next. They complement one another and build on the actions in the feet, legs, spine, and pelvic floor. When practiced together, they provide an excellent way to tap into the pelvic floor and Mūlabandha. As related poses, many of their alignment details are the same; these are described in detail for form A and then built on for the other forms. If practicing the different forms separately, follow the vinyāsas described in this section for entering and exiting the poses.

Prasārita Pādottānāsana A

1. Begin in Samasthitiḥ. On an exhalation, hop out to the right so that the feet are just over one leg length apart. Place the hands on the hips, and inhale fully to wake up the feet and legs, keeping the coccyx heavy. This allows you to establish a connection to the pelvic floor and tap into a sense of spaciousness in the hip joints as the crest of the inhalation lifts and spreads the core of the heart while elongating the spine.
2. On the exhalation, with the spine straight and the chin out, fold forward and place the palms of the hands on the floor between the feet. If necessary, bend the knees and rotate the feet inward (pigeon-toed) to reach the floor.
3. Keep the legs straight without locking the knees, and keep the feet evenly grounded. Especially as you enter the fold, watch carefully to keep the inner edges of the feet grounded. By reaching down through the mounds of the big toes and the inner edges of the heels first and

then grounding through the outer edges of the feet, the arches of both feet are invited to wake up. This is good.

4. Inhale and lift the head again, straightening the arms, lifting the chest, and reaching forward through the crown of the head to stretch the spine straight. On the next exhalation, contract the abdominal muscles as you fold forward, allowing the head to fall toward the floor. With the hands placed shoulder-width apart between the feet, press from the heels of the hands out through the fingertips to bring the head farther between the legs.
5. Keep the shoulders spreading and lifting away from the floor and the upper arms parallel as you gaze along the line of the nose. In all the forms, cultivate Uḍḍīyāna and Mūlabandhas by toning the PC muscle, connecting the ends of the breath and gazing at the tip of the nose. This will help you learn the true inner alignment of the poses. Hold the position for five breaths.
6. At the end of an exhalation, bring the awareness to the feet, legs, and center of the pelvic floor, while leaving the hands where they are. Inhale and lift the head, straightening the arms and spine so the back is approximately parallel to the floor.
7. Exhale and place the hands on the hips, pushing the skin of the outer hips back. As you inhale, straighten the spine to return to standing.

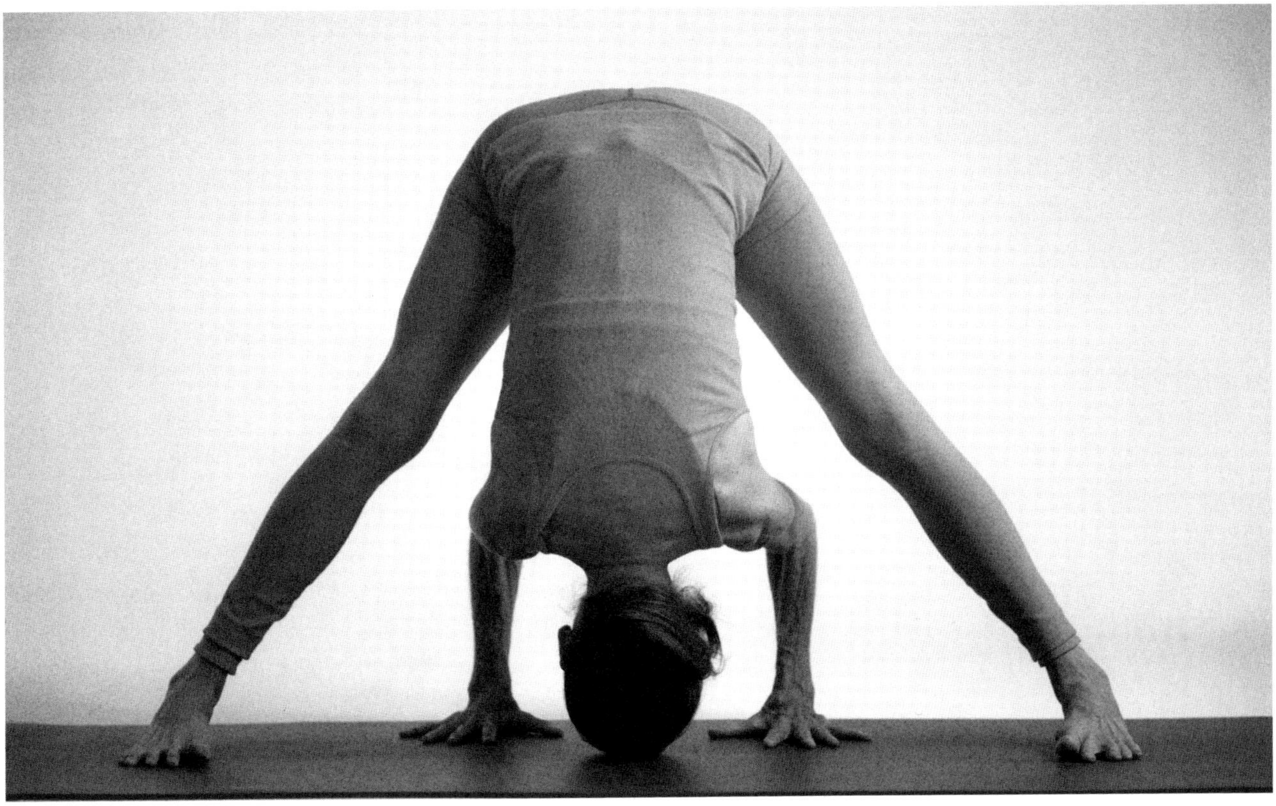

Prasārita Pādottānāsana B

1. Keeping the legs in a wide stance, exhale deeply to root down through the feet and legs. Inhaling, lift the arms straight out to the sides with a spin to encourage the feeling of the shoulder blades sliding down the back. Exhaling, place the hands on the hips, then inhale to lift the sternum and extend the spine as you use the first two fingers of each hand to apply gentle pressure to the lower belly at the area of the psoas buttons.
2. On the next exhalation, fold forward with the spine long, leaving the fingers in the low belly and allowing the elbows to reach evenly out to the sides. Keep the shoulders wide and pulled toward the hips, with the gaze steady along the line of the nose.
3. Soften the jaw and palate, and bring the awareness to the low belly (under your fingertips) and the connection of that part of the body to the pelvic floor. Hold the pose for five breaths, gazing along the line of the nose.
4. At the end of an exhalation, activate the legs, set the pelvic floor (holding the serpent's tail), and on the next inhalation, return to standing.

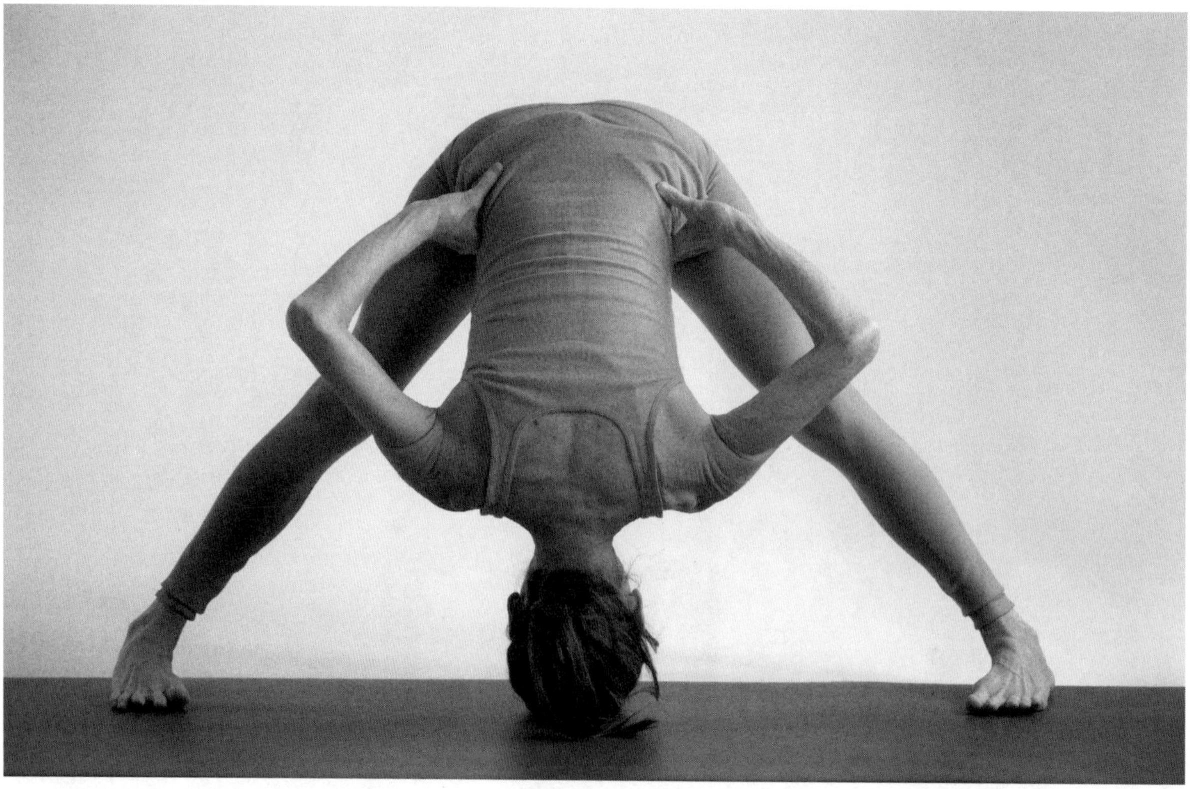

PRASĀRITA PĀDOTTĀNĀSANA C

1. Keeping the legs in a wide stance and the hands on the hips, exhale and ground through the legs and feet, making sure the arches of both feet are active. Before folding forward, inhale to straighten the arms out to the sides and roll the tops of the arms forward to facilitate clasping the hands behind the back; make the coccyx heavy to avoid collapsing the lumbar spine. The arms will bend slightly as you do this. Then roll the tops of the arms up, back, and out slightly as you straighten the arms.
2. On the exhalation, fold forward, dropping the clasped hands behind you and over your head toward the floor. The palms of the hands should face each other, and the shoulders should flow back and down. Don't worry if the hands don't touch the floor. Patience.
3. If you are flexible, you can try rotating the arms inward and flipping the hands over so the palms, still interlaced, are flat on the floor in order to make the pose more challenging. If you are new to the practice or tend to be stiff, you can hold a stick or strap between the hands with the thumbs pointing out to the sides to maximize the benefits from the pose.

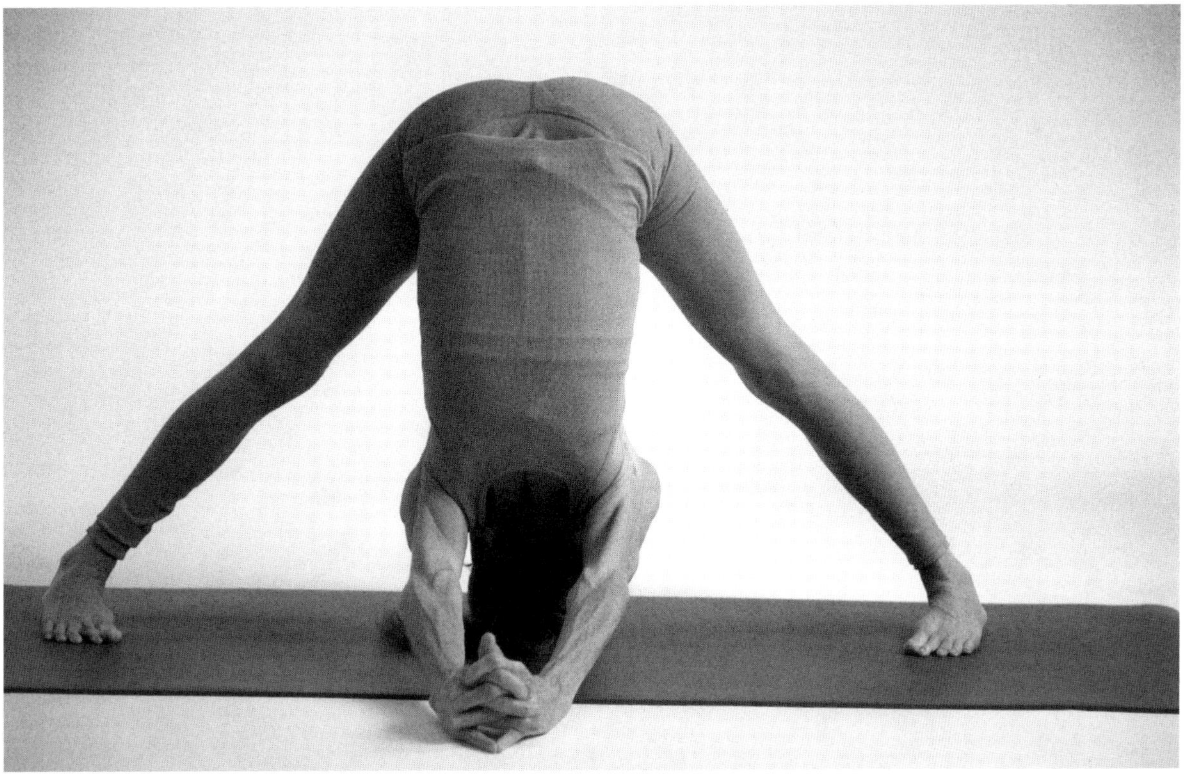

4. After five breaths, exhale fully, then exit to standing on the next inhalation. Exhale and place the hands on the hips again.

Prasārita Pādottānāsana D

1. Keeping the legs in a wide stance and the hands on the hips, inhale lifting the chest and heart. Exhale and straighten the spine as you fold forward to grab the big toes with the middle and index fingers of each hand. Pull firmly with the arms—without hunching the shoulders or straining the neck—as you reach out to the sides through the elbows. Allow the head to hang. Ground the mounds of your big toes in opposition to the slight upward pull of the fingers and make sure not to hyperextend or lock the knees. If necessary, you may bend the knees in order to hold the toes. Gaze softly along the line of the nose.
2. Hold for five breaths. At the end of an exhalation, strengthen the legs and activate the feet while leaving the hands in place. Inhale and lift the head, straightening the arms and lifting the spine away from the floor.

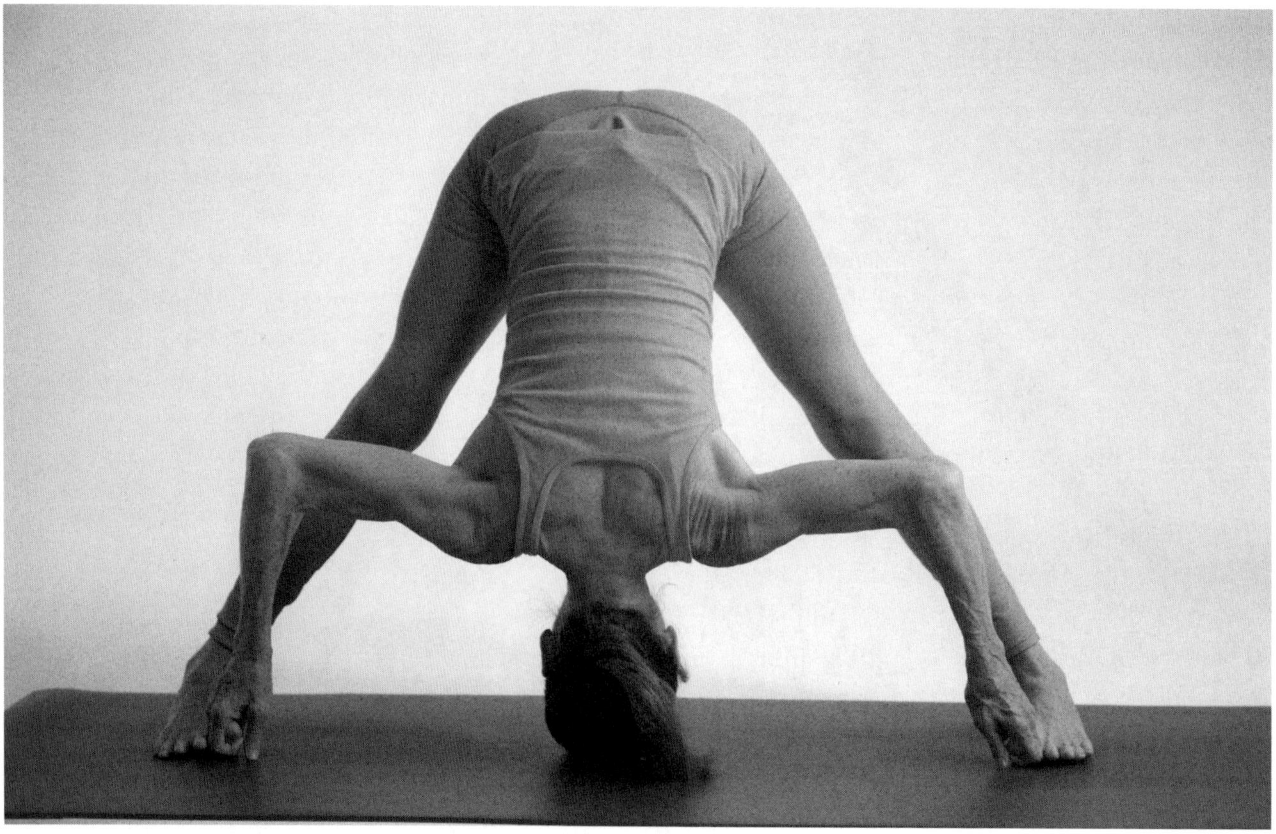

3. Exhale as you place the hands on the hips, pushing the skin of the outer hips back. As you inhale, return to standing with a straight spine.
4. If necessary, shift the feet together slightly to make it safe for you to hop back to the front of the mat, landing in Samasthitiḥ on an exhalation.

Pārśvottānāsana

Forward Bend to the Side Pose

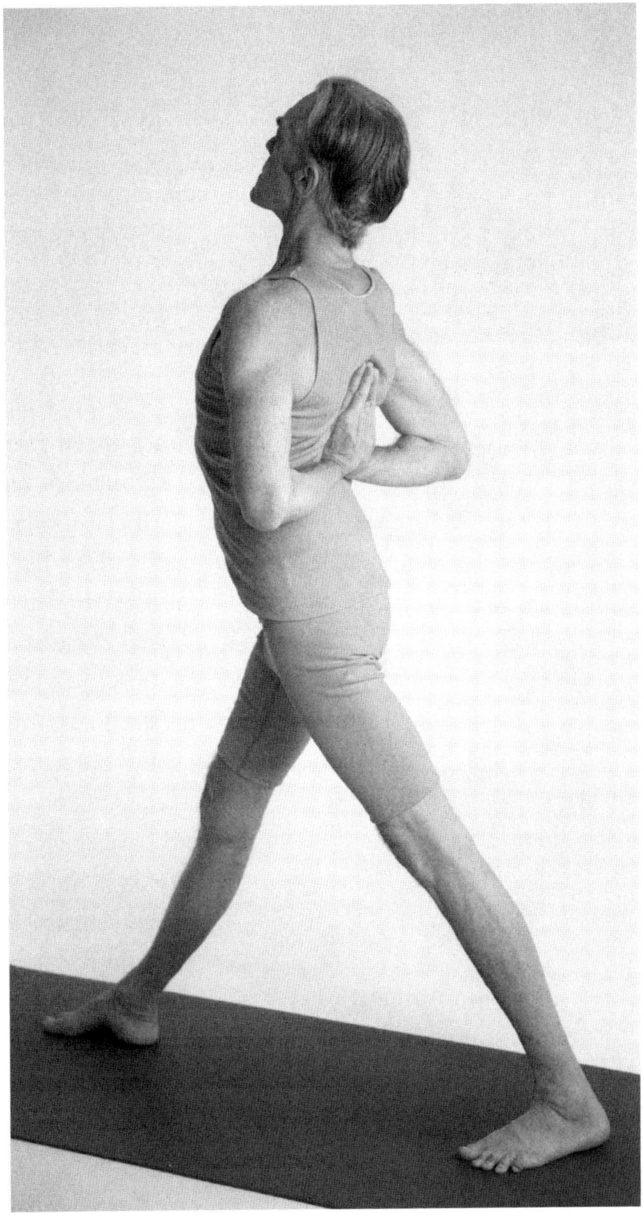

This standing pose is an example of an important twisting action from the kidney to the knee, which activates a line of connection diagonally across the front of the body from the serratus anterior muscle on one side through the external oblique muscles on that side to the internal oblique muscles on the opposite side. This valuable twisting action is found in a number of other poses and is a fundamental expression of the apānic form.

1. Start in Samasthitiḥ. As you exhale, hop out to the right toward the back of the mat so that the feet are about one leg length apart. Turn the right toes to face the back of the mat, and angle the left foot in about 40 degrees, squaring the hips to the right. Do not lock the knees or hips.
2. Roll the tops of the arms forward as you bend your elbows to place the hands behind your back in Añjali Mudrā. Once the hands are in place, roll the tops of the arms back, sliding the shoulder blades broad and dropping them down the back. If you are stiff, you can make fists behind the back and during the pose push the fists together so the elbows lift and the collarbones spread.
3. On an inhalation, work both legs and, keeping the kneecaps lifted, also lift the core of the heart. The hands will eventually be at the level of the thoracic spine, immediately behind the heart, so as you inhale, they can help to facilitate a subtle backbend. Gaze down the line of the nose.

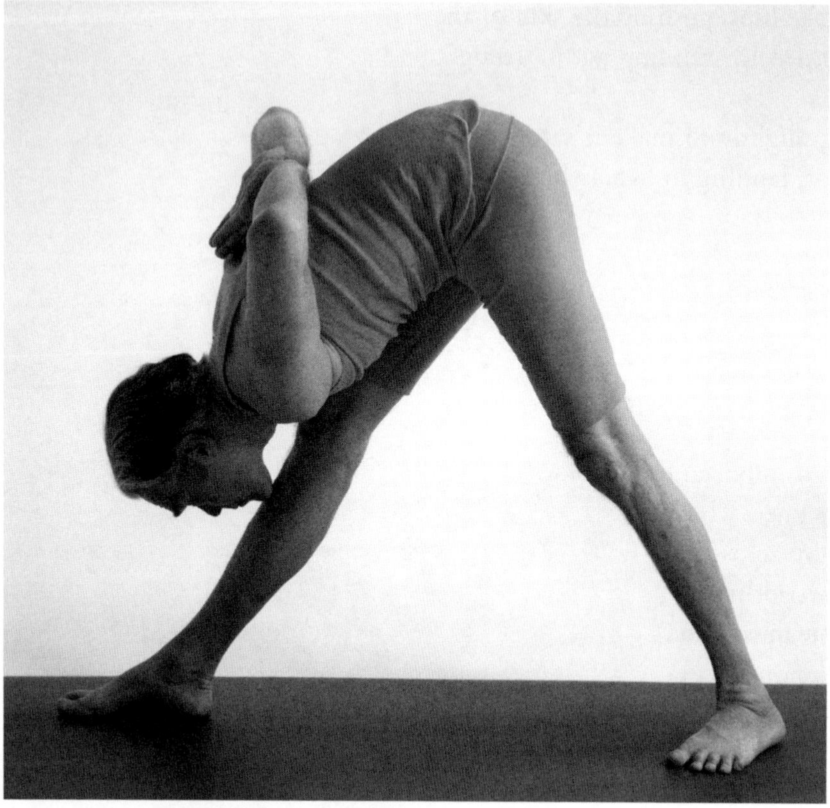

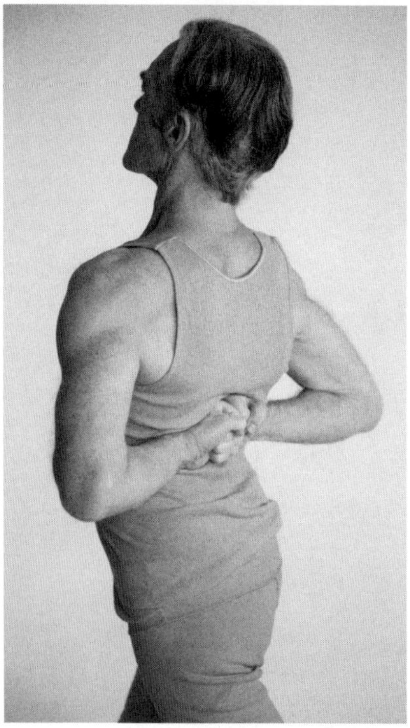

4. Be aware that arching back before the forward fold in this pose is an advanced move and is optional. It requires properly grounded feet, strong legs, and fully rotated hips.
5. Once fully extended on the inhalation, begin to fold forward toward the right leg on the next exhalation. Keep both legs activated and wrap the left kidney wing toward the right knee. Eventually the chin will come to the shin and you will be able to gaze at the nose. Until then, gaze at the right big toe as you fold and rest in the pose.
6. The inner edge of the right foot and the outer edge of the left heel stay grounded, especially when entering and exiting the pose. Keep the weight centered just in front of the heels. Notice the profound changes that occur within the pose with different distributions of weight in the feet. Lifting the elbows toward the ceiling can help to keep the upper body buoyant and the heart open.
7. Hold for five breaths. Inhaling with a heavy coccyx and using the heart and head to lengthen the torso, extend through the spine and return to standing with hands still in Añjali Mudrā behind the back.
8. Turn the feet to the other side and repeat the pose. After five breaths, return to standing on an inhalation. Turn the feet so they are parallel, release the hands from behind the back, and hop or step back to Samasthitiḥ at the front of the mat.

Utthita Hasta Pādāṅguṣṭhāsana

Standing Hand-to-Big-Toe Pose

This pose appears early in the Aṣṭāṅga Vinyāsa sequencing of poses and is, for many beginning students, the first major roadblock to moving through the series too quickly. It is an asymmetrical, twisting pose that also requires balance. Pattabhi Jois would often laugh and say, "Why dancing?" as his students hopped around the room to avoid falling over in this pose. It requires patience and concentration; even if you feel there's no hope, it will improve through practice.

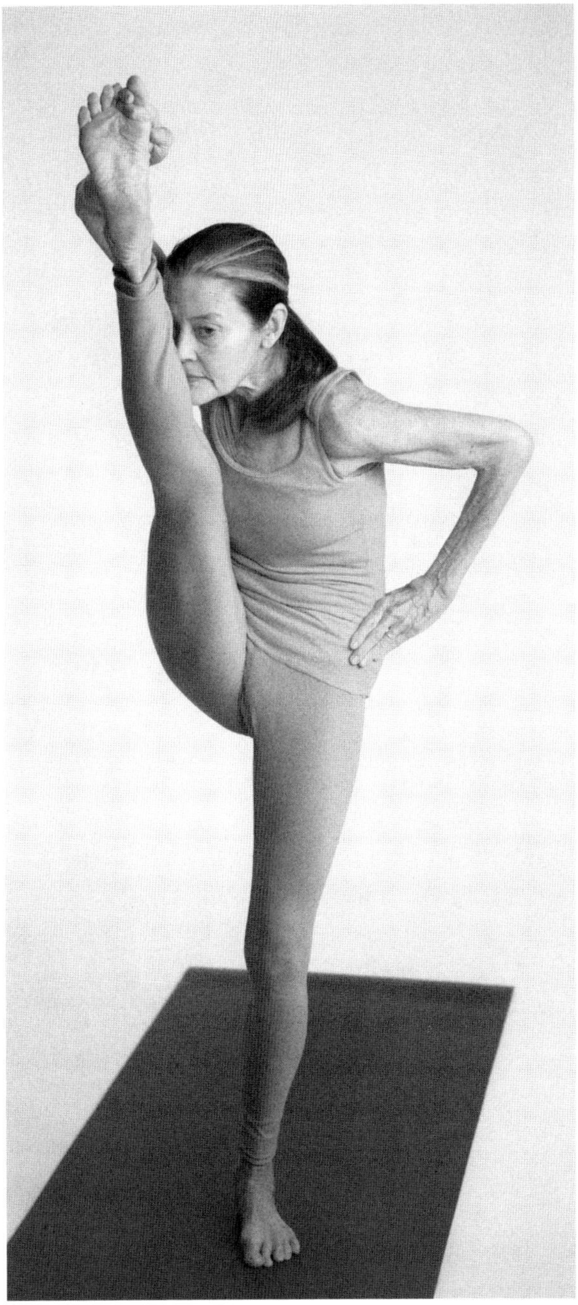

1. Begin in Samasthitiḥ. Grounding evenly through the left foot and leg, place the left hand on the waist. Lift and bend the right leg, rotating the femur slightly out to the side and taking the big toe firmly with the middle and index fingers of the right hand. Find a steady gazing point out in front of you on the floor along the line of the nose.
2. On an inhalation, press the right big toe against the fingers as you straighten the right leg and rotate the foot so it is reaching evenly out in front. Pull up on the toe with the arm slightly bent and a sense of the shoulder blades flowing down the back. At the same time, pull down through the right leg, as though trying to escape the grip of the right hand.
3. On the next exhalation, fold forward from the waist to put your chin on your shin. Wrap the left kidney wing toward the right knee, bowing to your foot and gazing gently along the line of the nose. Continue to pull up with the right arm as the heel pulls down toward the floor, facilitating the wrap and the bend. This complementary action between hand and foot actually makes the pose more stable.
4. Hold for five breaths, then straighten the spine and come out of the forward bend on an inhalation. On the next exhalation, open the right leg out to the side, dropping the outer right hip toward the floor and standing tall to resist puffing the left groin forward. Turn the head to gaze at a point on the horizon over the left shoulder. If you are a beginner, you may gaze at a point on the floor. Hold this position for five breaths.

5. On an inhale, draw the leg back to center, bow again for just one exhale, then stand tall on the next inhale. Lift the leg even higher and then release; while "fointing" (both pointing and flexing simultaneously) the foot, allow the leg to float for five breaths. Keep the heart area light and lifting up and your face free of tension. Hold for five breaths, then on an exhalation, return the right foot to the floor and do the pose on the left side. After practicing the pose on both sides, stand for one round of breath in Samasthitiḥ.
6. Beginners may use a wall for balance if necessary, placing the elbow of the arm that is not holding the leg near or barely touching the wall. This can overcome initial fear of the pose, but it can also become a habit. Better than using a wall is just holding the unengaged arm out to the side and possibly holding the pose for fewer breaths. Beware: using a wall does not force you to learn to balance. Remember, this

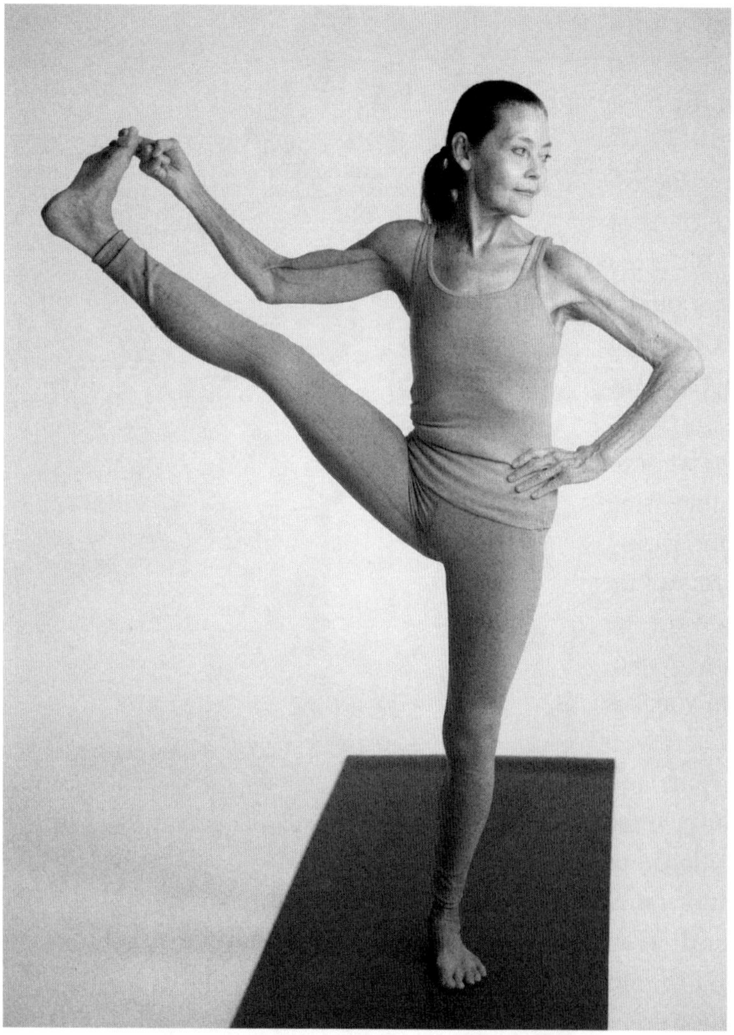

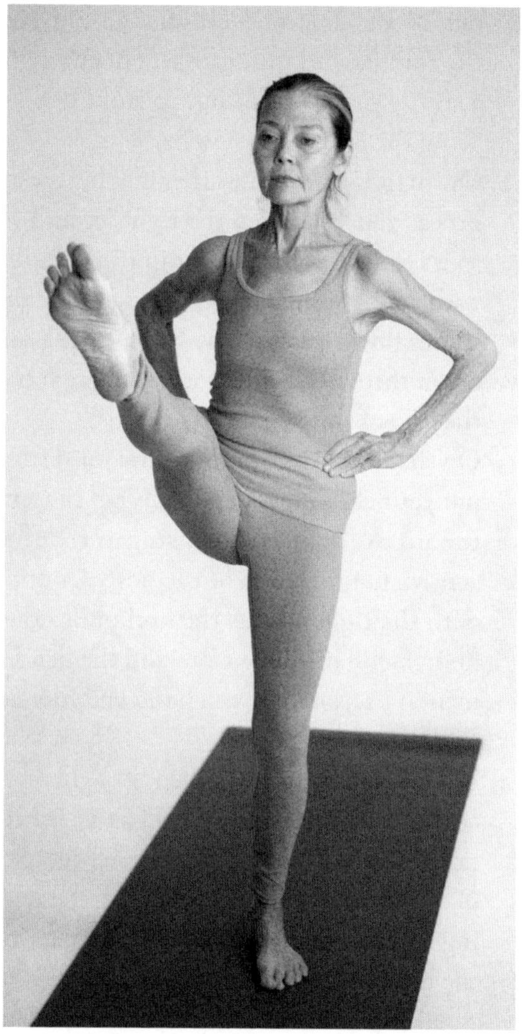

pose could well be called Humble Āsana! It is no crime to lose your balance and drop the floating leg back to the floor. Many people get frustrated doing this pose and may notice that breathing and emotional intensity increase while practicing it. This is perfectly fine. Emotions can give needed energy to the practice.

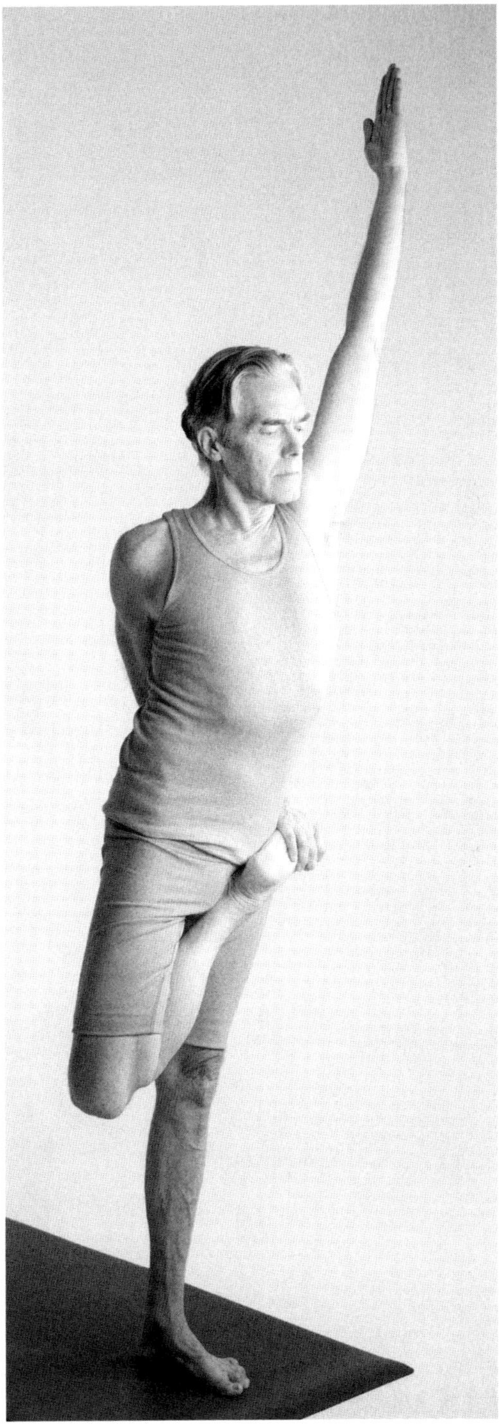

Ardha Baddha Padmottānāsana

Half-Bound Lotus Forward Bend Pose

Ardha Baddha Padmottānāsana, though practiced early in an Aṣṭāṅga Vinyāsa practice, is actually quite advanced. Not only does it assume the practitioner can take Half Padmāsana, but he or she must also have enough flexibility to hold the Padmāsana foot and fold forward while balancing. However, for some, jumping into the deep end of a pool is the best way to learn to swim! Even if the full form is not accessible, modifications and internal forms make it easier to learn, and the actions and counteractions, as well as the concentration skills required for this pose, are excellent for everyone to practice and refine. Those with knee injuries or tight hips and knees should be cautious and practice only the first preparatory position, working gradually into the pose over many weeks or months (or perhaps never).

1. Stand in Samasthitiḥ. Find a sense of strength and balance in the left leg, making sure the knee is slightly bent (micro-bent) to give stability to the pose as you exhale to ground into the pose. Inhaling, lift the right foot, bend the right knee, and externally rotate the femur as you lift the leg to draw the right heel toward the top edge of the pubic bone. *Carefully* press the knee down to point toward the floor.
2. Next, with an exhalation, reach around the back with the right arm to grab the right big toe. If you cannot reach the toe, don't worry. Use that hand to help you balance in the next phase.
3. Inhale and reach up with the left arm to stretch the psoas line and stabilize the pose, then bend forward to place the left hand or fingers on the floor as you exhale. Find a point on which your eyes can rest on the floor, and adjust the hips and knee as needed to fold comfortably and in order to square the hips and shoulders. Inhale and lift the head to

straighten the spine, and then fold deeply into the full form, placing the left hand flat on the floor beside the left foot.

4. Hold the pose for five breaths. In this final position, gaze at the tip of the nose. If you are flexible, you can look to the left big toe.
5. At the end of an exhale, tone the pelvic floor, and on the next inhale, lift the head and straighten the left arm to come halfway up. At first, look between the eyebrows as you lift the spine to a horizontal position.
6. Exhale completely again, staying in place to ground fully through the left foot and leg—making sure to keep a micro-bend in the leg. On the next inhalation, come up to standing. Release the right foot and place it back on the floor.
7. Repeat the pose on the other side, then return to Samasthitiḥ.

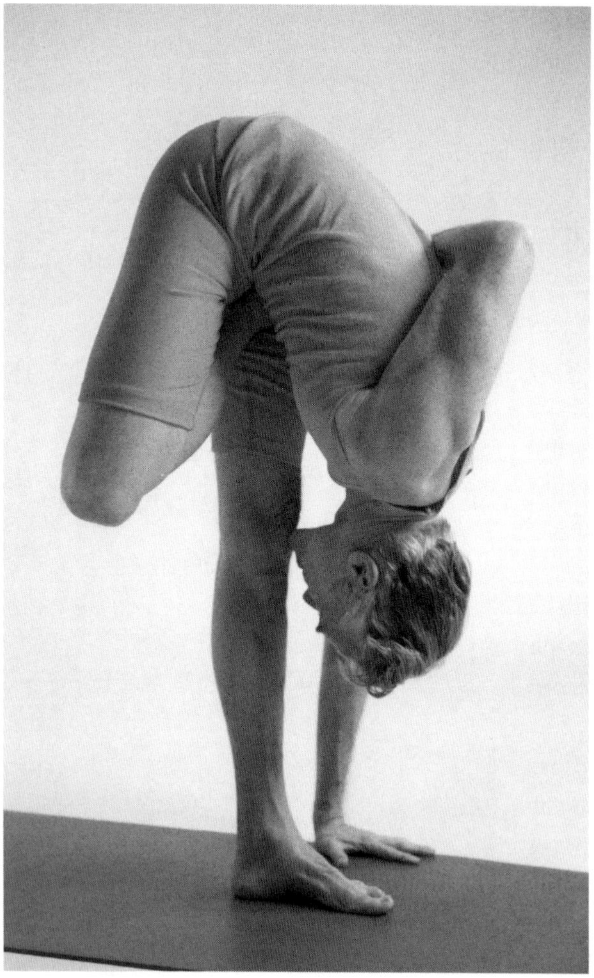

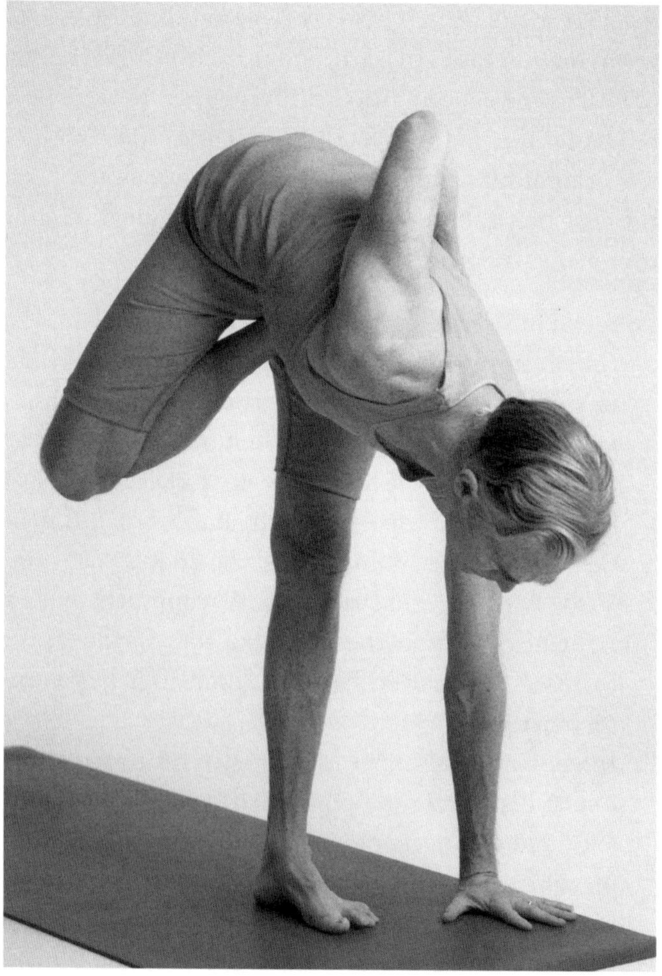

Utkaṭāsana

Difficult Pose

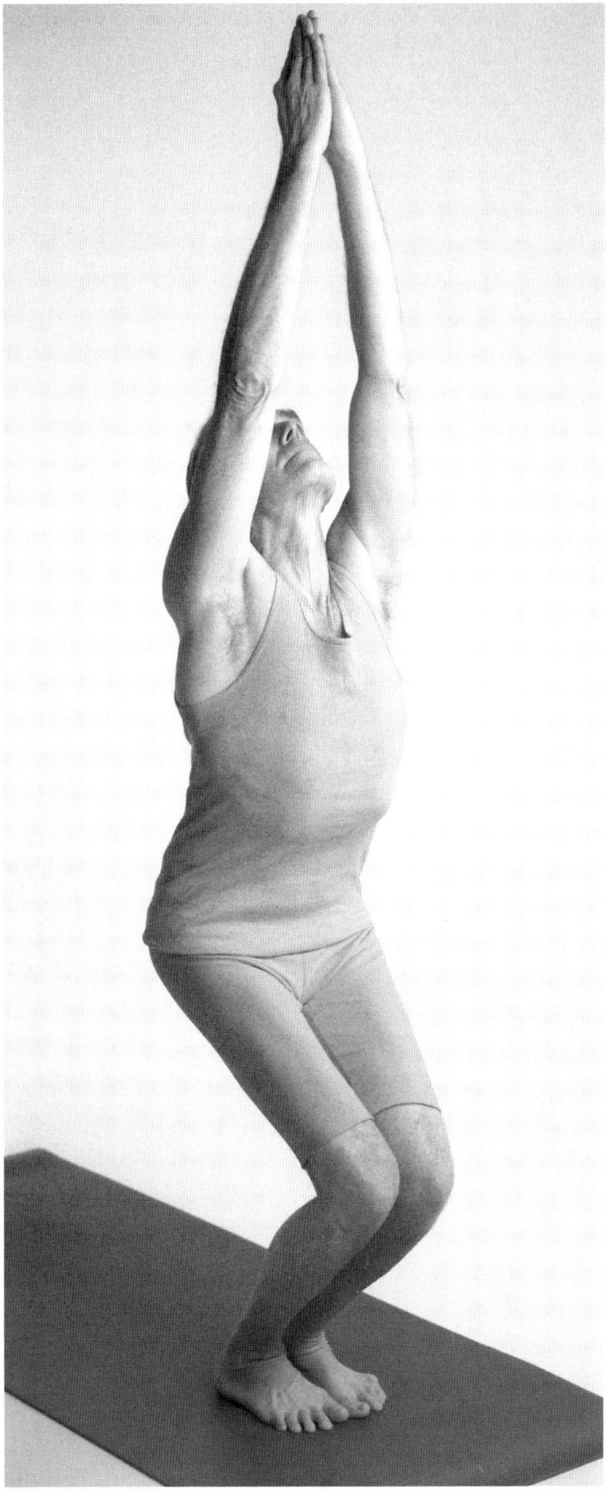

Sometimes also translated as Horrible Pose, Utkaṭāsana is an excellent way to experience Uḍḍīyāna Bandha while learning to keep the legs strong, the pelvic floor awake, and the shoulders protracted while reaching up. Don't shy away from bending your knees *deeply* to keep the pose alive, and remember to breathe fully—even as your arms are reaching enthusiastically up to the sky.

1. This pose is traditionally entered through a Full Vinyāsa. From Downward Facing Dog Pose, at the end of an exhalation, bend the knees, lift the head to look at the mat between the hands, and hop or step forward, inhaling just as your feet touch the floor. Bend the knees deeply as you land.
2. Keep the toes spreading, the heels down, and the inner knees touching as you drop down as if to sit in a chair. The coccyx should feel heavy. At the same time, draw back the lower belly just above the pubic bone. Do not tuck the sitting bones under! Draw them back and drop them down.
3. Keep the heart open, the fronts of the armpits wide, and the throat free of extraneous tension as you wrap the shoulders outward to lift the arms and reach up toward the ceiling. Reach up through the arms in front of the head with the palms touching, and do not crunch the neck. If putting the palms together is impossible, you may keep your hands slightly apart until you become more flexible. Do not strain your neck.
4. Look at the thumbs; because the hands are in front of the face, the line of the gaze is eventually *down* along the line of the nose.
5. Hold the pose for five breaths, then on an inhalation, push through the feet and legs to return to standing. Drop the arms along the sides of the body as you come into Samasthitiḥ, or move directly into a Full Vinyāsa.

Vīrabhadrāsana (Warrior Pose) A and B

Vīrabhadrāsana is a true expression of the union of opposites—the strength and vigor of a warrior and the centered, mellow feel of someone who is at peace within. That is the feeling we cultivate in this pose. By keeping the feet, legs, arms, and hands awake, space is created for the head, throat, torso, and pelvis to fully express stability. It is of particular importance to keep the gaze steady, the tongue soft, the palate released, and the breath free and easy. In the Aṣṭāṅga Vinyāsa form, Vīrabhadrāsana follows Utkaṭāsana with a Full Vinyāsa between, but of course it can be practiced by simply coming into it from Samasthitiḥ.

Vīrabhadrāsana A

1. From Downward Facing Dog Pose, at the end of an exhalation, bend the knees and lift the head to look at the floor between the hands. Turn the left foot in about 20 to 45 degrees and step forward into a lunge with the right foot. Ground through both feet as you inhale and rotate the pelvis and upper body toward the front of the mat, reaching up overhead through both arms.
2. As you reach up through the arms do not strain the neck. Lift the sides of the torso and the fronts of the armpits as you stretch the arms over the head. Gaze at the thumbs and soften the palate.
3. Do not allow the right knee to drift to either side, and do not drop down so far that the knee goes past the ankle. Keep the left leg very strong as you descend, increasing the distance between the feet if you need more stretch or more space so the right thigh can be parallel to the floor.
4. Keep the left foot grounded by making certain that the outer edge of the heel stays touching or near the floor. To do this, wake up the arches of the foot and spread the toes. Lifting the back edge of the foot will eventually injure the knee, and it encourages a collapse into the hip, which can cause an injury to the hip joint. The upper body should feel light, as if it is floating up and out of the pelvis as the inner left thigh draws up away from the floor.
5. Contract the pelvic floor as you draw the coccyx and sitting bones down. Gaze at the thumbs and hold the pose for five breaths. On an inhalation straighten the right leg and, leaving the arms and gaze up,

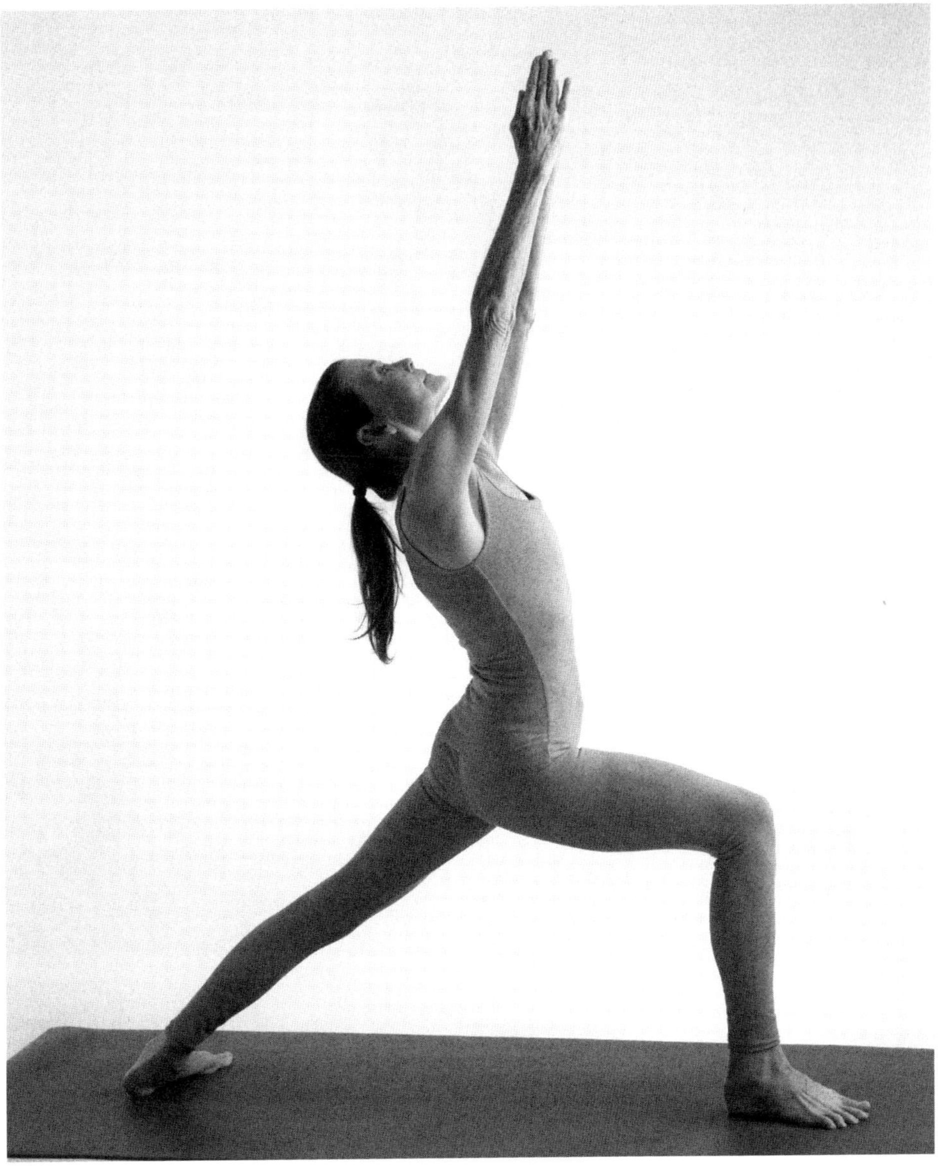

rotate the feet and torso to the left side and drop down, bending the left leg, to repeat the pose on the other side. After five breaths here, move directly into Vīrabhadrāsana B.

VĪRABHADRĀSANA B

1. On an exhalation, lower the arms halfway so they are parallel to the floor with the palms down; at the same time, rotate the torso and pelvis to the right. Reach out through the fingertips and drop the shoulder blades broadly down the back. Keep drawing down the

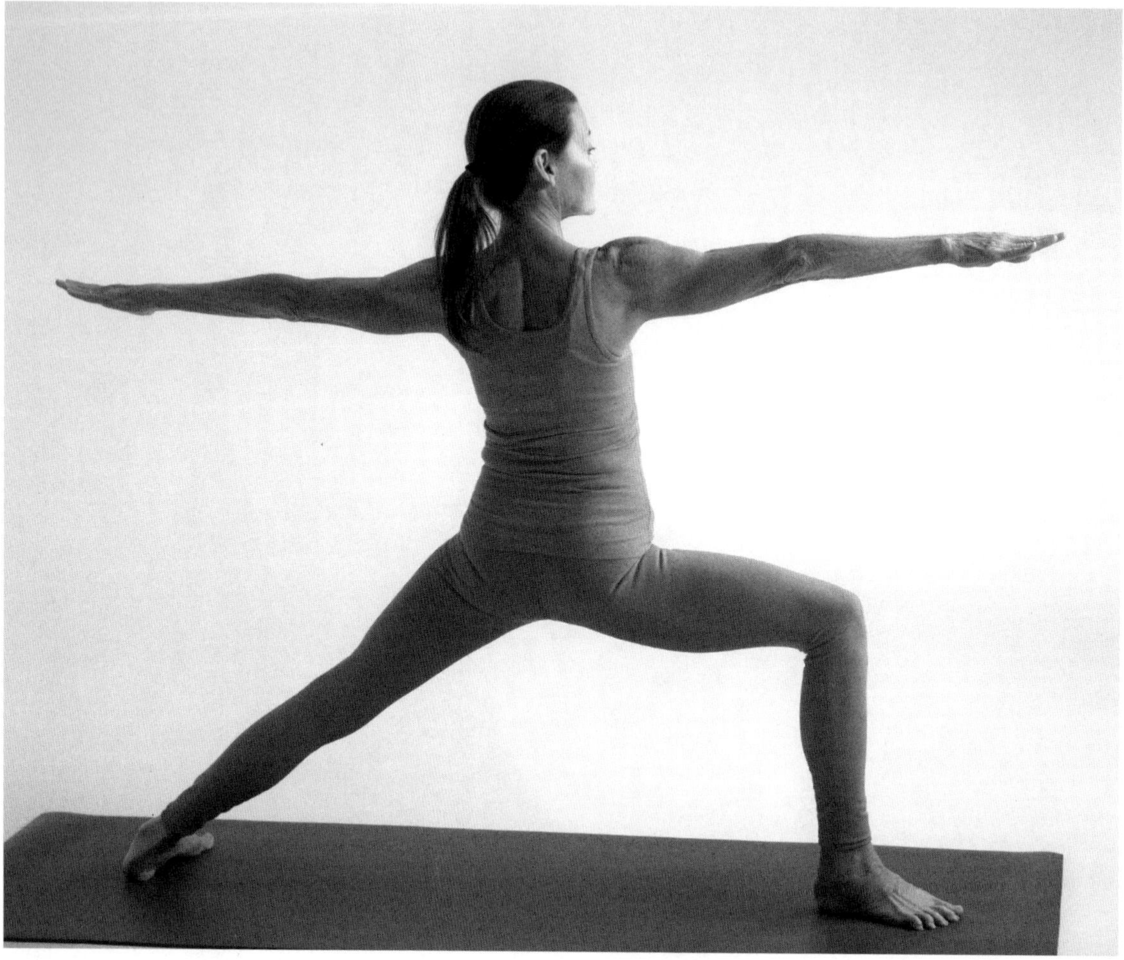

back surface of the body, while toning the pelvic floor. Keep the legs and feet strong and activated as you lift the front of the spine to prevent a sense of collapsing into the hip joints.

2. Ground the outer edge of the right heel and the inner edge of the left foot as you gaze out over the left shoulder at the middle finger of the left hand. Hold this position for five breaths. On an inhale, straighten the left knee, turn the right toes out toward the front of the mat, and angle the left foot in, then bend the right knee so you are in the pose on the other side. Gaze out over the right shoulder at the fingertips of the right hand, and hold the pose for five breaths.
3. Exit the pose by sliding the left heel back a couple of inches and twisting the pelvis around to face the right leg. You may reach up for one breath in Vīrabhadrāsana A or step directly back into the fourth position, Catvāri.

7

Forward Bends

WHEN WE CONSIDER THE PRIMARY SERIES, forward bending is the theme that comes to mind. Beyond those poses practiced as part of the opening sequence in the Sūrya Namaskāras and those found in the standing sequence—beginning with Paśchimottānāsana (Tuning Up the Back Pose) and ending with Ūrdhvā Mukha Paśchimottānāsana (Upward-Facing Forward Bend)—there are many forward folds. When practiced correctly, in sync with the internal cues to alignment and the patterns of Prāṇa, forward bends are incredibly grounding, therapeutic, calming, and integrating. If they are practiced aggressively or without attention to the internal forms that create healthy alignment, forward bends can contribute to shutting the heart area and a *tamasic* (apathetic, depressed) mind state. For those with tight hamstrings or an unstable lumbar region, bending forward without the internal cues of alignment can cause physical discomfort and injury. One popular criticism of Aṣṭāṅga Vinyāsa yoga, and the Primary Series in particular, is that Aṣṭāṅga practitioners are grumpy (closed-hearted and tamasic) and prone to hamstring and low back injuries due to all the repetitive movements into forward bends. These generalizations are based on a fundamental misunderstanding of the proper mechanics that help practitioners experience the benefits of forward bends. It's true that repetitive misalignment can cause problems, but with proper form, even those with physical limitations can actually practice forward folds over and over with no problems whatsoever.

The first vinyāsa of forward bends is that in order to rotate the pelvis around the head of the femur, we begin by inhaling to enhance the prāṇa pattern, which holds the spine straight and opens the heart area. To do this, scoop back under the lower belly using Uḍḍīyāna Bandha to guarantee the participation of the pelvic floor. This subtle, internal vinyāsa is so frequently overlooked that it could be considered the "secret" first step of folding forward. Once this foundation is established and the spine is elongated to let the prāṇa pattern shine out, rotate the pelvis passively around the heads of the femurs, gradually reintroducing the apāna pattern. This allows us to get into the pose intelligently and to exactly the right degree for our particular circumstances. The hip flexor muscles, such as the psoas muscle, should not be involved in a well-executed forward bend. Rather the opposing muscles of hip extension, which include the hamstrings, glutes, and occasionally the deep hip (lateral rotator) muscles, must stay alert and online—slightly toned—to give control and reversibility to the movement. But the basic movement of the pelvis around the heads of the femurs is a function of keeping the spine straight and drawing breath, awareness, and attentiveness up and out of the hip joints, so as we fold forward, we have a sense of elongation in the spine and a passive movement of the hips, which creates space in the hip joints and spine.

The next stage of the vinyāsa for forward bends is when, having closed the hip joints in the primary movement, the tensions around the hip joints slightly reverse so that in the end of the exhale counteractions come into play. This closes the hip joints; signals the pelvic floor to tone; and stimulates the apāna pattern, which guarantees that the hip flexors do not tighten unnecessarily. Remember that the hip flexors are involved in the prāṇa pattern, and the hamstrings are involved in the apāna pattern.

Forward bends in general allow us to enhance the quality of the exhalation because we are folding over the front area of the body, including the abdominal organs and particularly the lungs. Exhaling smoothly and fully makes it easy to find the appropriate fold in the hip joints and to release tension in the palate. Consciously releasing tension in the palate is calming to the nervous system and is essential for forward bends, because as we fold, the space available for air to be drawn into the lungs is constricted, making it impossible for them to expand, which may trigger feelings of fear. Once fear is introduced into any pose, the potential for meditative, liberating movements decreases. In forward bends we release the palate to keep the heart open as we let go of inhalation patterns that have opened spatially in and around the body. This makes these poses profoundly relaxing, and their deep therapeutic and restorative potential is revealed.

Once we are in the pose, its internal dialectic between action and counteraction begins, and we make fine adjustments in terms of the tone of the pelvic floor—front to back and side to side. Thus, the question of whether prāṇa or apāna is leading the pose can be considered, knowing that—as in all poses—both ends of the breath must work in tandem. Sometimes the heart has to move farther forward, and the pubic bone has to stimulate the poses. At other times the kidney area has to expand, and the coccyx has to show the way out of the pose by offering a sense of dropping and pulling to a point of solidity in the pelvic floor.

The final step in the vinyāsa sequence for forward bends is when these two patterns simultaneously awaken in the awareness; when that unification is stable, we can let go of both patterns. Coming out of the pose, we complete an exhalation to stabilize the pelvic floor and then, keeping the sense of an awakened and toned pelvic floor in the forefront of the awareness, the inhalation facilitates a spooning out under the belly (Uḍḍīyāna) that initiates the exit from the pose. Ideally we can exit the depth of the pose on the inhalation without losing the integrity of the apāna pattern.

Forward bends can be either symmetrical, as with Pādāṅguṣṭhāsana (Big Toe Pose), or asymmetrical, as with Jānuśīrṣāsana (Head-to-Knee Pose). In forward bends in which the folded leg is close to the midline in adduction, as in Jānuśīrṣāsana, the range of motion is much more restricted than when the folded leg is abducted, or angled out away from the midline, as in Upaviṣṭha Koṇāsana. Because of their even movement, symmetrical forward folds have the qualities of simplicity and purity. Tensions along the spine and the pelvic floor are uniform from side to side, so they encourage the apāna pattern to flow. This can be very relaxing and grounding. Symmetrical forward bends allow us to observe and breathe into the pose as we adjust for inherent asymmetries in the body, making it easy to experience the beneficial aspects of this family of poses. When we practice forward bends as part of smooth, pleasant breath cycles, we feel the natural rhythms up and down the spine and out from the central channel, and we can experience these patterns communicating with each other across the pelvic floor and palate. Tapping into this deep level of awareness is easier in symmetrical forward bends. Once we have a taste for the sensations associated with the depth of awareness experienced through these poses, the same sensations are more easily found in asymmetrical forward bends as well, demonstrating that paying attention to subtle levels of awareness and form is how the poses deepen and become most beneficial.

In some symmetrical forward bends in which the legs are close to the midline of the body, such as Paśchimottānāsana, it is important to understand that the hip joint can not close as deeply as it can when the legs are abducted in poses like Prasārita Pādottānāsana, where each leg is extended more than 30 degrees past the midline. This is due to the length and angle of the neck of the femur, which can be quite dissimilar in different people. If the neck of the femur is angled severely or is short, it can hit the labrum or the edge of the acetabulum, especially in the transitions in and out of the pose. This can also happen if the feet are wide apart and the legs abducted when folding, as in Prasārita Pādottānāsana if we attempt to put the head on the floor. (In Prasārita Pādottānāsana, the problem is exacerbated particularly when exiting the pose, so if the feet are moved in toward the midline of the body when exiting, impingement can be avoided.) Extreme movements in forward bends with abducted legs can eventually cause injury to the joint, but with close attention to anatomy and mechanics, the poses are very safe and healthy.

When forward bends are practiced incorrectly or inattentively, disk and spinal problems (particularly in the lumbar region) as well as overstretched hamstrings can occur. Although sometimes these complications have to do with unique individual structure, more often they are aggravated because the legs and feet are not engaging properly (which they must in all forward bends, even if the knees are bent), the hamstrings arc naturally short or tight, and/or the spine is not kept straight in the transitions into and out of the poses.

With regard to curving the spine as we fold or unfold, this is a pattern that may be habitual, as it is common in everyday activities; it's quite natural to look down at whatever has caught our interest as we begin to bend toward it. This automatically curls the spine, beginning with the cervical vertebrae, which almost magically tucks the pelvis under. The pattern can even approach a pure apānic coil, like a worm working its way out through the tip of the coccyx. Structurally the problem with folding forward in this way is that flexion of the spine automatically triggers the hamstrings and glutes to tone; this causes a posterior tilt in the pelvis, which may become locked in position. In either of these scenarios, the pelvis is not able to rotate passively around the heads of the femurs. To force a forward bend while the pelvis is locked, particularly if the legs and spine are not used intelligently, puts strain on the hamstrings and the lower back.

The role of the hamstrings in folding forward is also crucial. Depending on one's structure, hamstrings may be slightly longer or shorter—which gives more or less play before they reach their limit when bending forward with straight legs. Hamstrings can lengthen gradually through stretching, but they can also tighten due to certain activities such as running and biking or simply through lack of use. Because the hamstrings attach to the sitting bones, if they are tight and we fold forward with hyperextended or inactive legs, the sitting bones are pulled down and the pelvis rolls back along with them. So when we fold forward, especially if the spine is not straight, the low back can be compromised. If we push too hard under these circumstances, the hamstrings themselves can also be overstretched or strained, particularly at their attachments to the sitting bones.

Within the family of forward bends, there are two other general categories of poses. Those that are accessible and most beneficial when the spine is initially straight, especially during the entrance to and exit from the pose. Paśchimottānāsana, Baddha Koṇāsana, and Yoga Nidrāsana are examples of this form. There are also poses that are considered extreme forward bends, meaning the hip joints are deeply closed, but require extreme flexion of the spine initially. Poses such as Kūrmāsana and Dvi Pāda Śīrṣāsana fall into this latter category.

Forward bends that are not grounded in the full apāna pattern with its strong prāṇic complement can have the opposite effect of backbends and leave an emotional residue of depression or misery in the mind and body. When this happens, the area of the heart closes as a result of improper alignment; the internal breath is inhibited due to a lack of actions and counteractions in the pelvic floor, spine, and shoulders. It is not unusual for beginners to strain too much in forward bends, especially if they think there is something to accomplish. Touching the toes is a familiar goal we may struggle for, but putting too much effort toward that goal rather than tuning in to what's actually arising physically and mentally can cause the hamstrings to tighten even more, the result being that the "goal" is further away than it was at the beginning. Although we must push ourselves through our stuck patterns of resistance, if we exert too much grasping in any pose, it becomes increasingly difficult to observe the core of the body from the pelvic floor up through the head. When this happens in forward bends, and we tune out the feelings and sensations that are arising in the body, it is easy to undo the benefits of the pose. The sense of groundedness and of complete release disappear with each breath when we try too hard.

When practicing the seated forward bends as part of an Aṣṭāṅga Vinyāsa series, a Half Vinyāsa is taken between each pose; eventually, as strength increases and time permits, it is taken between each side of a given pose. For therapeutic reasons or if you have the desire (and the time) to do so, a Full Vinyāsa may also be practiced between seated poses. For this reason, this chapter gives instructions for entering and exiting the poses within a vinyāsa. When a pose is traditionally practiced without a Half Vinyāsa between it and the following pose, there is no mention of vinyāsa in the description.

PAŚCHIMOTTĀNĀSANA (TUNING UP THE BACK POSE) A, B, AND C

In the Primary Series, these three variations of Paśchimottānāsana are practiced in sequence, one immediately after the other, and each is held for five breaths. Though there are subtle differences between them, there are also some common internal and external forms. These commonalities are described for form A but apply to all three forms. Paśchimottānāsana is also included as part of the traditional finishing sequence.

Paśchimottānāsana A

1. From Downward Facing Dog Pose, jump through to a seated position with the legs stretched out straight in front of you. Exhale to bring awareness to the sensation of the sitting bones dropping into the earth. From this reference point, the following inhalation establishes a strong internal connection to the central channel of the body that reaches from the center of the pelvic floor up through the crown of the head.

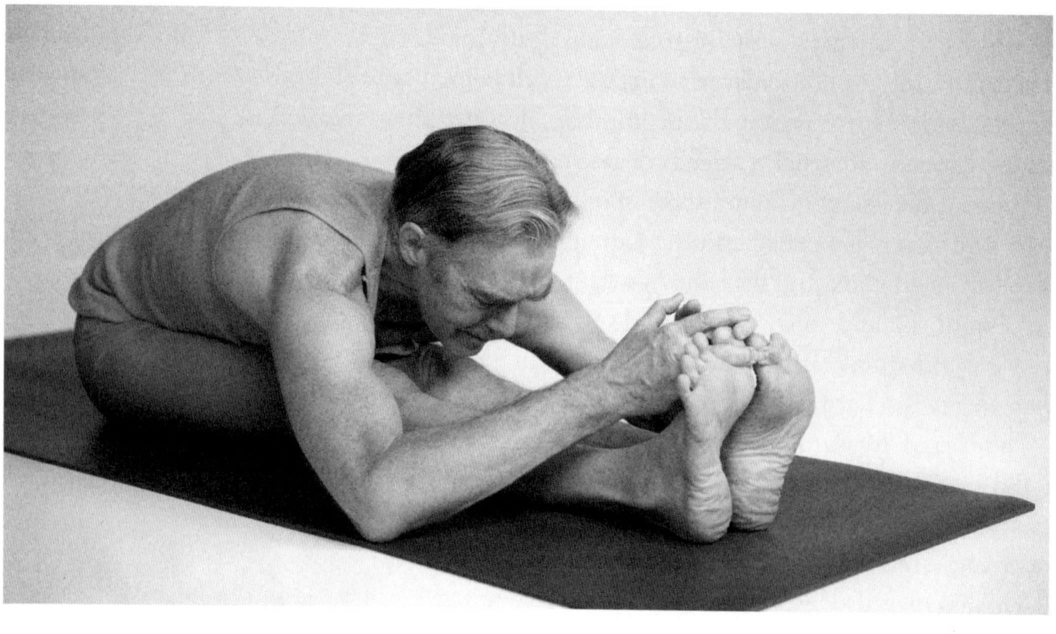

2. On an inhalation, reach the arms overhead to stretch the sides of the body and the psoas lines from the tips of the fingers down into the lower belly and the backs of the thighs.
3. As you exhale, fold forward to take the big toes with the middle and index fingers of each hand with the spine straightening. Extend through the spine and lift the belly up and over the tops of the thighs to allow the pelvis to rotate passively around the heads of the femurs.
4. If you cannot reach the toes, hold both ends of a strap, like a pair of reins that have been looped around the big toes, and/or bend the knees. It is far better to keep the alignment strong and active as you work to lengthen the hamstrings than to strain your back or hamstrings and collapse the heart area simply to reach the desired hand position. Patience is essential in all yoga āsanas, and especially so in Paśchimottānāsana.
5. Once you have the toes, activate the pose, moving in a sort of pulsating motion on the wave of the breath. On each inhalation, you may find that you come slightly out of the pose as you extend through the heart and the crown of the head, not trying to go down but reaching long and forward. On each exhalation, as you fold more deeply and drop into the pelvic floor, continue to pull back on the toes to encourage length in the spine and hamstrings.

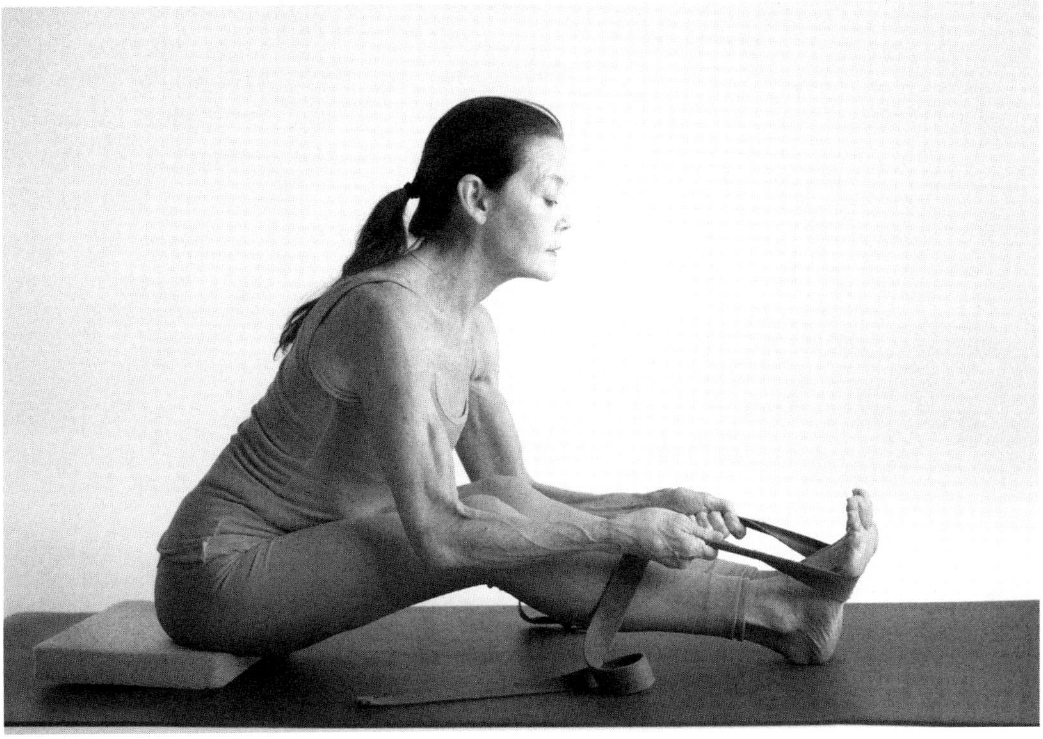

6. Keep the legs firm and straight with a slight inward rotation. This is expressed by activating the feet, which stimulates a feeling of pushing forward through the roots of the big toes as you spread all of the toes and square the bottoms of the feet to the front in response to pulling back on the big toes.
7. Before folding forward completely, draw up the front surface of the torso as the groins and the inner tops of the legs drop down. This action is done on the inhalation as you extend the spine and spread the collarbones to keep the heart open. Gradually deepen the fold around the hip joints by bringing the torso up and over the legs. As a counteraction pull the back surface of the body down, grounding the sitting bones. Do not hunch the shoulders or strain the neck.
8. Gaze softly at the tip of the nose. Eventually, when you have folded very deeply and are flat against the legs (closed like a large book), gaze between the eyebrows, but never strain the neck to keep the dṛṣṭi you imagine you should be taking.
9. Once in the pose, hold for five breaths. At the end of the last exhalation, bring awareness to the pelvic floor and ground down through the sitting bones. Inhaling, extend long through the crown of the head and rise back to a seated position.

Paśchimottānāsana B

1. Follow the same basic form as for Paśchimottānāsana A, but instead of reaching up with the arms to enter the pose, begin Paśchimottānāsana B just as you lift out of form A.

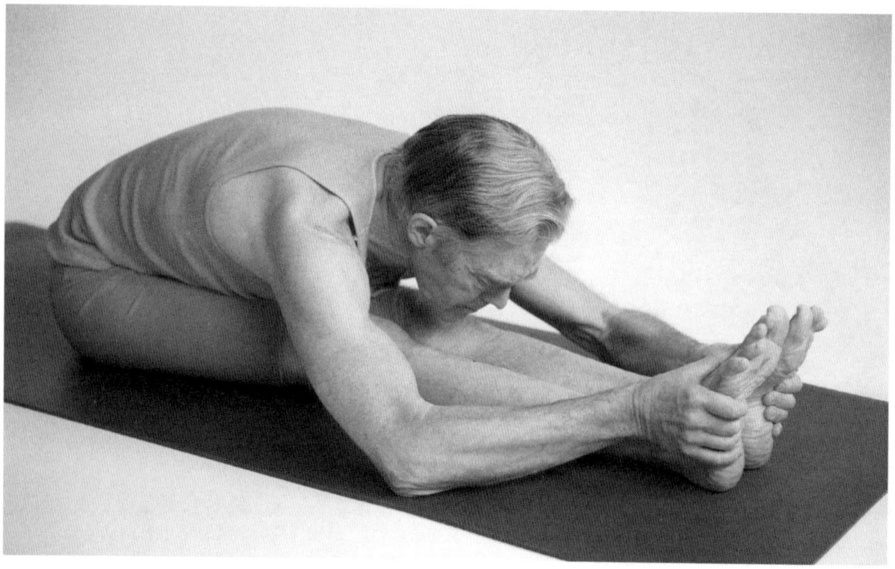

2. At the end of the inhalation that brought you out of the pose, switch the hand position to hold the feet with your hands. Curl your fingers around the sides of the feet placing thumbs on top of the first metatarsals (the top side of the mounds of your big toes). Push forward through the thumbs and spread the toes as you open the feet, and straighten the legs with a slight inward rotation.
3. Enter the full form on the wave of the breath (as in form A), inhaling one more time to straighten and then folding forward on the following exhale. Hold the pose for five breaths, gazing at the feet or along the line of the nose, depending on your flexibility.
4. If you cannot reach the feet, bend the knees and/or hold the ends of a strap looped around your feet for the pose. Even if you are doing one of these variations, you must still keep the legs and feet active and awake and work from a straightening spine. Just because the knees are bent is no reason for them to doze off!
5. After five breaths, exit the pose on an inhalation (as in form A).

Paśchimottānāsana C

1. Follow the same basic form as for Paśchimottānāsana A, but instead of reaching up with the arms to enter the pose, begin Paśchimottānāsana C just as you lift out of form B.
2. At the end of the inhalation that brought you out of the pose, switch the hand position so you are holding one wrist with the opposite hand on the far side of your feet. In time with the inhale, pull back on the feet through the backs of your hands, then fold forward coming

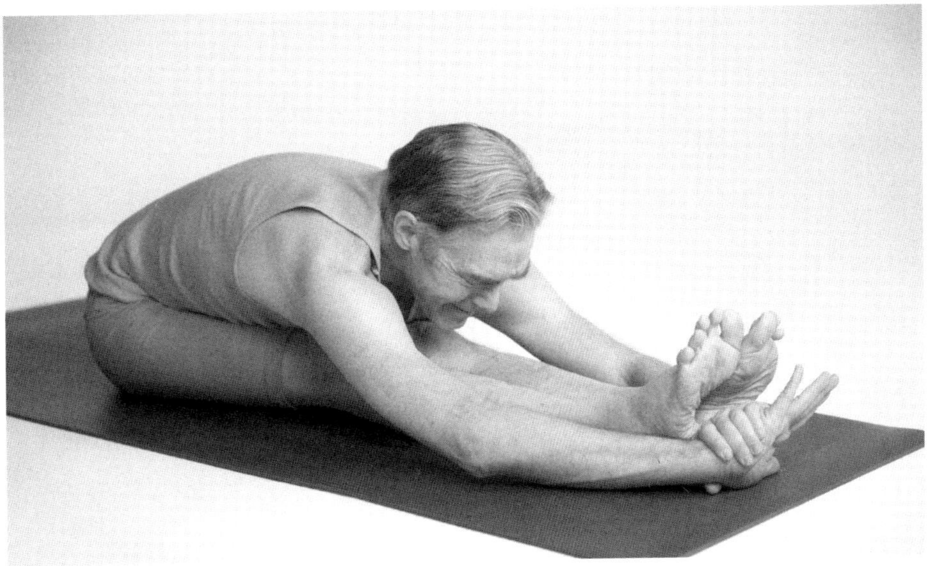

up and over the thighs to eventually place the ribs on the thighs. Bend the elbows out to the sides and push down slightly through the elbows toward the floor. Let the shoulder blades protract and move up to lengthen the arms. This stretches the latissimus dorsi, tracing the kidney wing pattern. Keep the upper trapezius muscles at the base of your neck soft, and release the tongue and palate.

3. After five breaths, exit the pose on an inhalation (as in form A).

Ardha Baddha Padma Paśchimottānāsana

Half-Bound Lotus Forward Bend Pose

Because Half Padmāsana is part of this pose, not all students are able to take this form; however, practicing variations that work with limitations is an excellent way to build confidence and hone the practice, even if Padmāsana never arrives! Those with knee injuries or tight hips should be cautious and may use a strap to hold the toes behind the back, use a block or blanket to elevate the pelvis, or practice only the first preparatory position for the duration of the pose. The ability to do the pose comes gradually as a result of all the other poses that *are* possible for the practitioner.

1. Come to a seated position with the legs stretched straight out in front of you. Fold the left leg into Half Padmāsana, placing the foot as deeply into the lower belly and left groin as possible. While entering Half Padmāsana, the pelvis may tilt back slightly at first, but once in

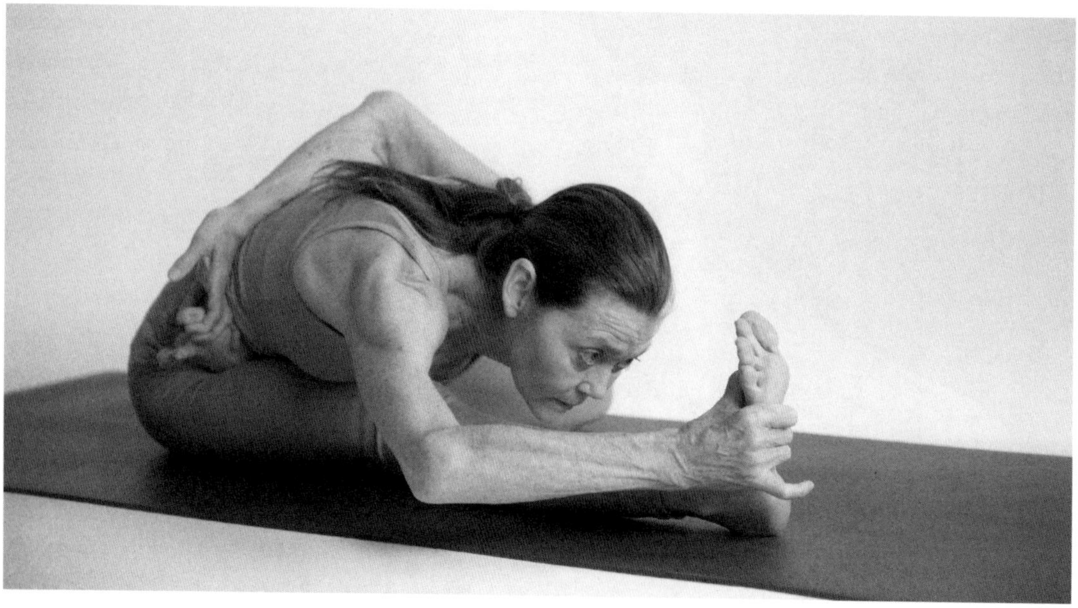

the fold, sit straight and turn the pelvis to bring the folded knee forward and down. The release of the hip and knee joint is facilitated by the Uḍḍīyāna Bandha action, which simultaneously lifts the front of the spine.

2. Keep the right leg awake, pressing the inner edge of the right foot forward through the mound of the big toe. There should be a twisting action in the hips, as you pull back the right sitting bone and bring the left leg forward. Press the folded knee down, creating an inward rotation in the femur.
3. Exhaling, reach behind the back with the left arm to grasp the left big toe. Inhaling, breathe up through the center of the body to straighten the spine and settle into the base of the pose in the pelvic floor. While holding the toe behind the back, do not hunch the shoulders toward the ears. If you cannot reach the toe, you may use a strap to loop around the toes. Alternatively, you can use the left hand to secure the folded leg. Proceed slowly if you are stiff! Some will need to only bring the heel of the folded leg back near the groins as in Jānuśīrṣāsana.
4. Still on the inhalation, reach up with the right arm, protracting that shoulder blade and stretching the psoas muscle on the right side. As you exhale, fold forward, reaching through the right arm and hand to hold the outer edge of the right foot. If you were unable to hold the toes in step 3 (above), instead of using a strap to hold the foot you may reach forward with both arms to grab the right foot with both hands. Once in the pose, inhale and roll the top of the left shoulder back and down, lifting the left elbow slightly to facilitate the action.
5. Hold the pose for five breaths. Begin to exit the pose on an inhalation, elongating the spine as you lift through the core of the heart. Once upright, release the left toe. Either switch legs to practice the pose on the other side, or preferably, cross the legs and do a Half Vinyāsa before folding the right leg into Half Padmāsana for the second side.

Tiryang Mukha Eka Pāda Paśchimottānāsana

One Leg Reversed Forward Bend Pose

This forward bend, found in the Primary Series, is an excellent example of the oblique line pattern of twisting—wrapping from the serratus anterior muscle on one side of the body to the obliques on the other. If folding the knee closed in Half Vīrāsana causes discomfort in the knee or hips, sitting on a blanket or block may help. To relieve discomfort

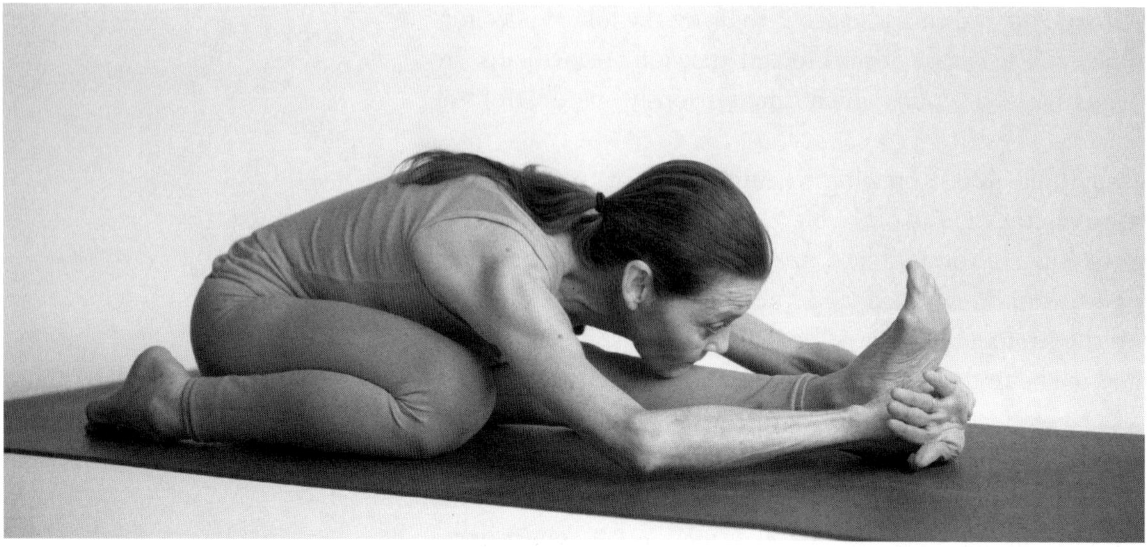

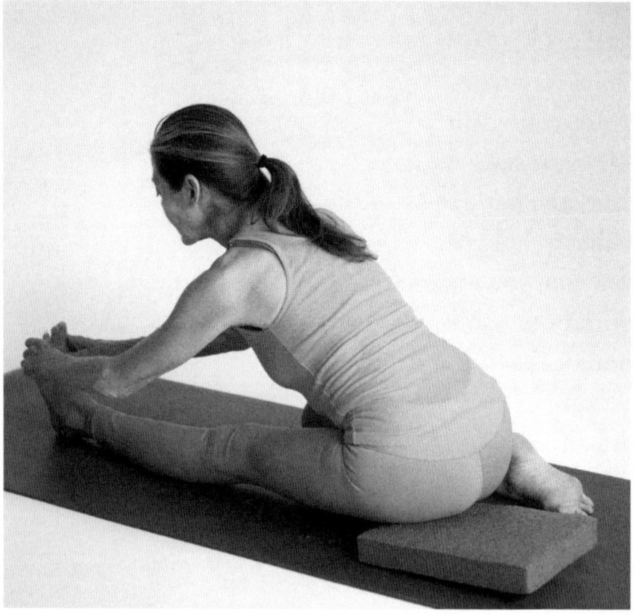

in the knee, a neatly folded hand towel placed behind the knee may also be helpful, as it makes more space in the joint. You may also experiment with the distance between the knees—it is not mandatory that the thighs be completely parallel and/or touching. In fact, this is an extreme pose, so like all poses you should work slowly, bit by bit, working the edge of sensation but not pushing into or through pain. The pose should feel open, free, and comfortable.

1. Float through from Downward Facing Dog Pose to a seated position with the right leg folded in Vīrāsana position and the left leg stretched straight out in front. Inhaling reach up with both arms, and exhaling fold forward to take the left foot with both hands. The right arm needs to reach so that it brings the right kidney area forward and down toward the left knee. The hips twist gently as they begin to square toward the left leg.
2. If you have stiff or injured knees, sit on a cushion or block so you will not be tilted to the side. It is often best to support only the sitting bone on the straight leg side with the prop, allowing the other sitting bone to drop down slightly so you can maintain more mobility in the pelvis while entering and exiting the pose.
3. If you experience pain in the right knee joint, be sure to roll the calf muscle out to the side and tuck the skin of the outer thigh down toward the floor.

4. Draw back the left sitting bone and attempt to ground the right one. This action may be facilitated initially by using the left hand on the floor as an "outrigger" to push into the floor on the left side of the body and help position the hips correctly. Pushing the tops of the toes of the right foot into the floor, as if flexing the foot, can also facilitate this action.
5. Bring the right kidney wing area firmly forward and then down toward the left knee. Use the pull of the arms on the left foot to help deepen the fold and set the twist in the pose.
6. Keep the left leg awake. Draw the skin of the inner thigh of this leg and the skin of the outer thigh on your right leg down toward the floor. Hold the pose for five breaths. To exit, place the hands on the floor by your knees, and on an exhalation lean forward and lift up, then step or jump back, straightening the legs into Catvāri. From Catvāri, transition through Upward and Downward Facing Dog Poses, then return to a seated position to do the pose on the other side.

Krauñchāsana

Krauñcha's Pose

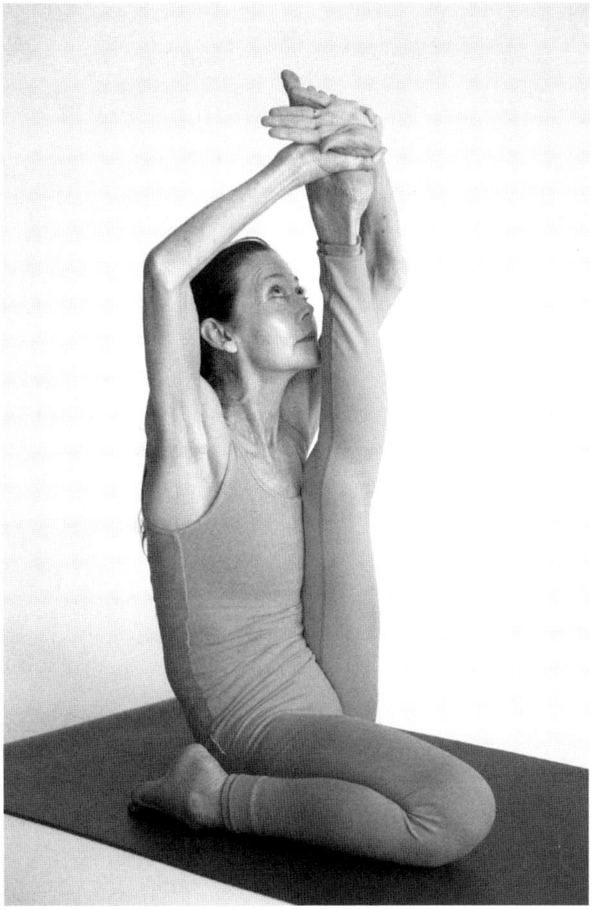

This āsana is named after the sage Krauñcha, who is said to have split open a mountain pass in the Himalayas to let the Himalayan geese fly through that middle path. When doing the pose, the uplifted leg feels almost like a mountain you must navigate around, and as you reach forward, there is a sense of splitting the mountain, starting in the pelvic floor and continuing up through the central channel. The pose appears in the Intermediate Series immediately following Paśāsana and also represents an element of conclusion or summary to the Primary Series. Like so many of the forward bends within the Primary Series, Krauñchāsana is another fine example of the oblique pattern of twisting while folding forward.

1. From Downward Facing Dog Pose, at the end of an exhalation, float through to a seated position with the right leg folded back in Vīrāsana position and the left leg straight out in front of you.
2. On the inhalation, bend the left knee and clasp the left wrist with the right hand beyond the sole

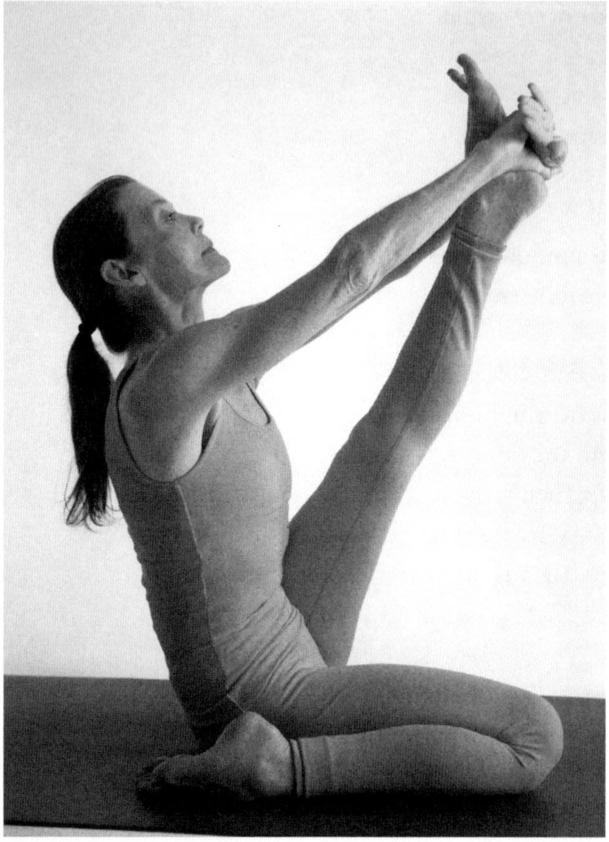

of the left foot. Through a sweeping action through the left foot, lift the left leg so that it is pointing toward the ceiling as you square the foot, reaching through the mound of the left big toe. To position the left leg correctly, allow a small external rotation in the femur, which involves bending the knee and dropping it out to the side while entering the pose. In this way, the head of the femur settles properly into place in the hip socket.

3. Straighten the left leg into the pose, emphasize a slight internal spin by reaching out through the big toe mound of the left foot. Resist the pull of the arms by pushing down toward the floor through the left heel. This wakes up the pose.
4. Lift the head as if to look at the big toe of the left foot, but gaze down the nose. Allow the shoulder blades to broaden and flow down the back; keep the tops of the shoulders away from the ears. Work the right foot as if to flex it; because the floor is in the way, the foot and muscles of the right leg will engage, stabilizing the base of the pose and signaling the right sitting bone to drop down toward the floor as the pelvic floor is activated. Keep the palate released and the tongue soft as you transition into the full form.
5. On an exhalation, bend the arms and draw the left leg closer to the torso, reaching up and forward through the upper body to place the chin on the shin as you wrap the right kidney area over toward the left knee.
6. Gaze up at the big toe and again activate the base of the pose. Hold this position for five breaths. On a final big inhalation, straighten the arms, still holding the foot, to return to the original position, then release the hands and jump back. Move through a Half Vinyāsa for the other side of the pose.

JĀNUŚĪRṢĀSANA (HEAD-TO-KNEE POSE) A, B, AND C

These three forms of Jānuśīrṣāsana are traditionally practiced one after another with a Half Vinyāsa between the individual forms. For more advanced students, a Half Vinyāsa is practiced between sides.

Jānuśīrṣāsana A

1. Come to a seated position with the legs stretched straight out in front of you. Fold the right knee closed and drop the knee out to the side with the sole of the foot near or touching the left thigh. Depending on your flexibility, the femurs should be at approximately a 90-degree angle. Pull back the left sitting bone as you press the right knee back and down with a slight inward rotation of the femur. This allows you to turn or square the hips toward the left leg as you enter the pose. The asymmetry of the action around the hip joints is the basic material of this family of poses.
2. Reach the arms over your head on an inhalation. As you exhale, fold forward and across the midline to hold the inner edge of the left foot with the right hand. Clasp the left wrist with the right hand.
3. The pelvis will naturally rotate to face the left leg. You may feel a slight lifting of the right sitting bone as you reach and lift up to fold, because the right leg has a primary inward rotation. As you deepen into exhalation and the fold, there is a counterrotation that drops that sitting bone back down toward the floor.
4. Wrapping the hands beyond the left foot and clasping the wrist takes time and flexibility, but working patiently and on the wave of the breath facilitates this action. Once in the pose, continue to unite deep internal actions and counteractions in the pelvic floor. Hold the pose for five breaths.
5. The counteraction of the left leg is an inward rotation with the inseam drawn down toward the floor. These leg actions will be facilitated if you keep the left leg awake and the left foot squared forward,

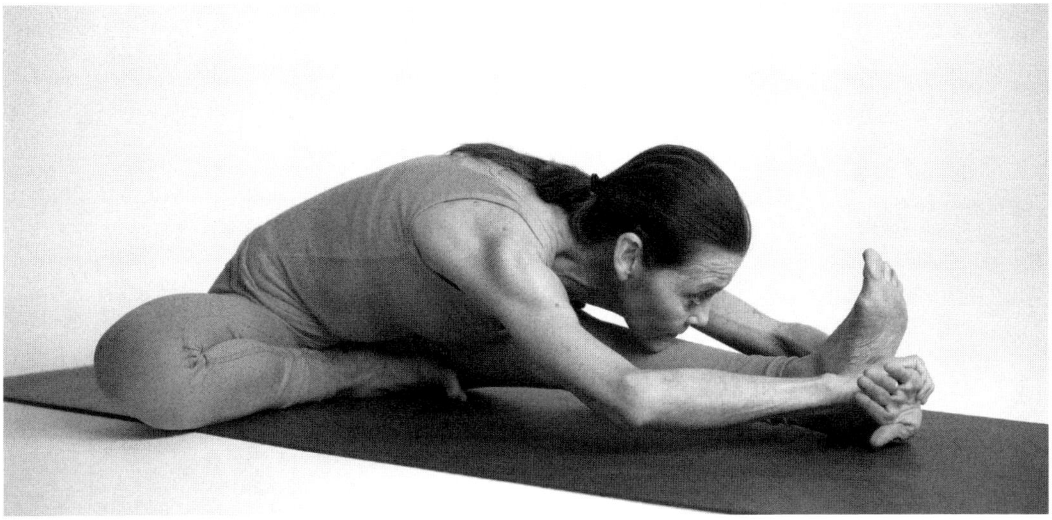

especially through the root of the left big toe. As in Paśchimottānāsana and other forward bends, work with the breath to enter and deepen the pose. Using the breath, play with alternating primary and counter-rotation patterns back and forth in the legs, feet, and around the hip joints. Their interplay can become even and refined as you learn the function of Mūlabandha.

6. At the end of an exhalation, ground the awareness into the pelvic floor. On the next inhalation, lift the torso and reach forward through the core of the heart as you straighten back to a seated position. Switch sides, or do a Half Vinyāsa before doing the pose on the other side.

Jānuśīrṣāsana B

1. Enter the pose as for Jānuśīrṣāsana A, beginning in a seated position with the legs stretched out straight in front.
2. Fold the right knee closed and sit up on the heel, placing it in front of the anus. Flex the foot (do not point the toes) so the inner edge of the right foot will eventually be visible along the inseam of the left thigh. Open the thighs to about an 65-degree angle (or to a lesser angle if you are stiff).
3. In this pose, you are sitting squarely on your heel so the sitting bones are approximately equidistant from the floor. Do not lean to one side!
4. On an inhalation, reach the arms over your head and, as in form A, fold forward to hold the sides of the left foot, or if you are more flexible, clasp the hands beyond the foot. Hold the pose for five breaths before transitioning to the other side, then do a Half Vinyāsa to Jānuśīrṣāsana C.

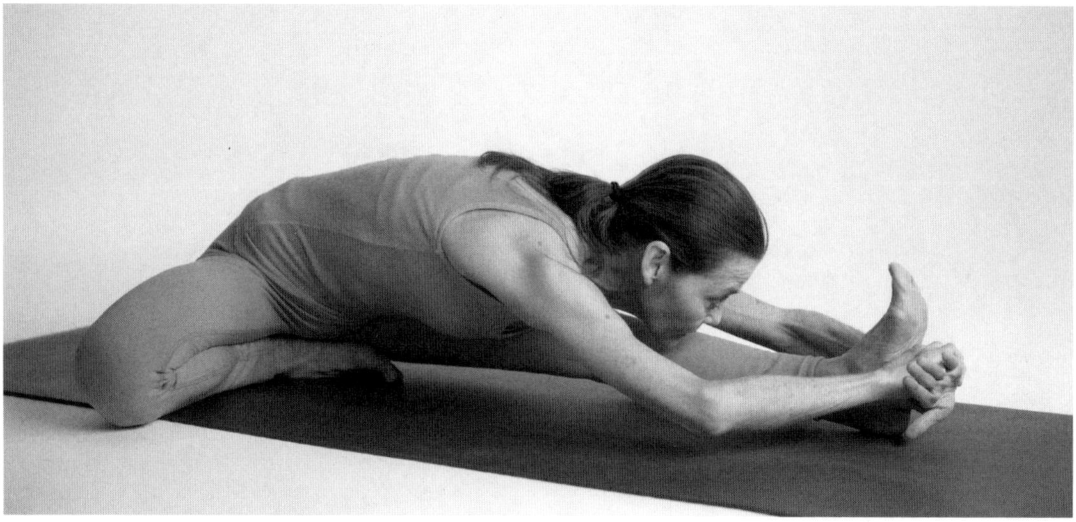

Jānuśīrṣāsana C

1. Enter the pose as for Jānuśīrṣāsana A and B, beginning in a seated position with the legs stretched out in front of you on the floor.
2. Fold the right knee closed and flex the foot. Bring the heel toward the lower belly and sit up straight. Turn the toes of the right foot down place them on the floor next to the inseam of the left leg. The right toes will eventually face squarely out to the right, and the sole of the foot will be perpendicular to the floor.
3. With the toes turned down this way, the right femur is encouraged to rotate inward as you start to lean forward into the pose. At this point, draw the right knee forward and eventually down to touch the floor, so the thighs form about a 45-degree angle. Be patient. If the knee does not easily reach the floor, do not push it. Remember to *flex the foot firmly* when entering the pose.

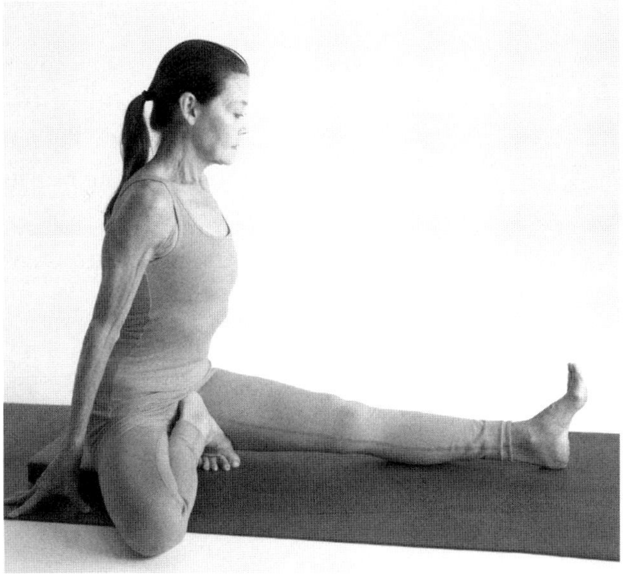

4. As in the previous forms of Jānuśīrṣāsana, reach up through the arms on an inhalation, and as you exhale to fold forward, draw the kidney area on the right side forward and clasp the hands onto the sides of the foot or hold the wrists beyond the foot. Gaze along the line of the nose, eventually at the toes.
5. Hold the pose for five breaths. Exit on an inhalation, as you sit up with a straight spine. Switch legs via a Half Vinyāsa or simply by changing sides.

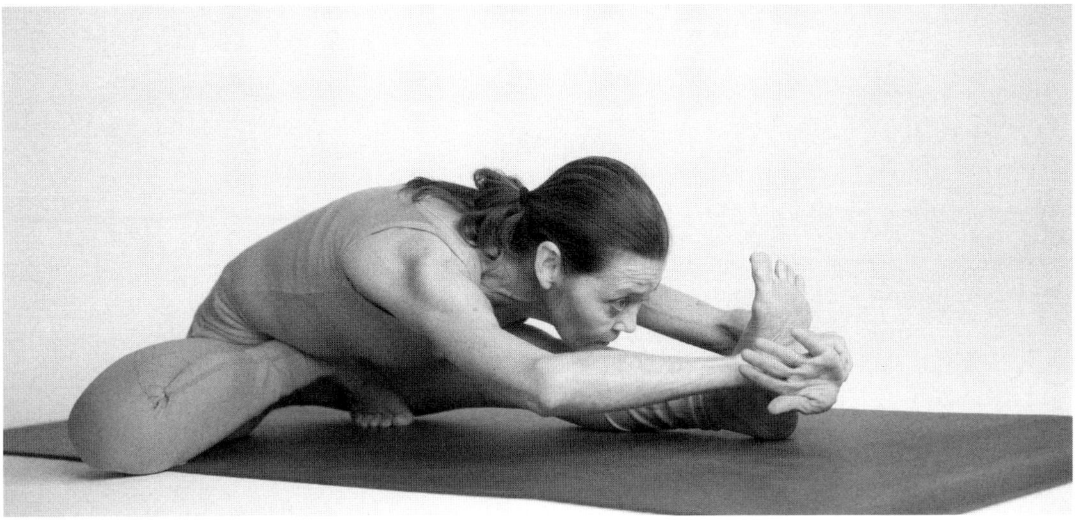

MARĪCHYĀSANA (MARĪCHI'S POSE) A AND B

Within the Primary Series, there are four forms of the Marīchyāsana poses, named after the sage Marīchi. The first and second forms (A and B) are forward bends, and the third and fourth (C and D) are twists. Although they are traditionally practiced as a continuous sequence (which is highly recommended), for the purpose of understanding the principles of the families of poses into which they fall, they are included in the forward bend section of this book.

Marīchyāsana A

1. From Downward Facing Dog Pose, float through to a seated position, bending the right knee and placing the right foot flat on the floor with the left leg straight along in front of you. Place the right foot about one hand-width from and parallel to the left thigh.
2. The right sitting bone will be slightly off the floor, as if you were squatting. When working into the pose and as you hold it, keep that sitting bone as low as possible, but do not collapse back onto the bone forcing it to come to the floor; this compromises the psoas muscle on that side and makes the upward spiraling lift necessary to exit the pose impossible.

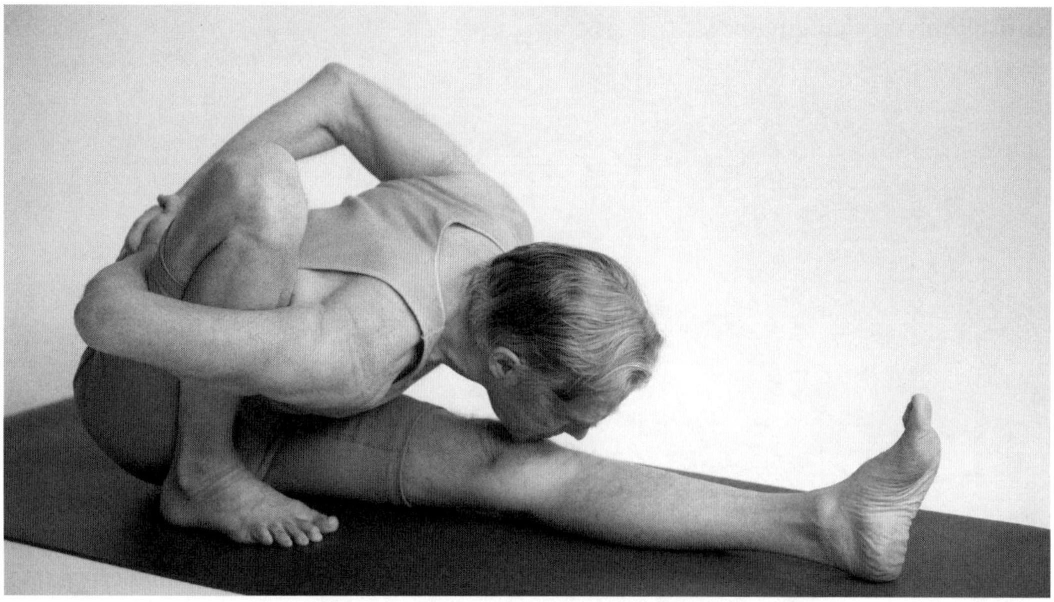

3. On an inhalation, reach up and forward with the right arm. On an exhalation, draw the right kidney area forward as you reach in the direction of the left foot, past the inner right thigh.
4. Lower the right shoulder as much as possible and wrap the right arm around the right leg, clasping your hands behind your back; use a strap if your hands won't reach. Once you have the bind, inhale and pull the clasped hands up the back, bending the right elbow slightly, which will help to keep the heart open. Exhaling, fold forward more deeply to put the chin on your left shin.
5. Gaze at the tip of your nose. If it is difficult to clasp the hands behind the back or to fold forward, gaze along the line of the nose and smooth out the ends of the breath. When the chin reaches the shin, gaze up toward the left big toe. Hold the pose for five breaths. On an inhalation, straighten up out of the fold and release the hands. Either switch sides or go through a Half Vinyāsa before returning to a seated position to do the pose on the other side.

Marīchyāsana B

1. From a seated position with the legs stretched out in front, fold the left knee and place the heel near the upper pubic bone, entering Half Padmāsana. Slowly release the flexion of the Padmāsana foot, and draw the right foot back to place it flat on the floor just outside the right hip, as in Marīchyāsana A.

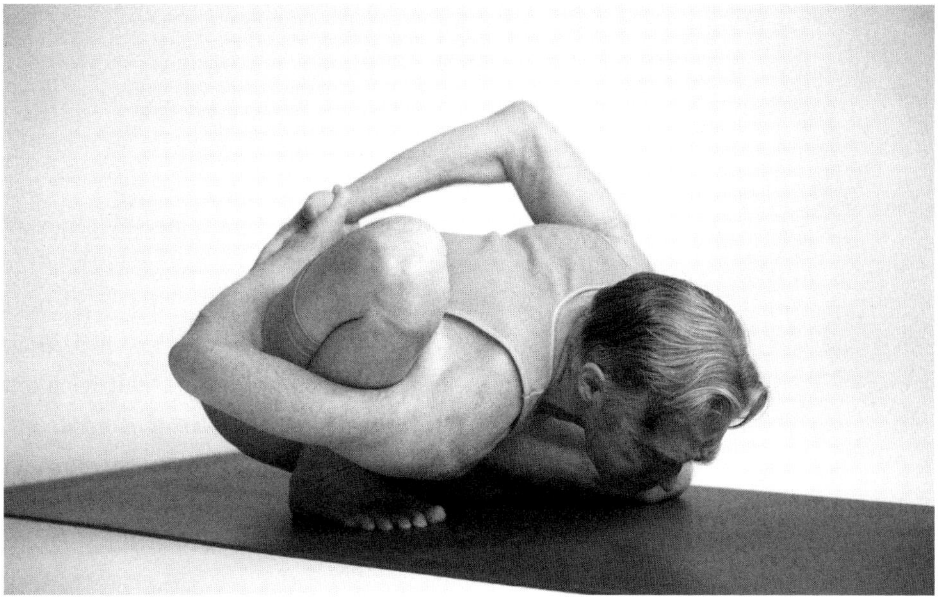

2. Press the left knee down toward the floor. On an inhalation, reach up with the right arm. On the exhalation, fold forward to reach the right arm out and wrap it around the right shin, clasping the hands behind the back.
3. If you cannot fold into Half Padmāsana, you may bend the left knee and place the heel in front of the right sitting bone. The right foot is then placed directly in front of the left ankle, with the right toes pointing forward. You may practice the pose in this form for a while and then gradually introduce the Half Padmāsana as flexibility increases. As with any variation, don't assume this is the final pose for you in this lifetime and become complacent in the form. Push yourself slowly, and gradually the full pose may be possible.
4. Once you are established in the preliminary seated position, inhale to reset the connection to the pelvic floor. On the next exhalation, begin to fold forward with the upper body, drawing the right kidney area toward the inside of the right leg, as in form A.
5. While folding forward, reach through the spine and the crown of the head rather than curling the spine to get the head to the floor. Eventually, your chin will rest comfortably on the floor. When you have reached the limit of your fold, lift the right elbow up and back, drawing the right shoulder slightly back and up behind you, and gaze down the nose. Once the chin comes to the floor, the gaze can be between the eyes. Hold the pose for five breaths. On an inhalation, sit up straight, unravel the legs or place the second leg into Full Padmāsana, and then jump back into Catvāri and complete the Half Vinyāsa to enter the second side (or simply switch sides).

Baddha Koṇāsana A, B, and C

Bound Angle Pose

This pose is one that many people throughout the world assume for sitting in a casual manner or for work, so for some Baddha Koṇāsana is quite easy. In the West, this sitting position is less common. After many years of sitting on furniture, the hips become less flexible, and Baddha Koṇāsana can be challenging. But with patience and practice, the pelvis can become more vertical in this pose, and the hips will slowly open. It may take some time to work into the pose, and it helps to sit in this position as much as possible while doing simple activities. It may take many months of practice for the hip joints to relax enough for the legs to descend, but it's worth the wait.

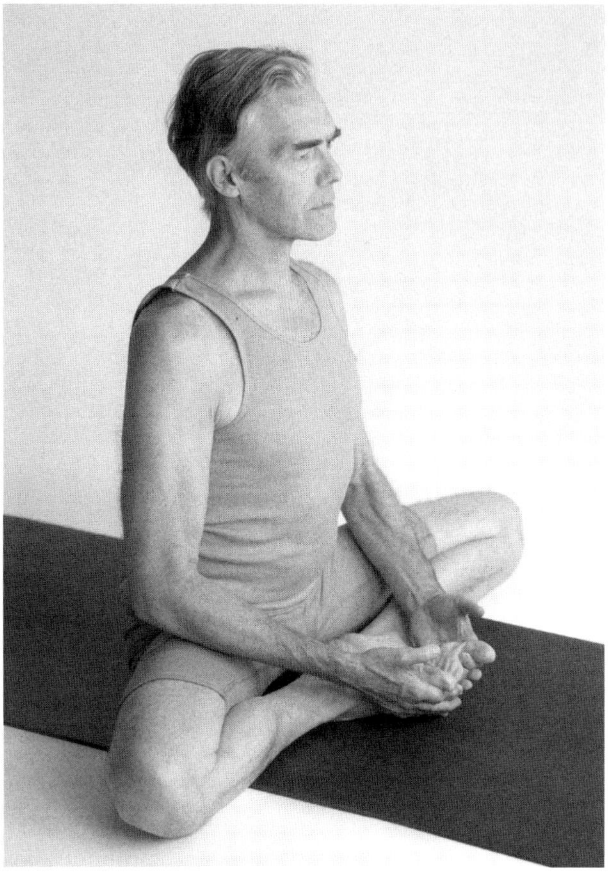

1. From a seated position, bring the heels together about 3 inches in front of the groins. Sit up straight by rolling the pelvis to point the sitting bones straight down to the floor. If you feel that you are falling backward and/or if your knees are more than 6 inches above the floor, place a blanket under the sitting bones to position the pelvis perpendicular to the floor. Rolling the pelvis to vertical is initially more important than bringing your knees down.
2. For form A, have the soles of the feet together and clasp the big toes with the middle and index fingers of each hand. Sit straighter and straighter by first dropping the pubic bone toward the floor and then dropping the coccyx as well. Dropping the pubic bone makes the heart float up (prāṇa); dropping the coccyx makes the kidney area float up (apāna). Ultimately, both patterns are wide awake and active in Baddha Koṇāsana.
3. Soften the tongue and release the palate as you gaze at the tip of the nose, cultivating Uḍḍīyāna and Mūlabandhas. Keep the heart lifted as the knees press gently toward the floor. Stay here for five breaths.
4. To enter form B, open the feet like a book, so the soles of the feet are facing the ceiling. Hollow back the lower belly, scooping out the cave of the sacrum. On an exhalation, with the spine straight via the prāṇa pattern, slowly fold forward to place the belly in the cradle of the feet and the chin on the floor. Gaze between the eyebrows or down the nose to create the internal form of this pose. The gaze should encourage the spine to remain elongating and should create no tension or strain in the neck, face, or jaw. Experiment with the relative "weights" of the coccyx and pubic bone by inverting the feet, pulling and pushing their inner edges away from and into each other. Do not depress the heart. If you cannot place the belly on the feet, maintain the same pattern of a straight spine and an awakened pelvic floor, folding forward just as far as is appropriate for you. Over time, the pose will evolve and deepen. Remain in form B for five breaths.

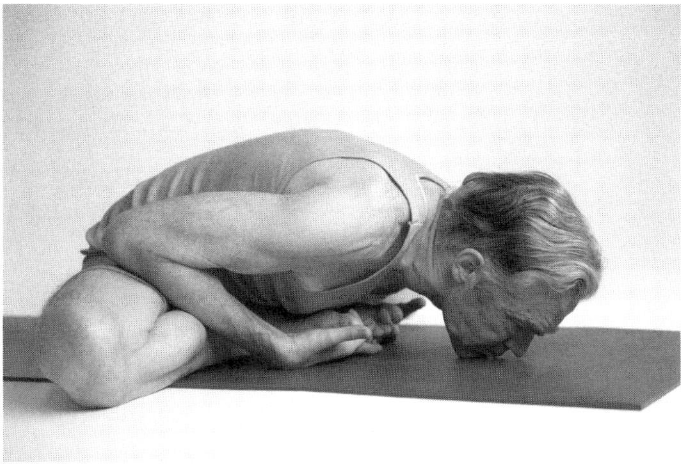

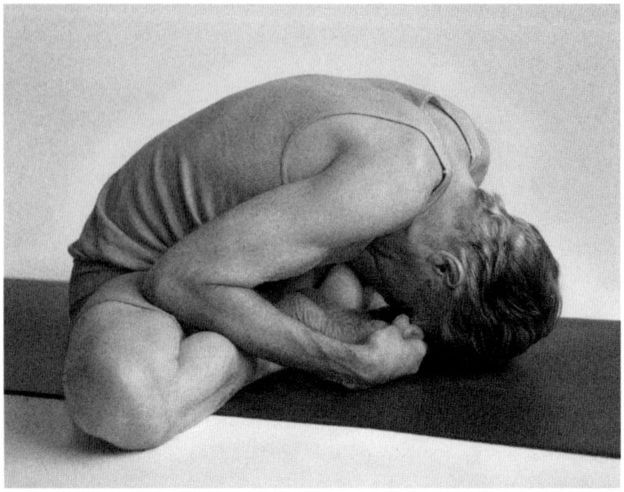

5. To exit, ground the awareness in the sitting bones and imagine that water is running down to the floor through gutters in the edges of your thighs. On an inhalation, with the spine straight and long, return to an upright, seated position based in the pelvic floor.
6. For form C, on an exhalation curl the spine forward, tucking the crown of the head down toward the soles of the feet. Broaden the kidney wings and rest in the pose for five breaths. Exit on an inhale as for form B, then lift up and jump back for a Half Vinyāsa, or simply move into the next pose.

UPAVIṢṬHA KOṆĀSANA (SEATED ANGLE POSE) A AND B

At first glance, this pose seems similar to Prasārita Pādottānāsana with the legs stretched out to the side during a forward bend. But because Upaviṣṭha Koṇāsana is a seated pose, and the feet and legs are not stabilized by the force of gravity from the upper body, the actions and counteractions in the hips, legs, and spine are quite dissimilar. Within the Aṣṭāṅga Vinyāsa system, the following three related forms of this pose are part of the Primary Series and are generally practiced in one flowing sequence.

Upaviṣṭha Koṇāsana A

1. If you are entering the pose from a Half Vinyāsa, jump through to a seated position and open the legs immediately to about a 100- to 120-degree angle. Otherwise, simply sit and open the legs. If you are flexible, do not spread the legs farther than this.
2. If you are less flexible, the pelvis is not vertical, and it is difficult to sit up straight, elevate the pelvis by sitting on a blanket or block. You may also place the hands on the floor behind your back, fingers pointing forward, and then draw your whole spine in and up. Even in this variation, keep the legs active and alive.
3. On an inhalation, as you ground down through the sitting bones, lift the core of the heart and straighten the spine. As you exhale, keep the spine straight and fold forward to clasp the sides of the feet with the hands. If that is not possible, hold your big toes or simply place the hands on the floor out in front of you. You may

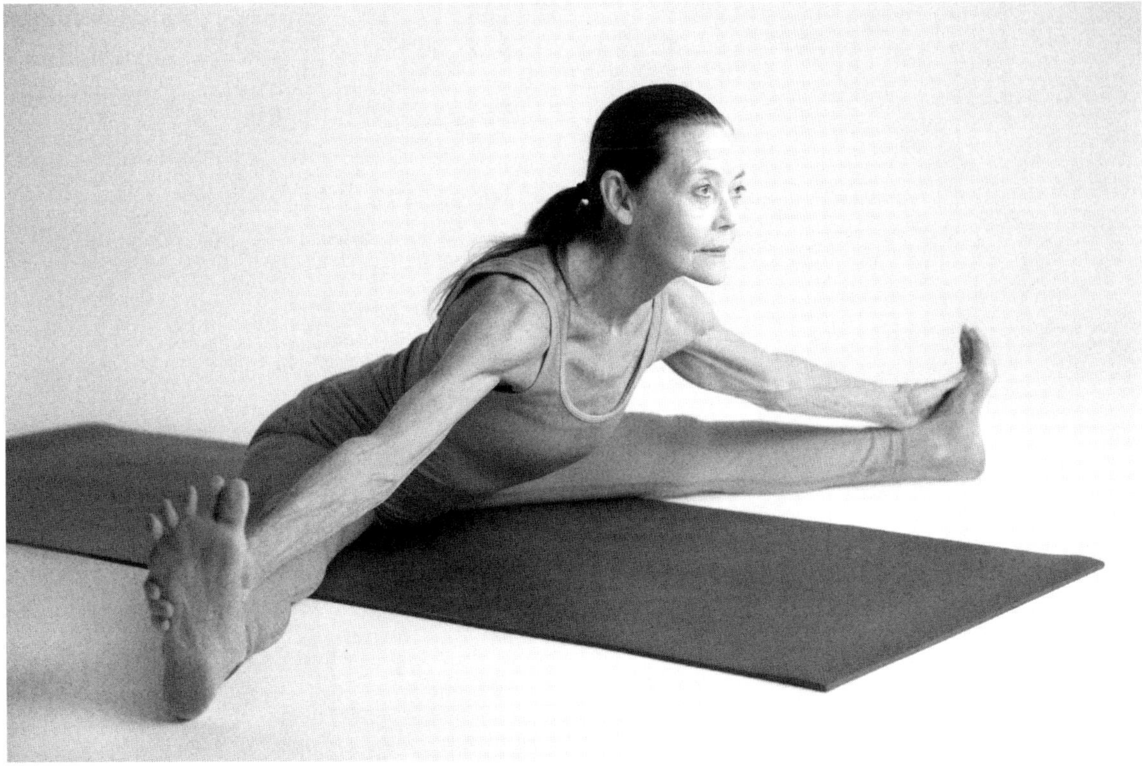

need to decrease the angle between the legs in order to fold correctly or to hold the feet.

4. On the next inhalation, again straighten the spine and pull yourself forward as you straighten the legs completely, drawing the upper inner backs of the knees toward the floor. If the hands are on the floor in front you, gently pull back through the hands toward your thighs, which can help to elongate and to pull the spine forward. Press out through the heels and keep the skin rolling up the front of the torso and pulling down the back of the body.
5. Folding forward, place the belly and then the chin on the floor, maintaining the hollow of Uḍḍīyāna Bandha in the forward bend. Throughout the pose, continue to lengthen the legs through the heels and maintain a grounded sense in the sitting bones. Gaze between the eyebrows. If you cannot fold completely forward, simply breathe into your circumstances, keeping the spine straight and all of the actions and counteractions of the pose awake. In this way, little by little you may find you are much closer to the floor than you ever thought imaginable.
6. Hold the pose for five breaths. On an inhalation, straighten the spine, return to an upright position, and draw the legs together. Either cross the legs and hop back for a Half Vinyāsa, or simply sit up for the next pose.

Upaviṣṭha Koṇāsana B

1. From a seated position with the legs wide (as in form A), reach forward to clasp the big toes. As you exhale, curl the spine forward to puff out your kidney area. Inhale, bend the elbows slightly, and pull back to bounce the calf muscles off the floor and lift the feet into

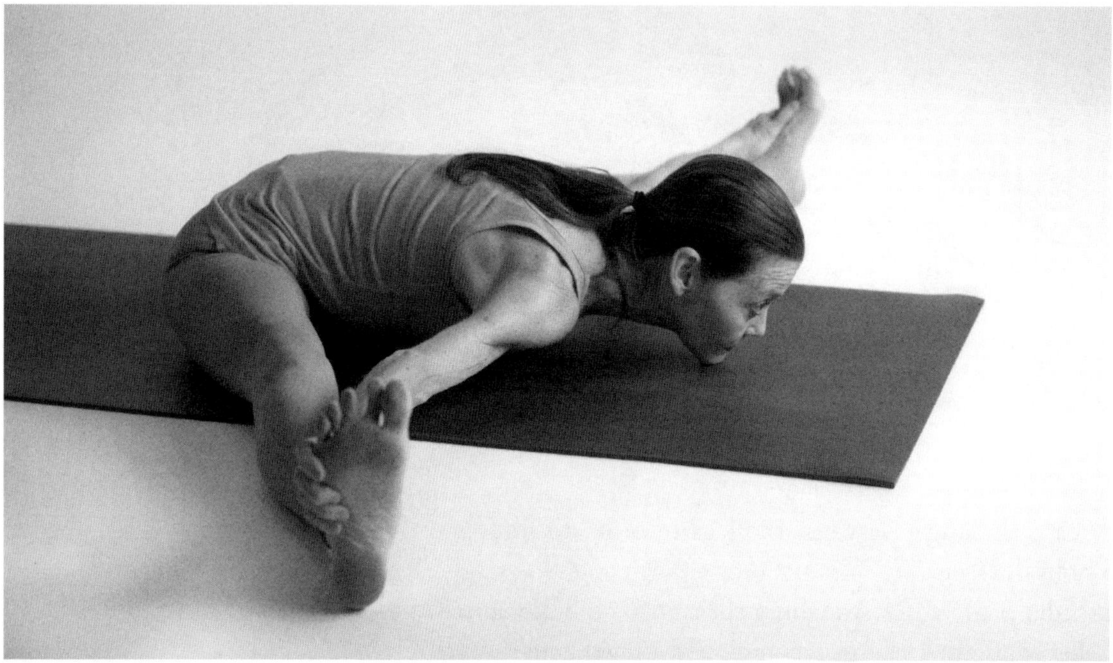

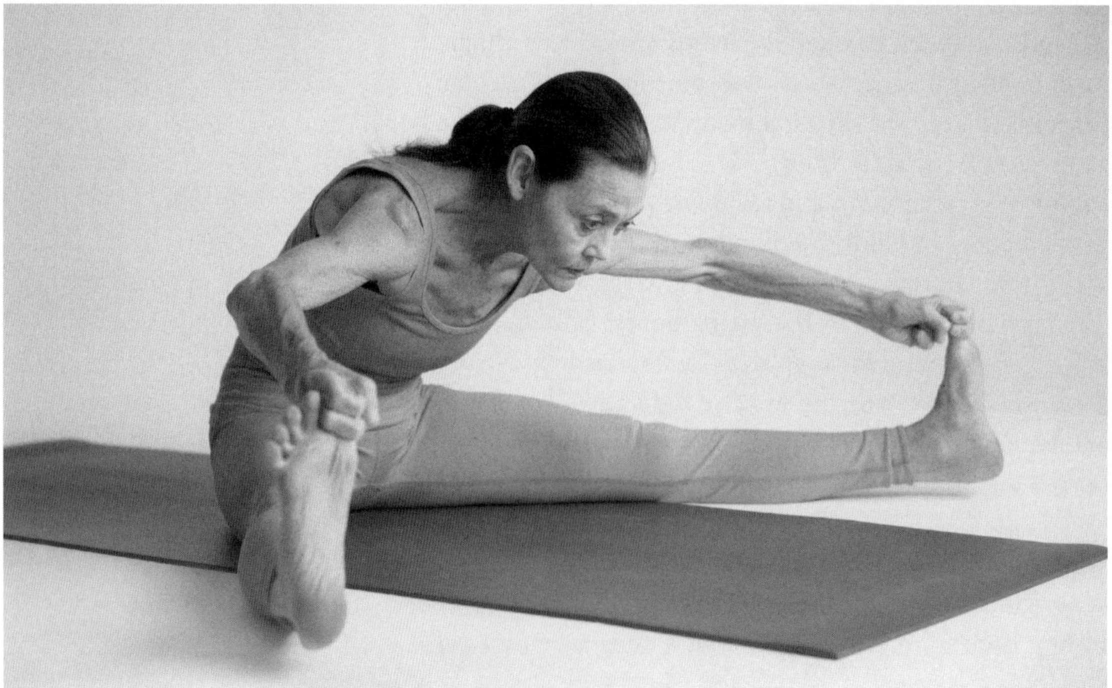

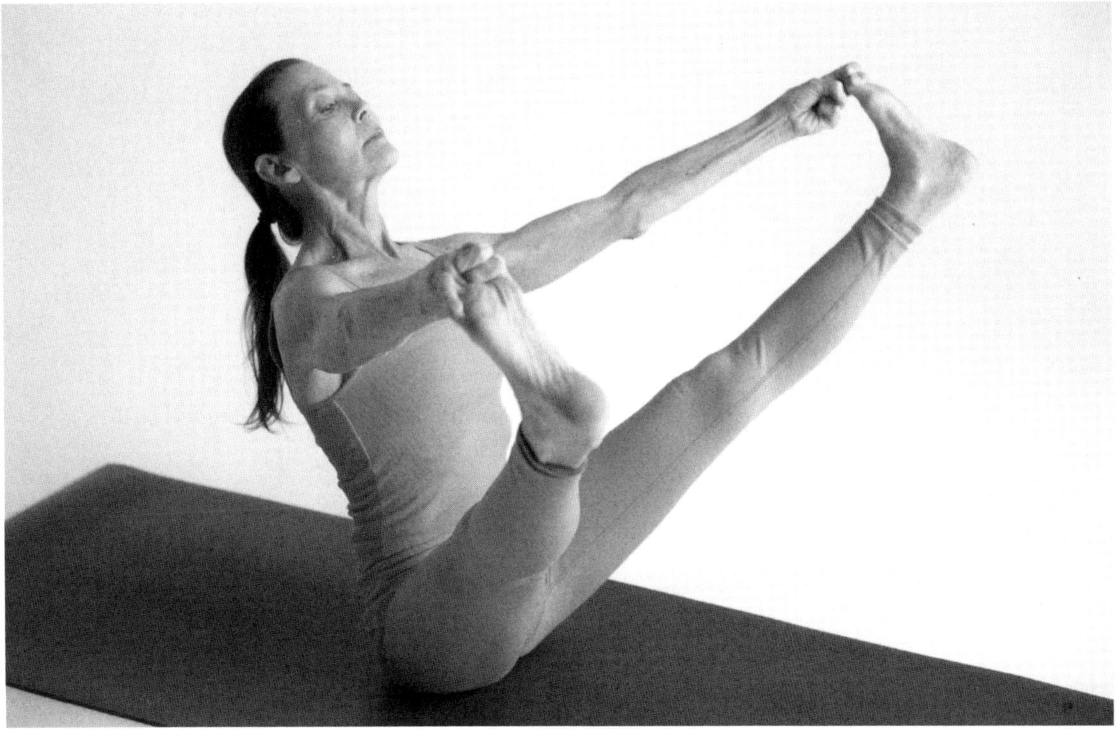

the air maintaining the wide spread of the legs. If this is impossible, try the bouncing action a time or two, then release the toes as you rock back to draw your legs up. Then reclasp your toes.

2. Balance on the back edges of the sitting bones, lifting the heart with the face parallel to the ceiling and gazing down along the line of the nose. Lengthen the inner edges of the legs and arms, lift the front edges of the armpits, and hold this form for five breaths.
3. To exit, on an exhalation drop the legs back down to the mat, cross the legs, and move through a Half Vinyāsa. Or simply take the next pose.

Supta Koṇāsana

Reclining Angle Pose

This version of Upaviṣṭha Koṇāsana begins by going into a wide-legged version of Halāsana (Plough Pose). As you rock up to a seated form, using the breath to control the movement, there is a brief pause before the legs drop gently to the floor. It takes practice, breath awareness, and a trust in the pattern of breath to do the pose correctly without slamming the heels down into the floor. To avoid the fear of hurting your heels while learning this pose, it can help to practice it on a thick carpet or, better yet, on a nice, thick lawn.

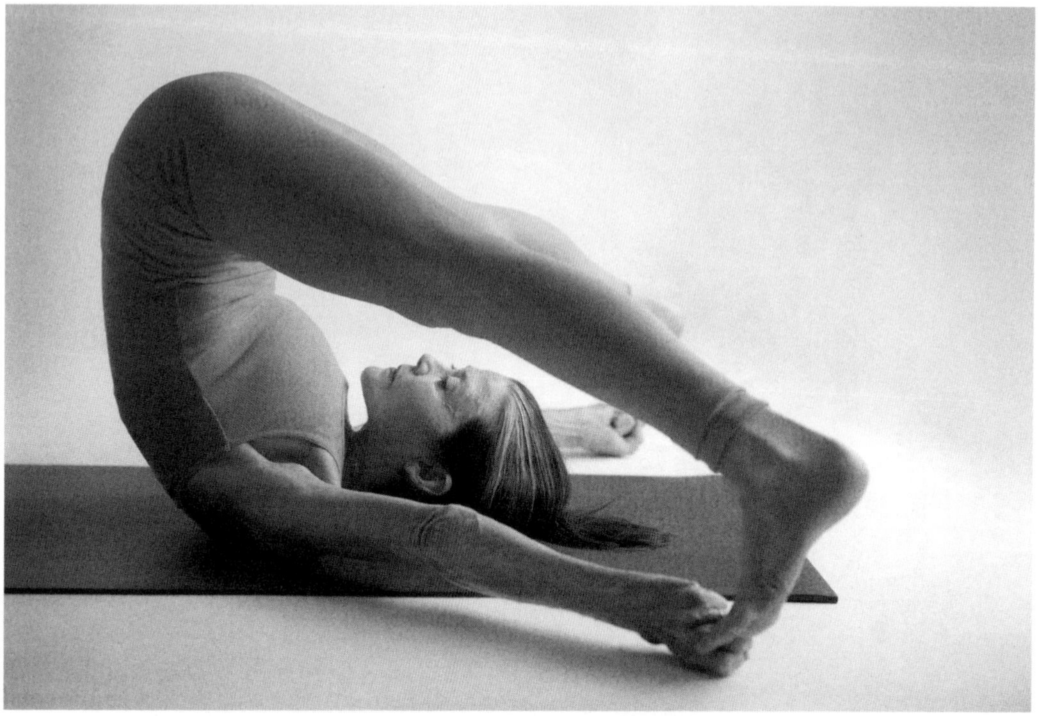

1. Lie on your back with the legs stretched out along the floor in Tāḍāgī Mudrā. At the end of an exhalation, empty of breath, begin to lift the legs, keeping them straight. When they have reached a 30-degree angle from the floor, inhale and continue lifting the hips to bring the feet over the head; place the toes on the floor. Reach the arms over your head as soon as the feet approach the floor, and clasp the big toes with the middle and index fingers of each hand. Spread the feet apart as for Upaviṣṭha Koṇāsana.
2. Gaze at the tip of the nose. Keep the legs straight, the pubic bone drawn up toward the ceiling, the throat soft, and the chin neutral (not pulled into the throat). This is an excellent position for Mūla and Uḍḍīyāna Bandha cultivation.
3. After five breaths in this position, you will rock up to Upaviṣṭha Koṇāsana B and then drop forward into Upaviṣṭha Koṇāsana A with the belly on the floor. To do this, first complete an exhale. Empty of breath and still holding the toes, begin to rock up toward the sitting bones, keeping the legs straight. Partway up, inhale and lift the heart to stop the movement. Do not inhale too soon, or you will not be able to rock up properly. Pause briefly, balancing on the back edges of the sitting bones, keeping the arms and legs straight with face lifted toward the ceiling and gazing gently down the nose. At the peak of the inhalation, in the gap where the breath begins to turn around, drop forward onto the calves, exhaling as you land. By lifting up away

from the floor through the arms and keeping the legs straight as you drop forward, you can avoid dropping heavily onto your heels.

4. These actions assume a lot—that your hamstrings are long enough to flow easily through the movements, and that the actions and counteractions of the prāṇa and apāna patterns are deeply rooted in your nervous system. Practice and patience, along with a sense of humor, eventually make this pose possible.
5. At the end of the exhalation that brought you forward onto the floor, immediately sit back up, release the feet, and through a Half Vinyāsa move into the next pose.

Ubhaya Pādāṅguṣṭhāsana

Two Big Toes Pose

Ubhaya Pādāṅguṣṭhāsana and Ūrdhvā Mukha Paśchimottānāsana are generally practiced in sequence, one immediately following the other. They are similar in that the setup for each is helpful in learning the correct shoulder action for Sarvāṅgāsana (Shoulderstand), and each places a strong emphasis on folding forward. Yet as similar as they are in form, holding the sides of the feet and the extreme fold of Ūrdhvā Mukha Paśchimottānāsana make it considerably more challenging for most practitioners.

1. Lie on the back in Tāḍāgī Mudrā. At the end of an exhalation, when you are empty of breath, begin to lift the legs. Inhale only when they have reached a 30-degree angle from the floor. Keep lifting the legs,

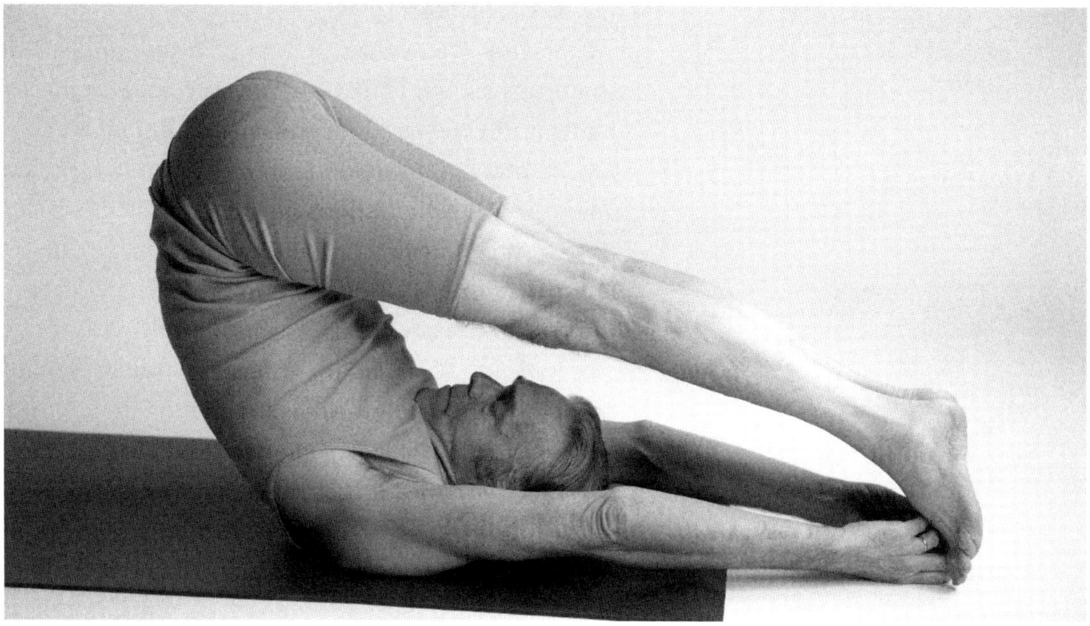

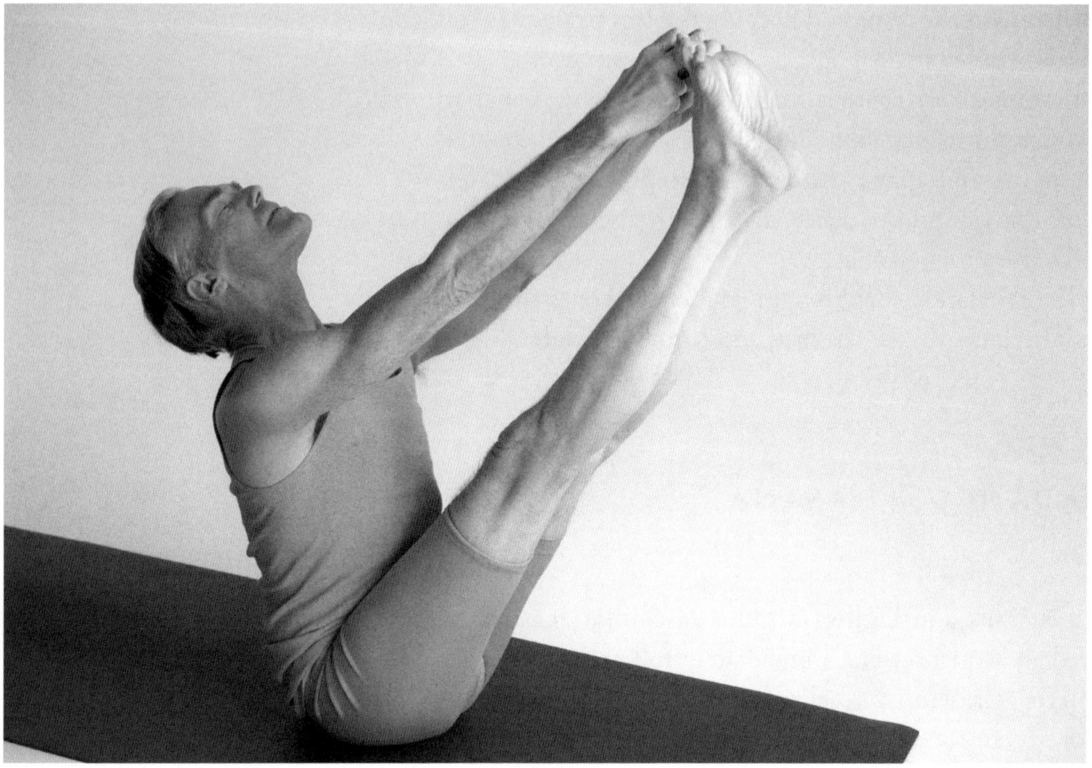

beginning to exhale as the feet are straight up in the air and as the toes come near the floor above your head. Exhale fully and reach up to grab the big toes with the middle and index fingers of each hand.

2. Draw the pubic bone toward the ceiling to straighten the spine and legs. Stay in this position with legs awake, softening the palate and focusing on smoothing out the breath for five breaths. Gaze softly at the tip of the nose.
3. At the end of an exhale, empty of breath and still holding the toes, begin to rock up. Halfway up, inhale, and lift your heart to stop the momentum forward. Keep straightening up through the spine, and also maintain an even pull between the arms and legs so you can balance on the back edges of the sitting bones. Do not curl the spine and rest on the sacrum.
4. Drop the shoulder blades down the back and feel the upward flow of the front surface of the body. Smile softly to empty the palate. The face looks up to the sky, but the gaze follows the line of the nose to the toes. This facilitates a feeling of broadening the skin on the back of the neck and head as the tongue, jaw, and palate soften. Hold this position for five breaths.
5. To exit the pose, on an exhalation, release the toes, cross the legs, and draw the knees up. On the inhalation, lift up and swing back through to Catvāri, then move through Half Vinyāsa to the next pose.

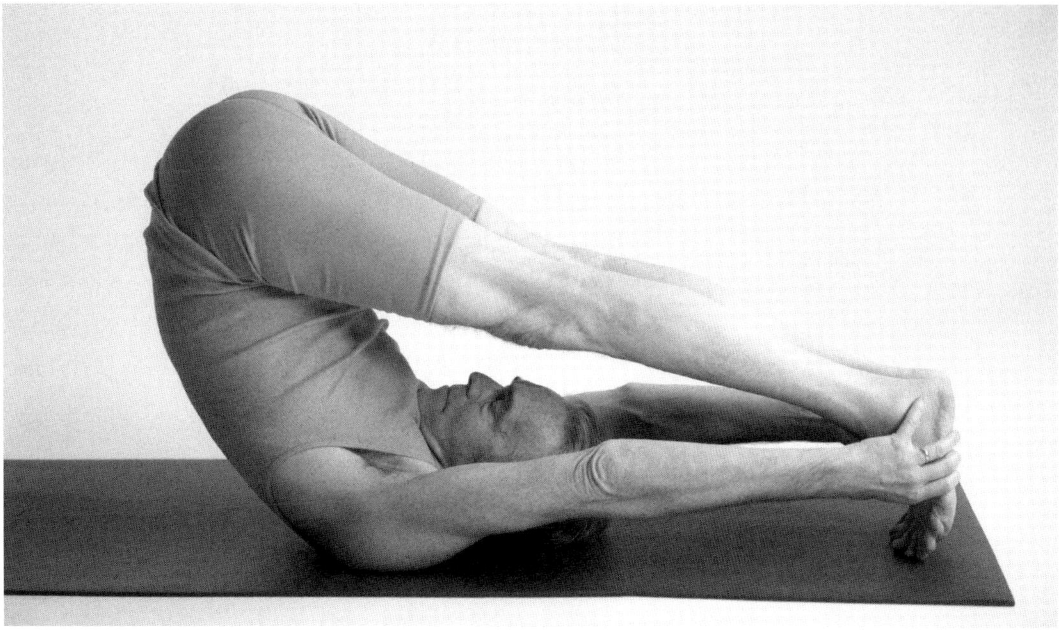

ŪRDHVĀ MUKHA PAŚCHIMOTTĀNĀSANA

Upward-Facing Forward Bend Pose

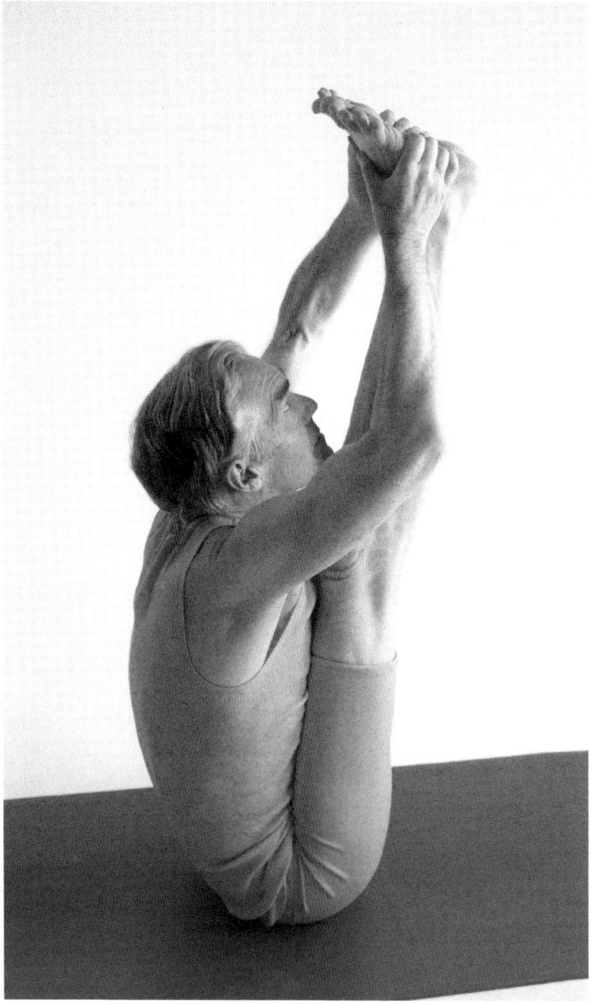

Patience and an acceptance of things as they are is the key to this pose. It is far more difficult to rock up here than in the previous pose, but what's the rush?

1. Enter the pose in the same way as for Ubhaya Pādāṅguṣṭhāsana, lifting the legs up from Tāḍāgī Mudrā and placing the feet on the floor over the head while moving on the wave of the breath. Take hold of the sides of the feet for this form.
2. Rock up and establish the same balance and upward lift as in step 3 of Ubhaya Pādāṅguṣṭhāsana with straight legs and, this time, holding on to the outsides of the feet. Once balanced, bend the arms partially and point the elbows out to the sides without hunching the shoulders.
3. Pull the legs toward a vertical position, and draw the chin toward the ankles. Do not drop the center of your heart. Gaze at the juncture of the big toes or between the eyebrows. Hold this position for five breaths. Then cross the legs and jump back for the Half Vinyāsa.

Nāvāsana

Boat Pose

Nāvāsana is one pose that people love to rush through or skip. But it is an excellent way to build stamina; embody actions and counteractions in the pelvic floor, abdominal muscles, and back; and to build heat within the practice. It's a pose to relish—or at least pretend to enjoy. Remember, *any* pose we want to avoid is most likely the one we should never skip as the mind is always looking to sabotage the practice.

1. Jump through from Downward Facing Dog Pose to land in a seated position with the legs lifted into the air at about a 45-degree angle from the floor. Or you may begin in a seated position and simply lift the legs. Be sure to balance on the back edges of the sitting bones in a way that makes you distinctly aware of the coccyx.
2. As you lift the legs, ground fully through the coccyx. Use the actions described in Chapter 3 for holding the tail of the serpent to stabilize

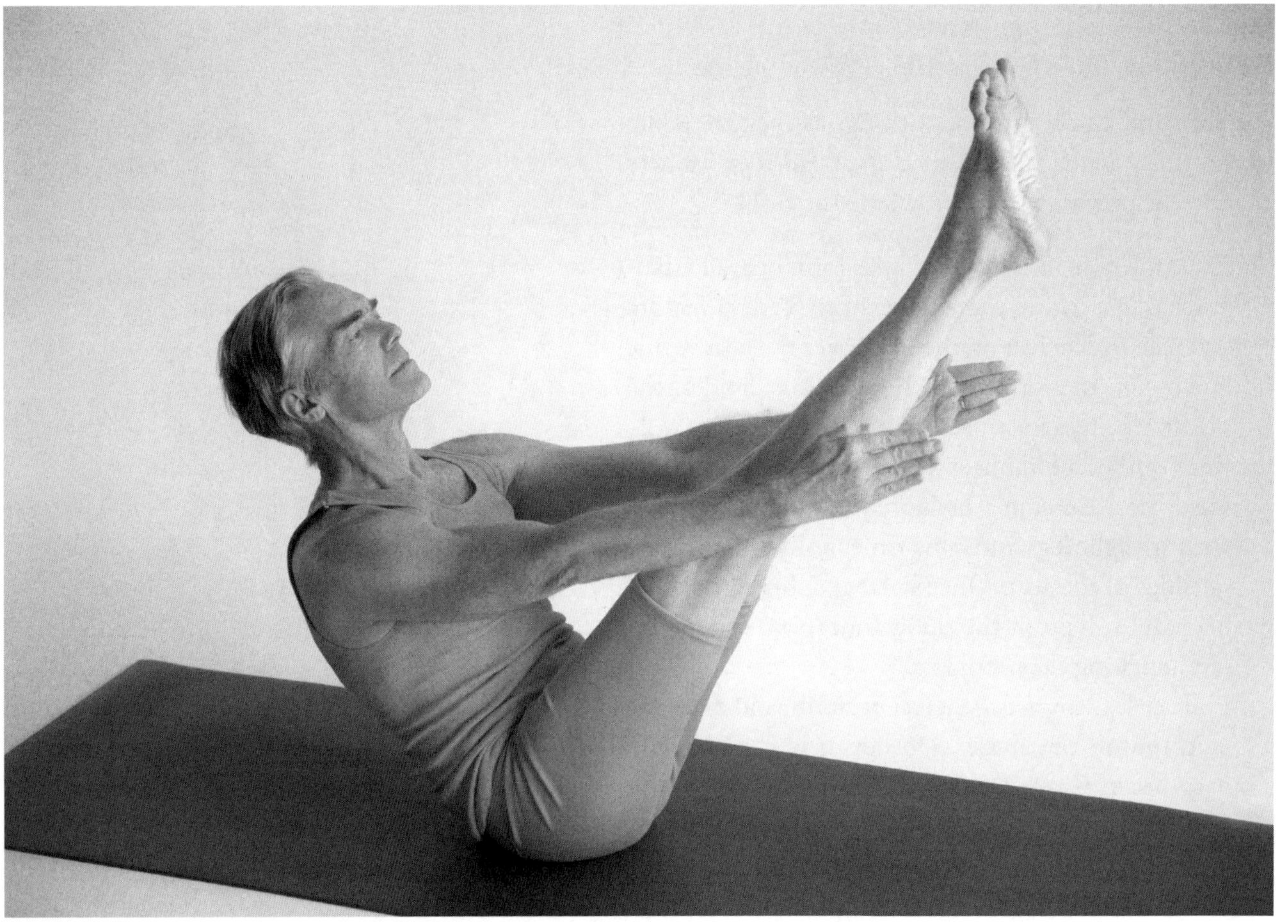

the base of the body and give you a point from which to extend through the core.

3. The legs should be strong, with a sense of pushing forward through them. Reach forward through the hands to straighten the arms on either side of the legs in front of you with the palms facing; keep the arms parallel to the floor.
4. Keep the heart lifted, the fronts of the armpits high, and the shoulder blades low. The abdominal muscles are toned, but the muscles that run along the spine—the erector spinae muscles—do not engage firmly. This will keep your spirits up even through five repetitions.
5. Press the inner edges of the feet forward, straightening the legs and gazing at the juncture of the big toes. After five breaths, lean forward, bend the knees to cross the legs on the exhalation. Inhale as you lift the buttocks off the floor and rock forward to balance on your hands as if to jump back, but then sit back down. When lifting, keep the shoulder blades flowing down the back. Advanced students can press up into Adho Mukha Vṛkṣāsana (Downward Facing Pose or a Handstand) between each set instead of simply lifting the buttocks off the floor.
6. Repeat Nāvāsana and the lift five times. After the fifth repetition, inhale and swing back through, exhaling into Catvāri for Half Vinyāsa, or proceed to the next pose.

Ardha Nāvāsana

Half Boat Pose

This version of Nāvāsana is good for training the apāna pattern, which can help eliminate lower back and SI joint pain.

1. Start in full Nāvāsana. On an exhalation, curl back so you are balanced on the sacrum, then lower straight legs until the heels are about 6 inches from the floor. Keep the head up, gazing at the toes.
2. At the same time, lower the shoulders to about 6 inches from the floor. Reach the arms along the sides of the body with hands resting on the sides of the thighs; the chin will be on or near the sternum.
3. Hold this pose for at least five breaths. It's easy to imagine the coccyx and sitting bones lengthening to become a long, strong dragon's tail. The abdominal muscles are strong and the PC muscle tones as the legs lengthen and reach out long.
4. At the end of an exhalation, lift the chest, straight legs, and feet, and inhale as you return to full Nāvāsana. This is like a straight-legged

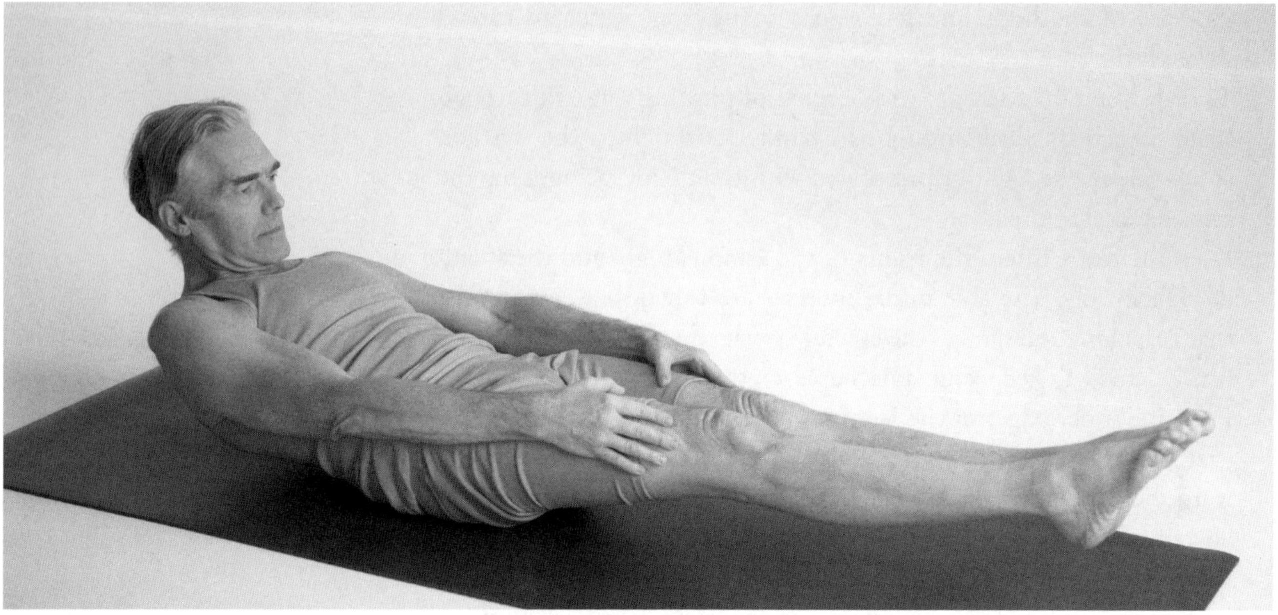

sit-up, so it takes focus and toning in the pelvic floor at the end of the initial exhalation. Cross the legs as for Nāvāsana and proceed through a Half Vinyāsa to carefully lengthen the abdominal muscles in Upward Facing Dog Pose.

Supta Hasta Pādāṅguṣṭhāsana

Reclining Hand-to-Big-Toe Pose

Very similar to Utthita Hasta Pādāṅguṣṭhāsana, this pose doesn't require the same balance. Both forms allow a clear focus on the rotation of the femur in the hip socket and the actions and counteractions that facilitate this movement. It is also important to pay attention to the rotations of the pelvis in relation to the straightened leg as it is dropped over to the side.

1. Lie on the back in Tāḍāgī Mudrā. At the end of an exhalation, empty of breath, lift the straightened right leg and take hold of the big toe with the middle and index fingers of the right hand. If you can't reach the toe, loop a strap around your foot and hold the ends with your right hand. Bend the right arm, bowing it out to the side in a plane perpendicular to the end of the mat. As you begin to sit up, wrap the left kidney toward the right thigh and pull the chin to the shin.
2. Keep the left arm straight, with the palm along the top of the left thigh. The left leg is straight with the toes pointed and the heel pushing into the floor.

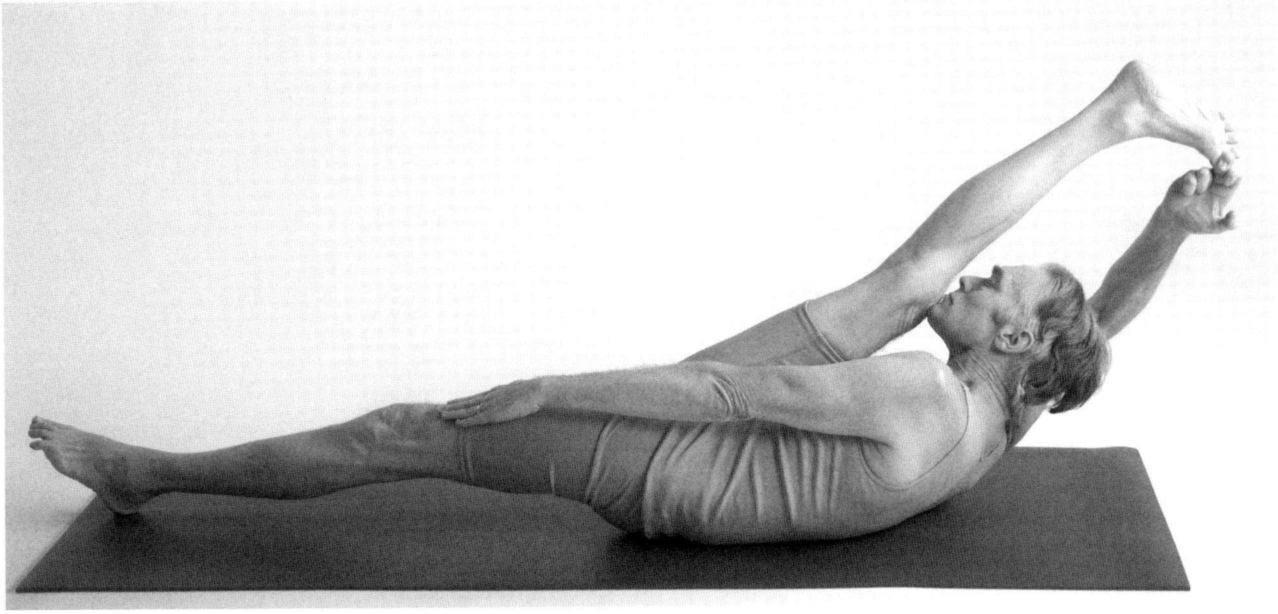

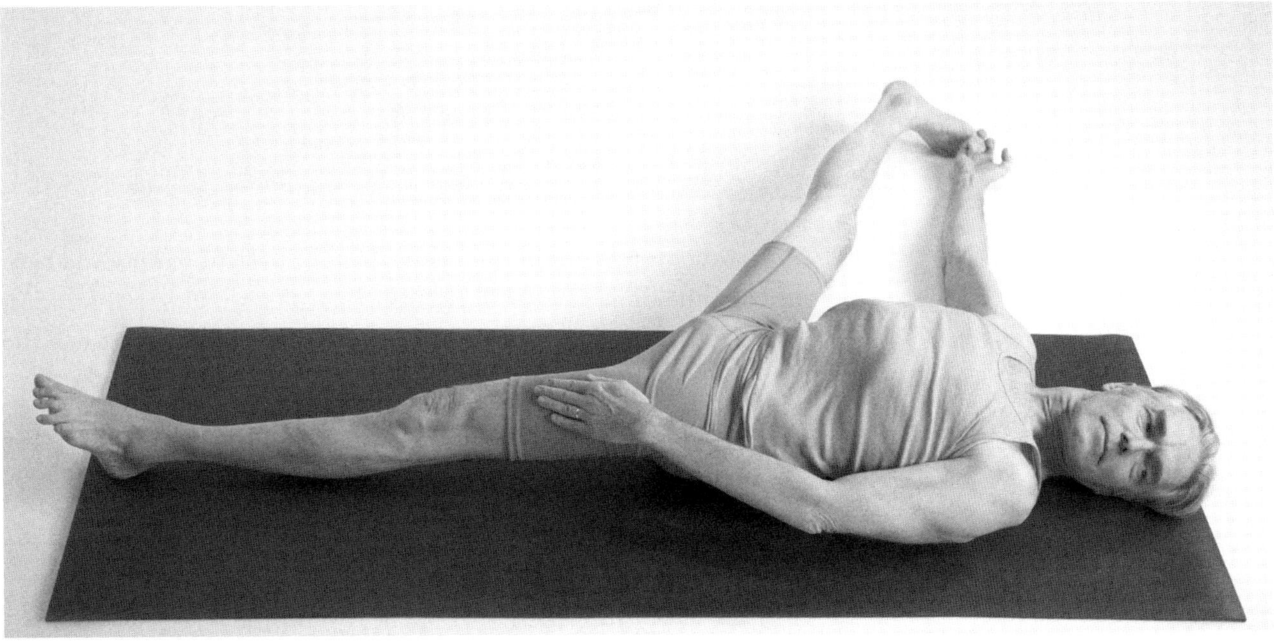

3. As you wrap the left kidney area toward the right knee, resist the pull of the arm through the leg by pushing the right heel toward the floor. Keep both shoulder blades flowing evenly down the back. (Advanced students can try lifting the back entirely off the floor.) Gaze along the line of the nose, and hold the position for five breaths.
4. Lower the head to the floor on an inhalation, then open the right leg out to the side on the exhalation. Keep the right arm slightly bowed as you lower the leg to the floor (use a strap to hold the foot if necessary, but still hold the strap with just the right hand). As the leg descends,

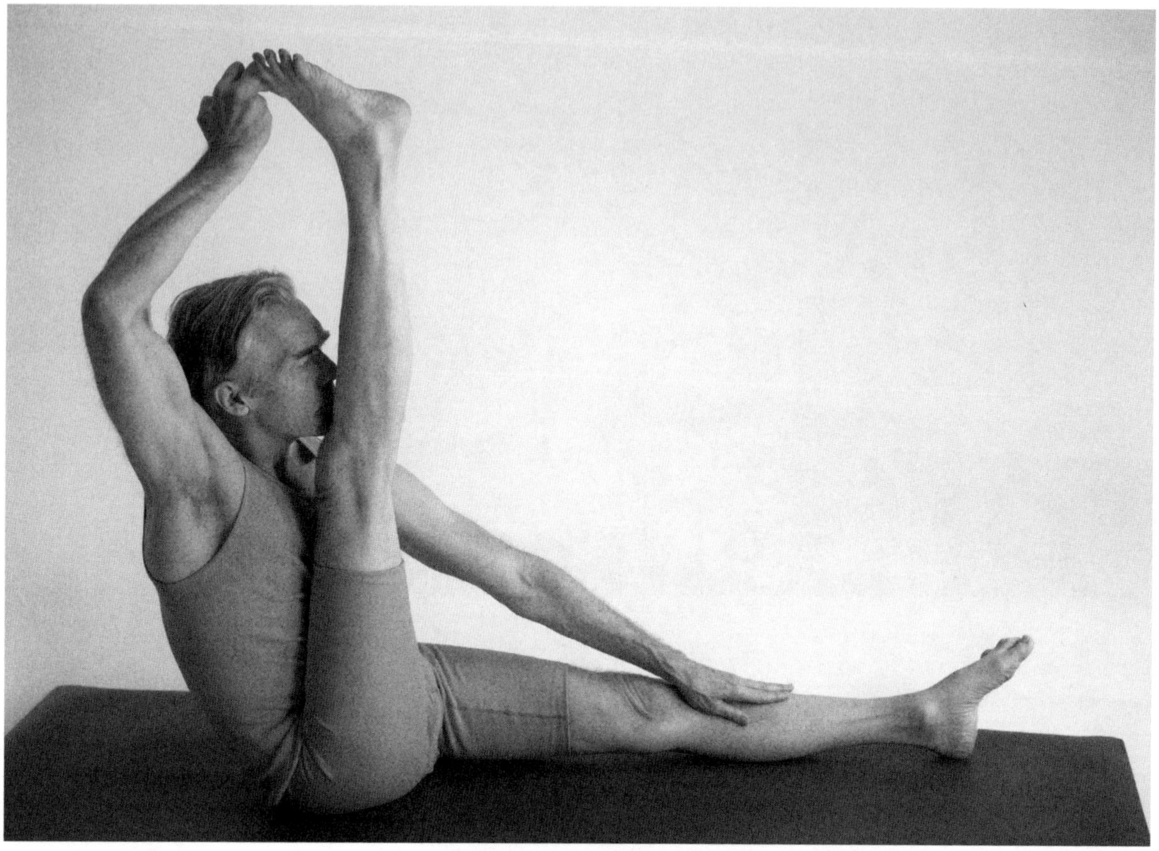

the toes come toward the floor first, then the heel drops once you have reached the limit of your flexibility. This allows the proper rotation of the top of the femur in the hip joint. If the foot does not reach the floor, no problem. Simply breathe into the sensations along the midline of the body.

5. Once the right leg is in place, accentuate the reach out and down through the left leg to even out the hips. Do not lock the pelvis as you enter the pose; the safest vinyāsa for entering this second phase of the pose with leg out to the side is to allow some mobility (and possibly a lifting away from the floor) of the hip on the straight-leg side of the body.
6. Turn the head to the left and gaze at a point along the line of the floor. Keep the right shoulder rolled back toward the floor with the right buttock down as well. Continue to reach out and down through the left foot. The key is to move evenly from the area 2 inches below the navel.
7. Hold this position for five breaths. Using the strength of the arm and lower belly, inhale and draw the right leg back up to center. As you exhale, lift the chin toward the shin and bow to the leg again, for one breath. Inhale and drop the head back to the floor.

8. Exhaling, lower the right leg down next to the left leg on the floor and repeat the pose on the other side. To exit the left side and the full pose, return to Tāḍāgī Mudrā, then flow through Cakrāsana and complete Half Vinyāsa in preparation for the next pose.

Garbha Piṇḍāsana

Embryo in the Womb Pose

To those who are not familiar with yoga, particularly the Primary Series, Garbha Piṇḍāsana may appear to be the most bizarre of all poses. It *is* quite unusual and can be challenging, but it's fun! The full form requires a safe Padmāsana and relies entirely on getting the correct vinyāsa of breath. Possibly one of the most beneficial aspects to this pose is that it is difficult, if not impossible, for the mind to wander, especially during the rocking phase of the pose. It is excellent training for learning to trust the intelligence of the breath while working through subtle layers of movement within the body.

1. From a straight, seated position, bring the feet into Padmāsana. Use the hands to draw the right foot back, bringing the heel toward the lower left side of the belly. Press the right knee toward the floor using

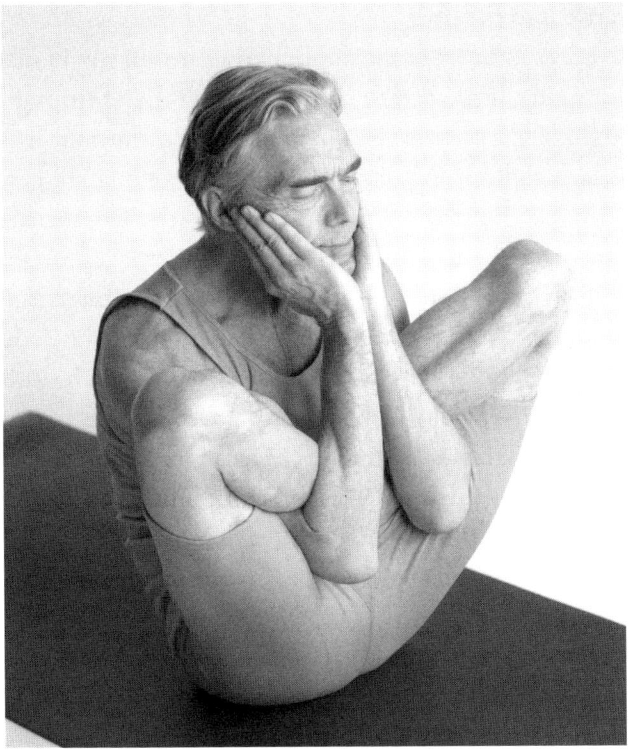

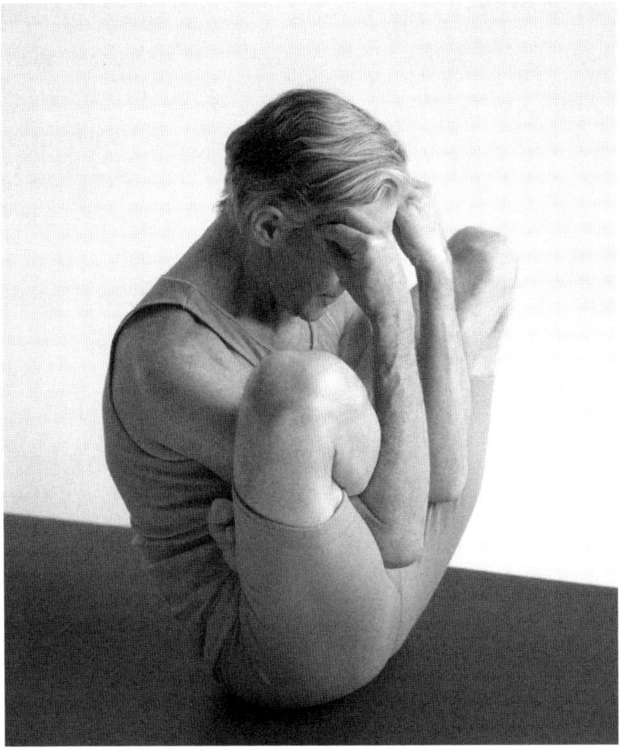

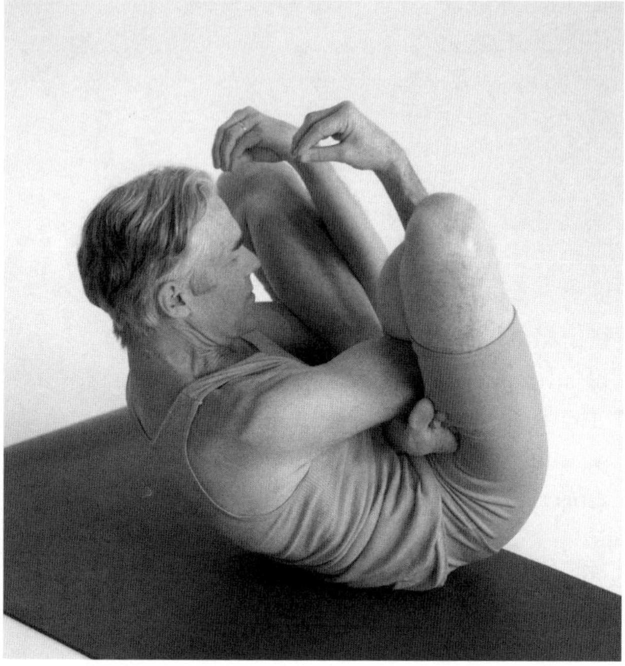

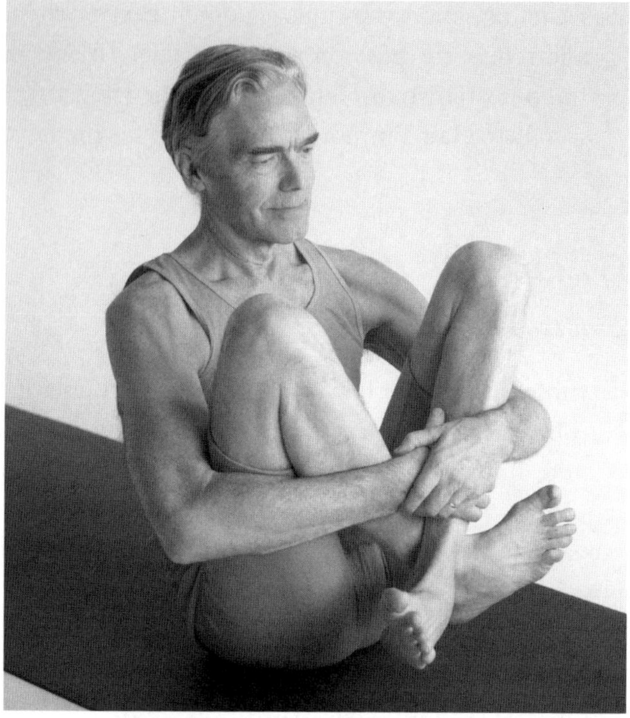

the hip muscles. Next draw the left foot in over the right leg, bringing the heel toward the lower right side of the belly so you are in Padmāsana. Once in Padmāsana at first, flex the feet so the ankles do not collapse. If you cannot manage Padmāsana, then just cross your legs. Exhale to settle into the pose.

2. Exhaling, lift the knees away from the floor, folding at your hip joints. On the next few rounds of the breath thread the right hand through the gap on the right side between the upper thigh and the calf. It is helpful to keep the hand flat. Move at an angle approximately parallel to the left shin so that the right thumb grazes the left shin as you push the arm through. When the forearm is halfway through, turn the palm of the hand toward your face to complete the insertion. Next, thread the left hand through the gap in the left side of the body between the upper thigh and the calf. Push both arms through until the elbows are beyond the shins. Use water to lubricate your skin if the arms don't slide through easily. Hold your face with hands cupped beneath the chin, gazing at the tip of the nose for five breaths.
3. If you are unable to assume Padmāsana and have crossed your legs, fold at the hip joints to lift the knees and wrap the arms around the outsides of the knees. Clasp the hands together and draw the knees in toward your chest, then hold for five breaths.
4. On an exhalation, rock backward onto your upper back while maintaining a curled spine and keeping the hands tucked in toward the

forehead. On the next inhalation, rock partway up, approximately to the sacrum, using the abdominal muscles to navigate a turn to the right. Repeat this rocking and turning nine times to make a complete circle. On the final inhalation, rock forward onto the hands and into Kukkuṭāsana (or with the hands on the floor outside the upper thighs if you are not in Padmāsana). Hold for five breaths with the face lifted and gazing down the line of the nose.

KUKKUṬĀSANA

Cock Pose

This arm balance is typically practiced immediately following Garbha Piṇḍāsana and relies fully on coordinating the wave of the breath with the pattern of movement within the form. You must exhale fully as you rock back to facilitate an inhalation that is grounded enough in both the core of the body and the pelvic floor to bring you up to balancing.

1. Enter the pose from step 4 of Garbha Piṇḍāsana; you are still in Padmāsana with the arms through your legs and the hands on the floor in front of the upper shins. On the inhalation and the final rock, continue to draw your chest and hips forward and up to balance on the hands in Kukkuṭāsana. The hands should be flat on the floor and well articulated, the arms straightening, and sitting bones lifted off the floor. Turn the head up, and focus the gaze slightly down along the line of the nose.
2. If when rocking you were unable to balance on the hands, sit back down, lift the knees as you exhale to rock forward. As the hands come to the floor work the abdominal muscles to lift the legs and buttocks off the floor. Inhale and look between the eyebrows when the center of gravity comes over the hands.
3. If you are not in Padmāsana after completing Garbha Piṇḍāsana, rock forward and lift the buttocks off the floor, balancing on the hands. Lift the face toward the ceiling while gazing down along the line of the nose for five breaths, then lower down to sit on the floor.

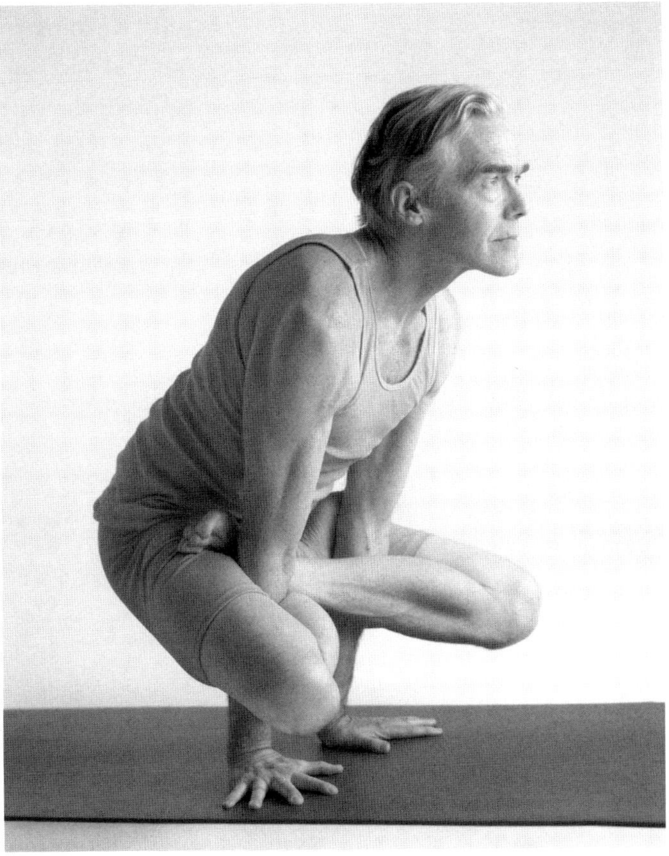

4. Remove the arms from between the legs. Move through a Half Vinyāsa either keeping the legs in Padmāsana or uncrossing the legs before jumping back.

Kūrmāsana

Turtle Pose

The turtle figures prominently in Indian mythology as the support of the universe. Like other āsanas named after animals, it can be helpful in Kūrmāsana to imagine yourself as a turtle with the curve of the back and the arms around the body representing the turtle's shell. This pose requires considerable flexibility in the hips and spine. It is one that also demands patience and consistency to move into fully. Nonetheless, if you take it step-by-step, the form unfolds with time.

1. At the end of an exhale jump forward from Downward Facing Dog Pose so the feet land on the floor outside the arms, with the thighs beginning to wrap around the arms. Sit down.
2. Hook the inner knees as high up on the arms as possible, exhaling, and allow the feet to be out in front and just a little wider than the hips. Keeping the arms threaded under the legs, straighten the arms out and back on the floor with the palms facing down. Be careful not to place the thighs directly on the elbow joints, particularly if your elbows tend to hyperextend. Work the pose so there is no strain in any joints.
3. As you exhale, gradually push through the heels to extend the legs forward and out to the sides slightly until they are flat on the floor.

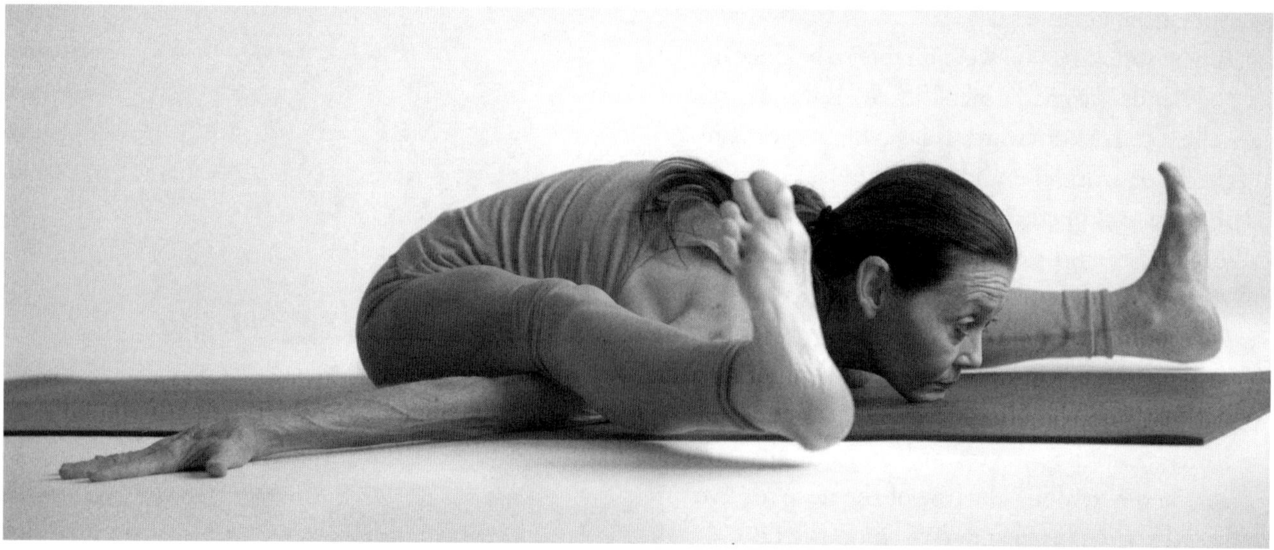

The feet will move apart as this movement deepens, and the chest will automatically drop toward the floor.

4. When the belly is on the floor (or you have reached your limit of flexibility), gaze up between the eyebrows to maintain the internal lift of the heart. By straightening the legs as much as possible, the heels will eventually pop up off the floor automatically.
5. Hold this position for five breaths. On an inhalation, release the pose and return to a seated position. Release the arms and unwrap the legs, then move directly into Supta Kūrmāsana.

Supta Kūrmāsana

Reclining Turtle Pose

This pose represents a turtle withdrawing into its shell and into the calming flexion of the spine and a strong expression of the apāna pattern. It appears in the Primary Series and is an excellent preparatory pose for those working toward the Eka Pāda family of poses.

1. Reclining, with the legs wrapped around the upper arms and bent at 90-degree angles, bring the heels together and cross the right ankle over the left.
2. Rotate the arms inward. Drop the shoulders to reach the arms under the thighs and around the back. Clasp the hands behind the back, pulling them up the spine. Gaze at the tip of the nose, and hold this form for five breaths.
3. If you are a beginning student, you can work with the pose by simply bringing the heels together instead of crossing them. Then reach the

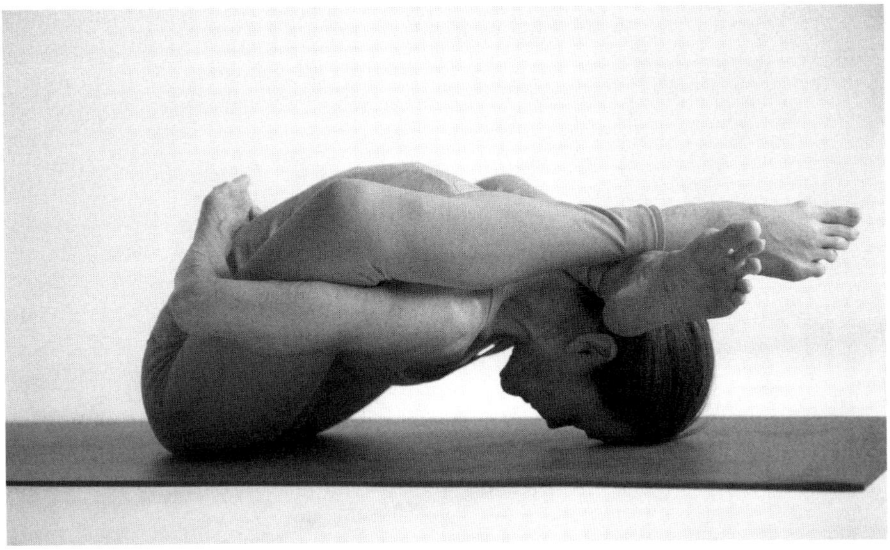

arms under the thighs, reaching out and slightly back behind you (as far as flexibility allows) and if possible touch your head to the floor. If you are an advanced student, you can cross the ankles or shins behind the head or neck while sitting (as in Dvi Pāda Śīrṣāsana) and then lower forward to the floor. In this case, look between the eyebrows.

4. Hold the pose for five breaths. To exit either release the hands and use them to push yourself up to seated, lift up, unravel the legs, and come into Ṭiṭṭibhāsana, then move through Bakāsana into Catvāri, or simply release hands and ankles, sit up, and jump back into Catvāri. From Catvāri unroll into Pañca, and then roll back into Ṣaṭ.

Eka Pāda Śīrṣāsana

One Foot Behind the Head Pose

For many Aṣṭāṅga Vinyāsa practitioners, the Eka Pāda family (which actually begins with Kūrmāsana in the Primary Series) is both daunting and strangely attractive—like those relatives who are eccentric and nobody outside the family can really tolerate or understand, but everyone in the family loves. These Eka Pāda poses can be considered forward bends in that they involve extreme flexion in both the hip joints and the spine.

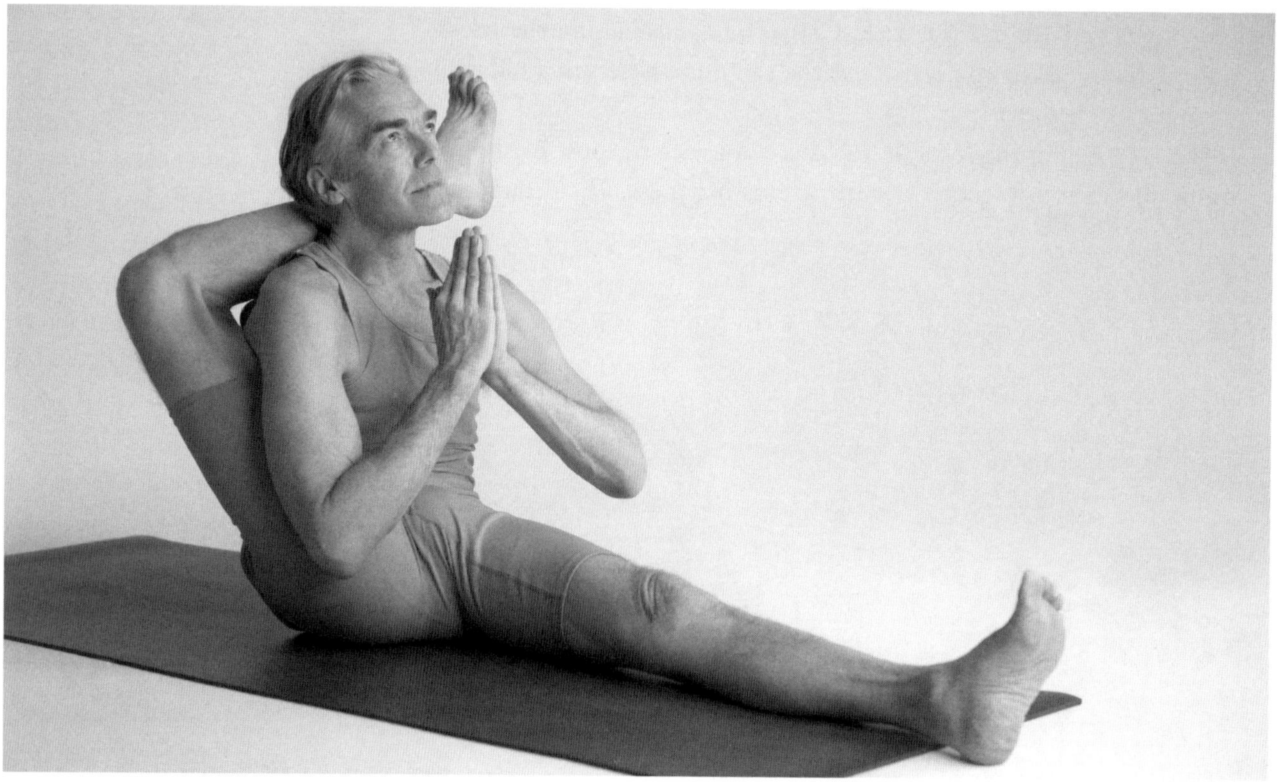

It is important to work slowly and in stages to keep the lower back safe. Although for first-timers it can be a thrill to get the leg behind the head, blowing out a disk to do so is not worth it. Be patient and work only to your limit, without pain and with great integrity.

1. From Downward Facing Dog Pose on an exhale, hop forward to a seated position with the right thigh wrapped around the right arm. Or simply begin the pose from a seated position and wrap the leg around the arm. Roll back on the pelvis, bending the right knee to take the right foot in your arms, as if cradling a baby. Leave the left leg stretched out in front of you, but do not rigorously engage that leg or foot while working into the pose.
2. Lace the right arm under the right thigh, rolling the right calf toward the back of the body, and as you exhale work the leg as far up the arm as possible. On another exhale, take the right shin behind the neck, and position the foot near the left shoulder, toes pointing to the ceiling.
3. Keep the spine flexing and the outer right hip relaxed, with the abdominal muscles toned but not fully engaged. Deepen the position of the leg by working the right shoulder down and through beneath the calf. Twisting the upper body to the left and pulling with the right hand on the left thigh can facilitate this.
4. Once the leg is in position, inhale and sit up a little more straight, then straighten the left leg by reaching out through the mound of the left big toe to create an inward rotation in the leg. Fold the hands in front of the heart in Añjali Mudrā. Gaze softly along the line of the nose at a point on the floor, and hold the position for five breaths.

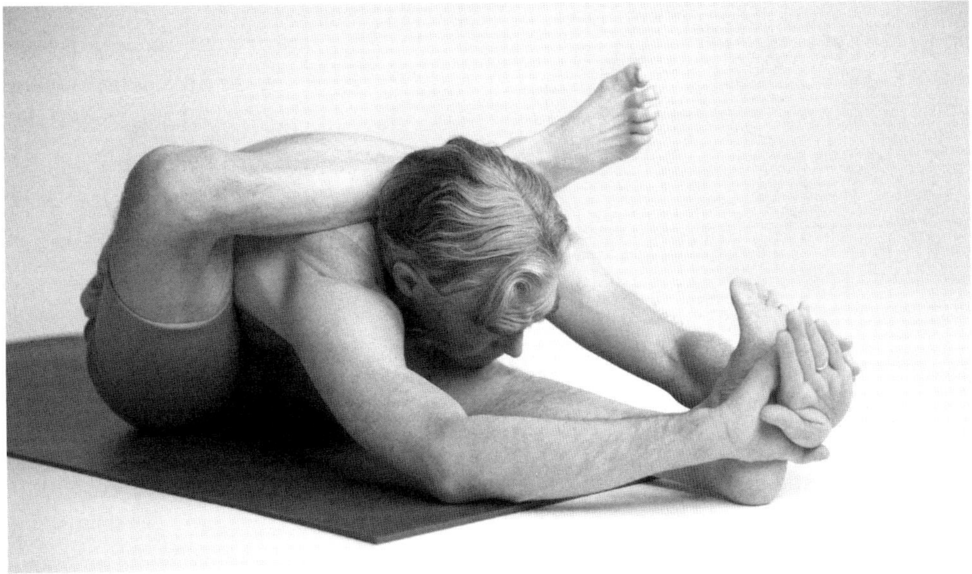

5. Release the mudrā, and on an exhalation, fold forward to place the chin on the left shin, stretching the arms out in front and clasping the left wrist with the right hand beyond the left foot. Gaze along the line of the nose or at the left big toe as you hold the position for five breaths.
6. On an inhalation, release the clasp of the hands and sit up. Exhale and with the right leg still behind the head, place the hands beside the hips. On the next inhalation, lift the hips up off the floor, pointing the left leg straight up with toes pointing to the ceiling and gazing at the left toes. On the following exhalation, swing back into Catvāri, then move through a Half Vinyāsa before doing the pose on the other side.

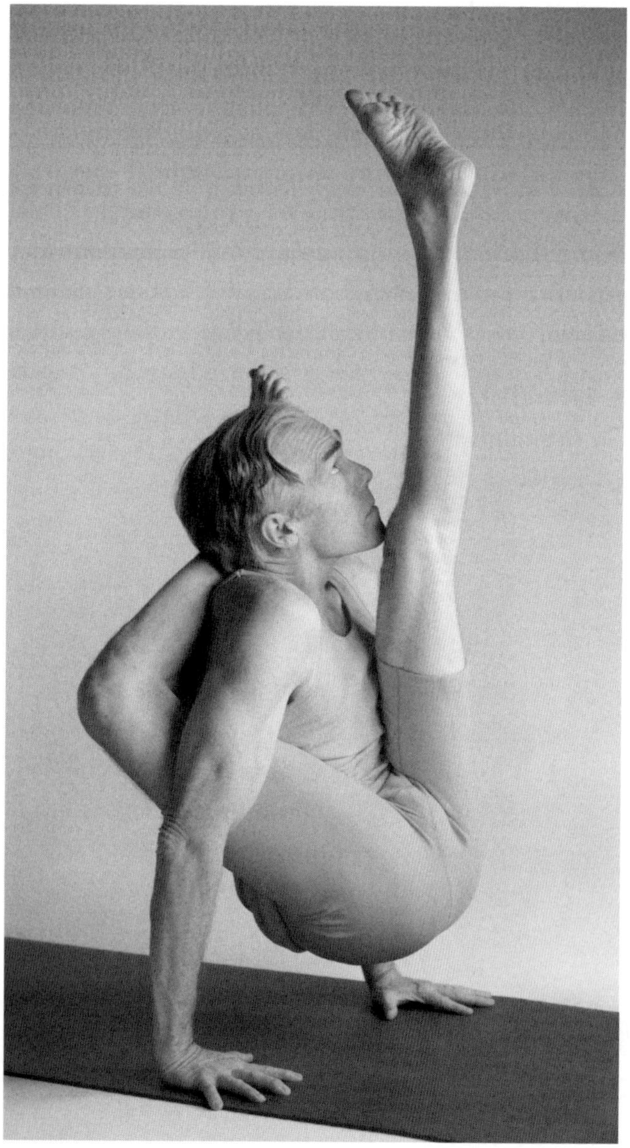

Cakorāsana

Moonbeam-Drinking Bird Pose

This pose strongly contracts the abdominal muscles and gives a sense of lengthening and complete action in the pelvic floor and coccyx. At the same time, it opens the heart so that it floats upward with the prāṇa opening fully in the presence of strong apāna. Cakorāsana is used as a transition when moving out of many poses in the Eka Pāda family and is also a separate pose in and of itself.

1. Follow steps 1 through 3 for Eka Pāda Śīrṣāsana, with the right leg behind the head. Bring the chest forward and draw the right leg down behind the lower neck so the neck can straighten and the head can roll back.
2. Place the hands on the floor next to the hips and exhale completely. While empty of breath, lift the hips up off the floor and reach up through the left leg to a vertical position, pointing the toes. With practice, the chin will touch the upper shin of the left leg. Gaze optimistically upward like the *cakora* bird as it's approaching the moon for its nectar.
3. Hold the pose for five breaths. This position really works the rectus abdominis muscles and activates the apāna pattern based in the pelvic floor, while keeping the heart open.

4. On an exhalation, rock the pelvis forward and then back slightly using that momentum to help you swing back through into Catvāri, and do a Half Vinyāsa before practicing the pose on the other side.

Dvi Pāda Śīrṣāsana

Two Feet Behind the Head Pose

1. From Downward Facing Dog Pose at the end of an exhale, hop forward to land standing with bent legs, with the feet beyond the hands and the thighs wrapped around the arms. Sit gently, leaving the legs beyond the arms.
2. Sit up as in Eka Pāda Śīrṣāsana. Wrap the *left* leg behind the head first. Once it is securely in place, draw the right leg back, hooking that ankle outside the left. Work the upper arms through the thighs and

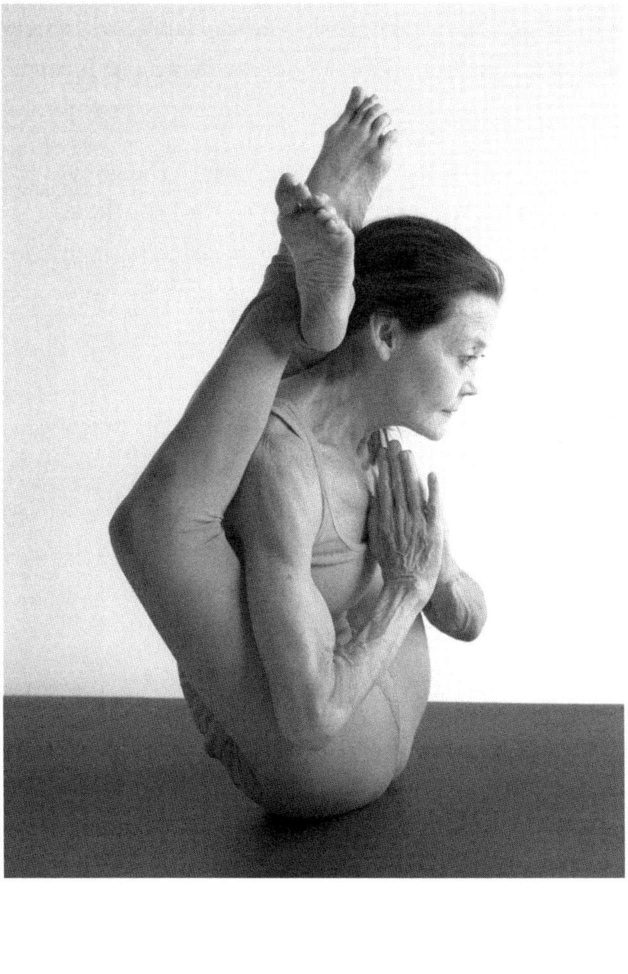

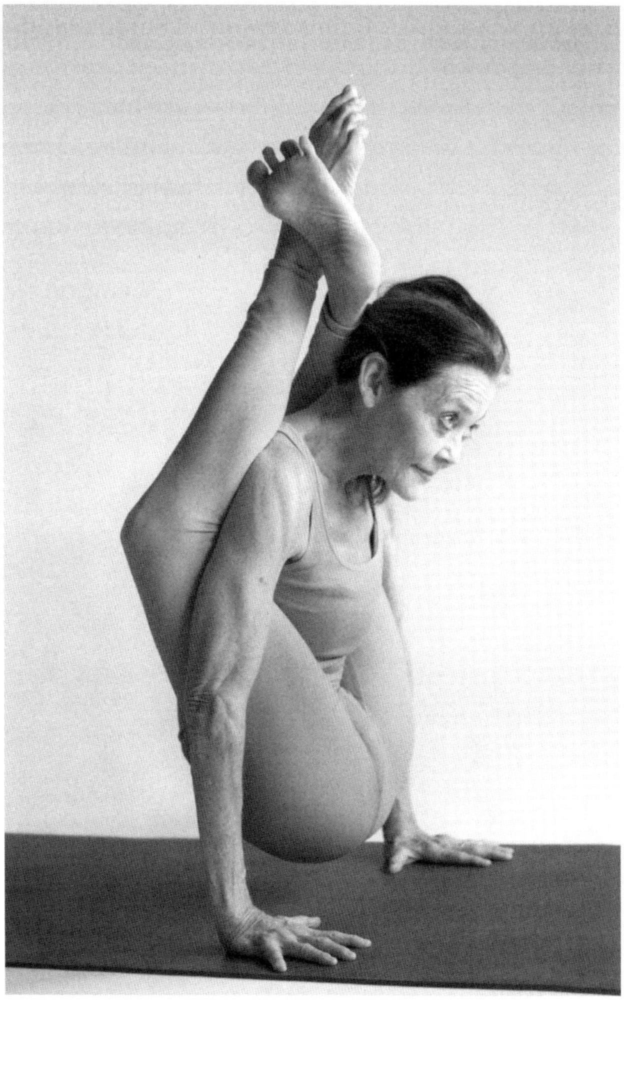

the legs as far down the neck and back as possible and draw the ankles and feet slightly apart.

3. Fold the hands in front of the heart in Añjali Mudrā, and gaze gently down to the floor along the line of the nose. Hold this position for five breaths.
4. Place the hands flat on the floor beside the hips. On an inhalation, lift straight up, balancing on the hands so your hips are off the floor. Hold for five breaths, still gazing ahead softly.
5. Unhook the feet and lift the hips away from the floor, pushing down through the arms and reaching out through the legs into Ṭiṭṭibhāsana (Small Water Bird Pose). Hold this for only one breath and then jump back (via Bakāsana, if possible) into Catvāri and do a Half Vinyāsa.

Yoga Nidrāsana

Yoga Sleeping Pose

Very similar to Dvi Pāda Śīrṣāsana but in a prone position, some practitioners find this pose far more accessible than the upright form. Because the back is supported by the floor in Yoga Nidrāsana, there is far less risk of overpushing and injuring the spine or disks, so this is a good pose to experiment with if Dvi Pāda Śirṣāsana does not come easily and as preparation for that pose.

1. Lying on your back, bring both legs up and out toward the sides of the body, bending the knees and pointing the toes toward the floor.
2. As you exhale, wrap the left leg behind the head (as you did for Dvi Pāda Śirṣāsana) rolling the left calf back toward the floor and

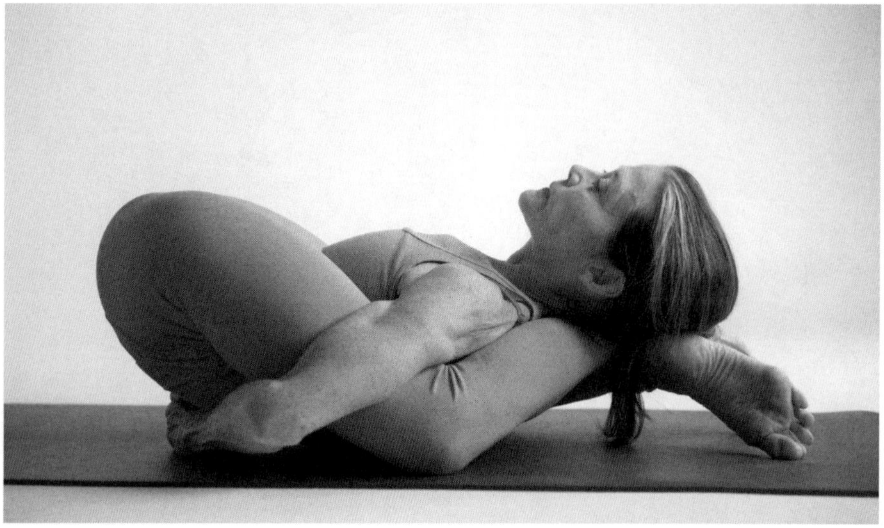

wrapping the left shoulder through the leg. Move the left leg and foot down the back with the foot as far over toward the right shoulder behind the neck as possible.

3. Next wrap the right leg behind the neck, moving the right shoulder through and positioning the right ankle outside the left, close to the floor. The ankles should overlap, and the toes should be pointed.
4. Wrap the arms around the sides and clasp them behind the back. Gaze gently down the line of the nose; make the heart float with the prāṇa pattern while releasing the jaw and palate. Hold the pose for five breaths.
5. To exit, release the arms and legs, straighten the legs, and roll through Cakrāsana into Catvāri and Half Vinyāsa.

8

Backbends

FOR SOME PRACTITIONERS, BACKBENDS ARE THE glory poses—coming from being stuck in the mud to rise up and stretch the rays of intelligence and enthusiasm out in all directions. For others, backbends are the nemesis; they're frightening, miserable, and to be avoided at all costs. From either of these disparate perspectives, it is quite easy (if not inevitable) to injure yourself practicing backbends, unless you pay attention to the internal actions and counteractions of the apāna and the prāṇa as you move in and out of the poses. Perhaps you get a free pass from either extreme view for a number of months or years before an injury occurs. However, if you repeatedly ignore the internal essence of the form—maybe because it feels kind of good to stretch the abdomen and fold deeply in the lower back; or maybe it seems safe to grit the teeth and push through pain with grimly determined muscle power—at some point, either during a particularly stiff practice or when the mind wanders one day, you are likely to experience an injury. Fortunately even at that juncture, it's not too late, and the internal forms are there to save you, presenting backbending benefits for your particular circumstance.

The odds of being injured in backbends without good alignment are higher than those in most other families of poses primarily because we find ourselves in Upward Facing Dog Pose (a rather advanced pose) many times during any given practice. Chapter 5 covers Upward Facing Dog Pose and variations that teach proper alignment because they are so central to every practice. So not only are there innumerable opportunities to drop deeply into the intricacies of the form, there are just as many chances to move by rote or in extreme ways and wind up with an injury. With practice though, almost everyone can learn to get into and out of backbends deeply and safely.

Backbends are the epitome of the prāṇa family, expressing a sense of extension and expansion up and out. Just as we know when we've been overemphasizing the apānic pattern without its beloved prāṇa present in forward bends—because we feel physically and emotionally shut down, defensive, and despairing—we also have an internal barometer that lets us know when we've gone too far with the expansive prāṇic pattern as well. Apāna gives a visceral sense of impermanence and interconnectedness to forms projected into the sense fields opened by the inhaling prāṇa pattern. When we ignore this grounding, stabilizing aspect of apāna in backbends, a sense of an asymmetrical, manic "hyperprāṇa" arises in which it is difficult to focus the mind, and an underlying sense of anxiety arises. We may be overwhelmed by waves of emotion or we may feel spacy or ungrounded in our day-to-day interactions with others. Unfortunately, because many of these manifestations of excessive prāṇa are intoxicating and ego building (rather than depressing like the overly apānic patterns of poorly balanced forward bends), they are easy to overlook. Consequently, we may not recognize overly prāṇic patterns, and even if we do, we may not see the need to adjust the practice to come back down to earth to an interdependent and healthy existence with other beings.

To bring balance into backbends, it is important to focus and refocus on the complementary opposite patterns of movement within the Prāṇa that fully engage us in the poses. In this way, the poses naturally unfold as deeply as is appropriate not only for our body, but also for our mental and emotional states on any given day. Because a central physiological aspect of backbends is that we literally "open the heart" to do the poses, taking care not to overdo this physical pattern when we are feeling emotionally unsettled or vulnerable is very important. Sometimes, even for those who can do extremely deep backbends, it is not advisable to go to the body's limit; it is better to maintain smooth and even breathing while taking the pose just a bit less deep.

For all backbends the underlying pattern is that as we inhale and consider the pose, we then ground fully on the exhalation to set the apānic pattern solidly in the pelvic floor as the base of the pose. This allows us to experience backbends as integrating poses that bring intelligence and protection to the lower back and groins. The apānic pattern, connecting to the coccyx while toning the pelvic floor and then spreading and lifting the kidney wings, grounds us so the prāṇic pattern can stimulate and passively stretch the hip flexors and groins. Once the complementary patterns are in play, backbends will manifest naturally and safely. They will deepen just the right amount as we do our part to allow the conversation between prāṇa and apāna to evolve into an affectionate embrace.

As novices we may think that backbends are just that—bending the back of the body, particularly the spine, backward. Though that is correct up to a point, the way to go deeply into backbends and really feel their benefits is to work up and through the body—to lengthen and stretch the *front* of the body from the pelvic floor and to avoid compression of the vertebral facet joints in the back of the spine. Although the natural S shape of the spine does allow for easy extension in the areas of the lumbar and cervical spine, it soon becomes apparent from this internal perspective that extension of the whole spine is vital and more important to healthy backbends than is extreme extension of the spine at only a couple of spots. Moving from the deadened spine rather than the pelvic floor and full body usually causes pain and injury because we fold into the easily bendable areas—compressing the lumbar vertebrae, pressing the kidney wings closed at T12, and collapsing the head back on the atlas in the cervical region. When practicing backbends in a more integrated manner, we flow on the wave of the breath, lengthening top to bottom through the central channel and up the front of the body. We must also tone, extend, and open the structures in the front and the back of the body—the hip joints, the psoas muscles, the back of the diaphragm, the full thoracic and the lower cervical vertebrae—to ensure a spacious and stable backbend. Moving on the wave of the breath makes these individual actions natural and nonaggressive. They are difficult when not hooked together in a wave.

Most backbends involve a deep opening and extension of the front of each hip joint, often referred to as the groin. This extension is an apānic movement because actively, in its purest manifestation, it employs the abdominal muscles, hamstrings, and buttocks muscles. At a certain phase as we move into backbends, the muscles associated with the apāna family (hamstrings and gluteus muscles) cause a release of the hip flexors through reciprocal inhibition. This can be understood initially as an active tail-tucking pattern, which slows down extension of the spine and defines a stable root from which the prāṇa pattern can unfold symmetrically. Tail tucking, like everything else, can be overdone, causing external rotation of the femurs, narrowing of the pelvic floor, and ejection of the pubic bone from the narrowed pelvic floor. This is where Mūlabandha allows the essential counter-counteraction of the prāṇa to come into play, so there is a sensation of the coccyx lengthening and moving forward toward the pubic bone as the sacrum lifts up and in toward the lower belly.

Because it is so stimulating to open the chest, diaphragm, and throat, it is challenging to find, let alone move from, the pelvic floor. Yet awareness of the pelvic floor, the presence of the coccyx, and the opening of the kidney wings are the counteractions that deepen the poses and protect the SI joints, the lower spine, and the lower ribs so the expansive prāṇic patterns can unfold fully. If we become accustomed to being overly prāṇic in backbends, the extreme ungrounded version of this pattern can invade many other poses and ruin their contemplative effects on both body and mind.

In more extreme backbends, such as Ūrdhvā Dhanurāsana (Upward Bow Pose), it is also important to engage and position the shoulders correctly to support the bend in the upper lumbar and lower thoracic spine. Even though the backbending pattern is often perceived as most pronounced around the area of the heart (the part of the body that opposes and complements the thoracic area) and in the upper spine, the lower thoracic region can be compromised if the shoulders are misaligned. Learning the correct protraction of the shoulder blades and then the art of extending the upper spine from the heart area up through the head, without compressing the vertebrae and without breaking the rhythmical sequence of extension that is rooted in the pelvic floor, is essential while backbending. Proper shoulder alignment is also dependent on opening the kidney wings to get the belly to stretch and lengthen without losing the apānic tone into a sort of *psychic hernia* that expands out from the line of the spine through an overstretched solar plexus or overly flaccid buttocks. This misalignment splays out the intelligence into a multiplicity of options and divides the subtle aspects of uniting prāṇa and apāna along the midline of the body.

In backbends, we must also pay close attention to the position of the head, the gaze, where in the body the pose is physically connected to the earth, and finally the relationship of the open palate to the pelvic floor. These more subtle aspects of the poses may be considered separately, but it is most effective in terms of supporting internal patterns of the form to study them in relationship to the body as a whole and through a sense of overall movement of the spine.

For most practitioners, the easiest place in the spine to fold backward is in the area of the upper cervical spine. If you tilt your head back to look up, you're doing a backbend in the cervical spine. Because looking up is so much a part of day-to-day life, we may not realize the impact that an unconscious folding of the uppermost cervical spine (the atlanto-occipital joint) has on a full backbend; it actually stops the flow of Prāṇa from top to bottom and tends to perpetuate an ungrounded feeling. The head and neck can either intelligently express a rhythmical extension from the heart through the crown, or the head can act as a heavy weight that simply falls back habitually, with the occiput dropping back onto the atlas. So as we move into backbends, if we can imagine the feeling of extension up through the core of the body from the chest (or better yet from the pelvic floor through the chest) and out through the crown of the head, we can begin to avoid dropping the head back unconsciously and overextending the cervical spine. The head is always the last component of the spine to roll back in healthy extension. This action of gradual extension from lower to higher in the cervical spine and full expression of the backbending form may be facilitated by dropping awareness deep into the center of the pelvic floor where we can feel the connection to the midline of the body. If we then imagine the central channel from top to bottom as smooth, luminous, and long, curving backward on the wave of the breath as if the breath were a fountain of movement up, back, up and over, then the backbend comes naturally. This feeling can be supported by tuning in to a sense of lifting and spreading the kidney wings and also paying attention to sensations in the skin of the throat and the back of the head; consciously softening and broadening and gently lifting all these areas of the body.

It is also important to cultivate a soft, downcast gaze as we move into backbends. When we look up, the posterior suboccipital muscles under the back of the skull are signaled to contract in direct response to the eye movement. This usually also translates into a contraction of the erector spinae muscles. If we look up as we move into backbends, both of these groups of muscles are likely to fire, automatically causing the head to fall back on the atlas. This stops extension in the lower cervical and upper thoracic areas. In addition, engaging the posterior suboccipitals has the powerful effect of triggering larger patterns of hyperextension throughout the body, such as closing the kidney area and releasing the pelvic floor. On the other hand, looking down as we enter backbends contracts the anterior suboccipital muscles, which tilt the head forward on the atlas and prevent it from falling back. So keeping the dṛṣṭi down along the line of the nose—without tension in the eyes—is integral to healthy backbends. It makes us extend the cervical spine from bottom to top after opening the upper chest and heart area.

A curious aspect of practicing backbends is that even though naturally flexible practitioners can extend and get into backbends with seemingly little effort, and we would expect them to benefit greatly from the poses, this is not always the case. Having arrived in the territory of the backbend, it still requires a great deal of internal and meditative focus to actually turn a gymnastic position into a fully functioning yoga pose and receive the benefits of that pose. Because those who are naturally flexible arrive more easily in the pose, they also run a greater risk than stiffer individuals of becoming intoxicated by the waves of expansive, prāṇic residue that may sweep through the body in the initial stages of the pose. So paradoxically, it is not unusual that stiffer practitioners taste the benefits of backbends first.

Śalabhāsana A and B

Locust Pose

This is not a glory backbend—one that impresses friends and family members who don't think too much about yoga but love to watch you try extreme poses. Imagining yourself as a locust flying close to the ground can make the pose more enjoyable and also informs the alignment well. Śalabhāsana is an active backbend in the sense that it relies on muscles along the back of the spine and body (hamstrings and buttocks muscles) for its form, whereas in more flashy backbends, like Ūrdhvā Dhanurāsana, these muscles are eventually softened at different phases or throughout the pose. Forms A and B may be practiced separately; however, it is part of the traditional Intermediate Series to practice them together and also makes sense physically, as there is just a simple movement of the hands that allows the posture to deepen and that separates the two variations of this pose.

1. Lie on the belly with the forehead on the floor, the legs together, the toes pointed, and the arms stretched down along the side with the palms facing up. Lift the tops of the arms away from the mat about 2 or 3 inches, being careful not to pinch the shoulder blades together.
2. Exhale fully, then as you inhale, begin lifting the head, shoulders, chest, and legs away from the floor. Bend the elbows slightly, pushing the backs of the hands into the mat to aid in the lift.
3. Keep the legs engaged, the jaw soft, and the gaze steady as you reach back through the inner edges of the feet. Do not sickle the feet so that the toes touch and heels spread apart; keep the feet parallel or with the sides touching. It can be helpful to hold a block between the feet or ankles to prevent external rotation of the legs and to accentuate this foot action.
4. This is form A. Hold it for five breaths, gazing along the line of the nose with the head, chest, and legs lifted.

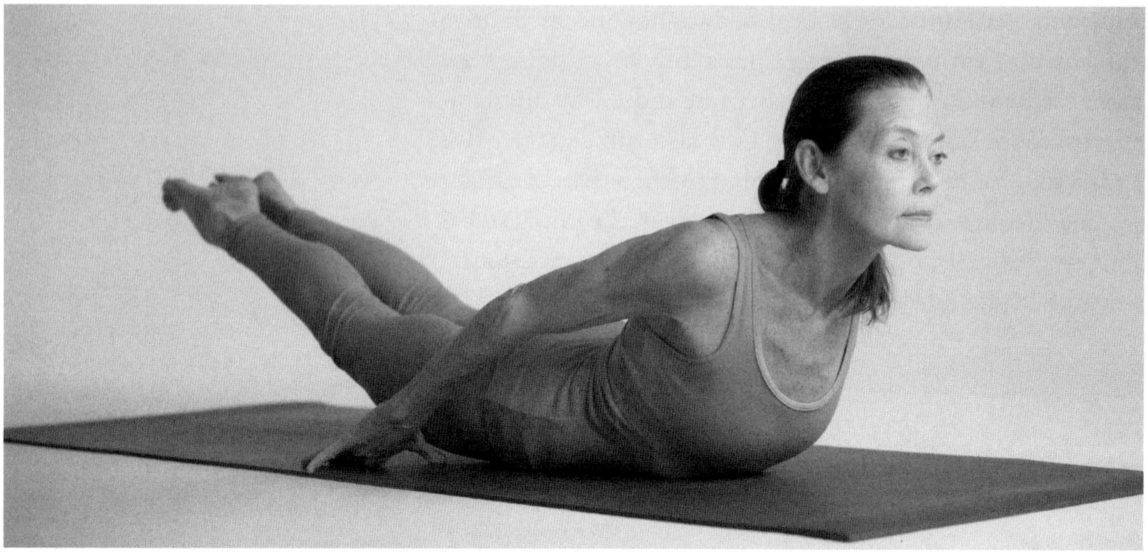

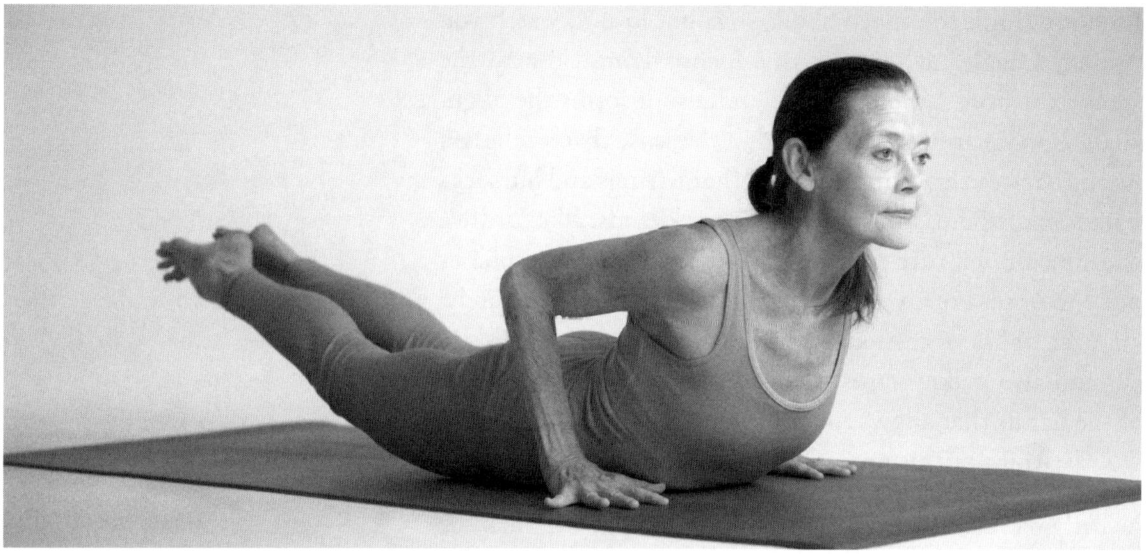

5. On an exhalation, place the palms of the hands on the floor next to the waist. As you inhale, push gently to lift the chest a little more. This is form B. Hold it for five breaths, then move the hands along the side of the body next to the heart, and on an exhalation, turn the toes under and push with the arms to pop up into Catvāri. Move through a Half Vinyāsa into the next pose.

Pūrvottanāsana

Stretching Up the Front Pose

This is the perfect counterpose to Paśchimottānāsana and is the most obvious embodiment of the tail of the serpent. It wakes up the hamstrings

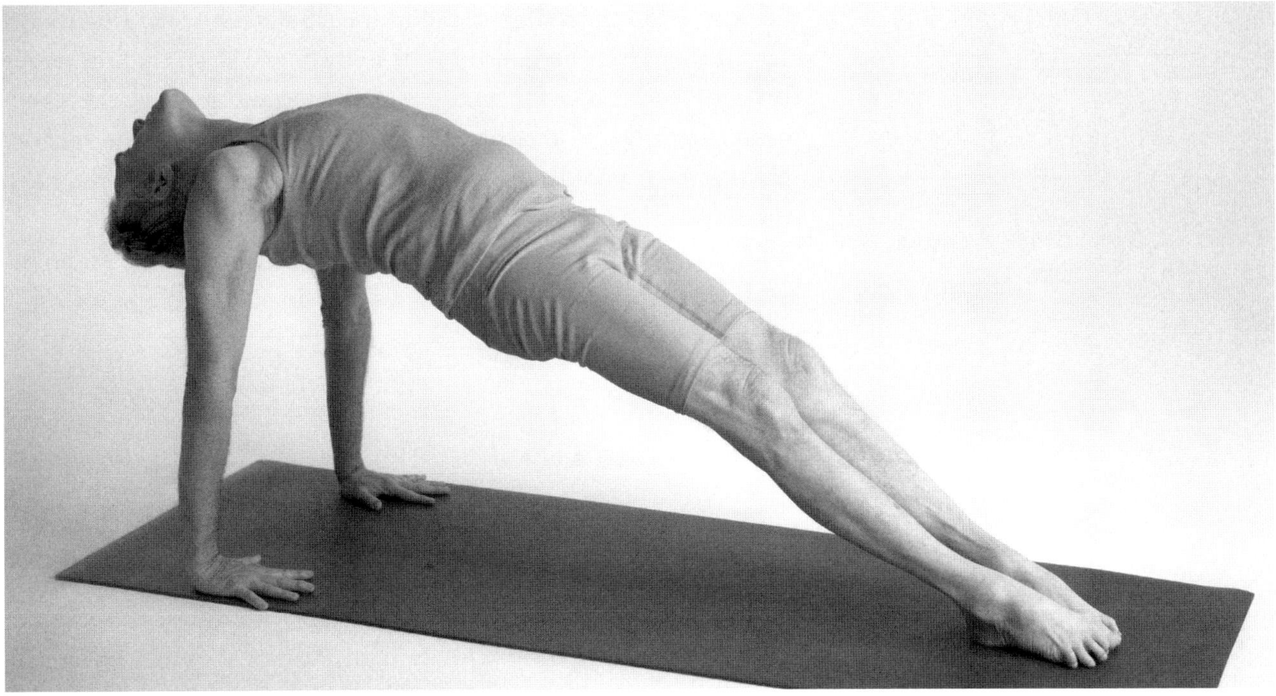

and is very beneficial if the hamstrings are either tight or overstretched at their attachment points because it requires the belly of the muscles to engage. All backbends are actually a stretch of the front of the body, and no pose underscores this stretch more than Pūrvottanāsana.

1. Enter the pose from Downward Facing Dog Pose, jumping through to a sitting position on the end of an exhalation with the legs stretched straight out in front. Inhaling place the hands about 8 inches behind the buttocks, with the fingers pointing toward the front of the mat. Drop the chin down near the upper sternum, and roll the shoulders back and down. This is similar to Daṇḍāsana.
2. Bend the elbows as you exhale, and strongly curl the coccyx as you lengthen out through the legs. This movement is the epitome of the tail of the serpent movement. Lean back and start to lift the hips, still curling the coccyx as if to collect and hold the uniting of prāṇa and apāna. Imagine lengthening the coccyx all the way to the feet.
3. While inhaling, draw the sacrum up as you straighten the arms. Unroll the spine bottom to top, lifting the heart and gazing down the line of the nose. Remember that the head should be the last part to roll back.
4. Keep the legs engaged as you enter the pose, at first reaching through the balls of the toes and, as you reach the full lift, pointing the toes toward the floor. Keep the apānic grounding firm during the entire pose. Be sure to roll the shoulders back and down as you enter

the pose, and keep a slight bend in the elbows while holding it. The sacrum should lift up and into the body as you keep the legs strong throughout the pose. It is also very important to keep the hands pressing evenly and intelligently into the mat, keeping the roots of the fingers—especially the index fingers—firmly rooted to the earth throughout the transitions and while in the pose.

5. Hold the pose for five breaths. Lower back to the floor on an exhalation, keeping the legs strong as you do so and prepare for the next pose.

Supta Vīrāsana

Reclining Hero Pose

It can be helpful in backbends to stretch the quadriceps. Within the Intermediate Series, Bhekāsana does just that. For those who are not ready for Bhekāsana or those who want an additional quadricep stretch, Vīrāsana and Supta Vīrāsana are excellent poses to explore as well, even though they are not officially part of the Aṣṭāṅga sequences. In all of the movements of this pose, move on the waves of the breath, and breathe fully and evenly throughout.

1. From a kneeling position, lower the pelvis to the floor between the lower legs, imagining the sitting bones plugging into the floor. As you position the body in this sitting position, use the hands to gently rotate the calves out to the sides and guide the skin of the outer thighs in and down toward the floor. If you experience discomfort

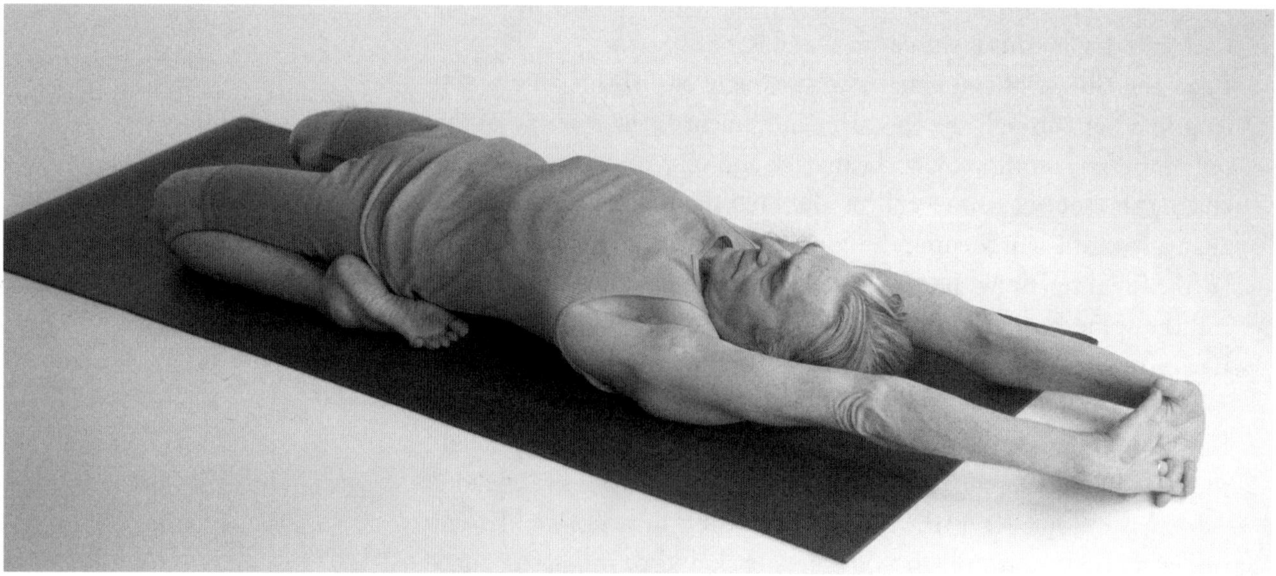

in the knees or hips, support the sitting bones with a blanket or block. Place a blanket beneath the knees and ankles if the ankles are uncomfortable. You should feel no pain in the knees, ankles, or hips.

2. This is Vīrāsana and may be used as a form for sitting meditation or simply sitting during the course of the day. It is even and stable, and some practitioners find it easier to keep the pelvis vertical to the floor in Vīrāsana than in simple cross-legged forms. Because the legs are folded back, the quadriceps are naturally stretched and begin to lengthen.
3. To increase the stretch, after a few breaths, begin to lean the torso back, as if to lie down. If you are very flexible, this may be easy; if you are not, it may seem impossible. Find your limit and do not overstrain in this pose. It is most beneficial as a preparatory stretch and to aid digestion, so you may practice it after eating and before beginning a practice.
4. If it is difficult or impossible to lie back on the floor, arrange bolsters or blankets behind your body on which to lie. If lying back is easy, do so slowly, keeping the lower body toned but not gripped. If it is not comfortable to lie back, you may lean back placing the hands on the mat behind you with fingers pointing toward the front of the mat.
5. Once back as far as you can go (without overstraining), place the arms along the sides of the body. If you are using the hands behind you as support, simply keep them there. To experiment with the stretch, gently lift the pelvis off the floor and tuck the coccyx up toward the pubic bone. This will cause the femurs to rotate outward, and the knees may move apart slightly.
6. Next drop the pubic bone down toward the coccyx, tilting the pelvis down slightly, which will cause the knees to move closer together as the femurs rotate inward.
7. For a more extreme stretch if you are lying down, reach up along the floor over your head with both arms, spinning the arms so the palms face the midline of the body as the shoulder blades protract.

Bhekāsana

Frog Pose

It may be difficult to imagine ourselves as frogs until we find ourselves in Bhekāsana, simultaneously "spring-loaded" and "stuck in the mud," which provides useful perspective for evaluating other difficult situations that arise in life. Bhekāsana is practiced early in the Intermediate Series as a preparatory pose for the more intense backbend sequence. Lying on the

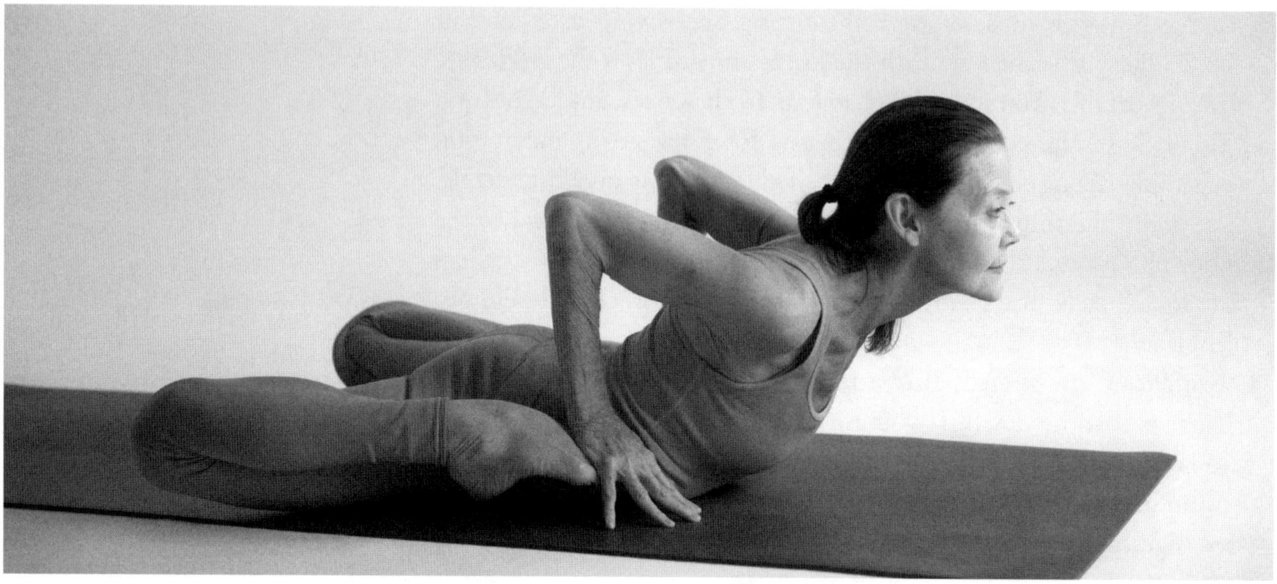

belly with the legs in reverse Vīrāsana and the chest lifted, the quadriceps and psoas muscles are stretched, the arms and shoulders are positioned to engage the serratus anterior muscles, and the shoulder blades are positioned as support for the thoracic spine.

1. Lying on the belly lift the feet to bend the knees. Reach back and clasp the fronts of the feet, rotating the hands so the fingers point in the same direction as the toes. Position the upper arms approximately parallel to one another.
2. Exhale fully, then on an inhalation, lift the shoulders and chest as you push the feet down toward the floor outside the thighs. Keep the upper arms parallel and reach out through the sternum and crown of the head as you gaze down the nose. If possible, flatten the soles of the feet on the floor, but do not strain and injure the knees. The thighs may roll out to the sides slightly, but do not let them move too far apart.
3. Hold this position for five breaths, gazing down the line of the nose and breathing smoothly. On an exhalation, release the feet and place the hands flat on the floor next to the heart as you straighten the legs back down to the floor, with the feet flexed. Push into Catvāri on the next exhalation, move into Upward Facing Dog Pose on the next inhalation, then go through a Half Vinyāsa into the next pose.
4. If it is too difficult to clasp both feet at the same time, a preparatory version of this pose may be helpful. Lying on the belly, lift the upper body as if moving into the Sphinx Pose or Bhujaṇgāsana on the elbows. Place the left arm out in front of the body with the forearm pointing straight ahead and the elbow just beneath the left shoulder.

Bend the right knee and clasp the top of the foot with the right hand; point the fingers forward if possible. Breathe into the pose, increasing the stretch in the leg and upper body on the inhalation and releasing it slightly on the exhalation. After five breaths on the left side, repeat this form on the other side. Then exit the pose as for full Bhekāsana.

DHANURĀSANA

Bridge Pose

This pose is delightful, with a sense of liberation and freedom—even for beginning practitioners. It is a traditional part of the Intermediate Series, but those who are not quite ready for the full series can experiment with it as a means of learning the internal actions and counteractions that inform all backbends.

1. Exhaling, lie down on the belly. Place the top of the forehead on the floor while gazing softly down toward the tip of the nose. Use the same position as described for the beginning of Śalabhāsana.

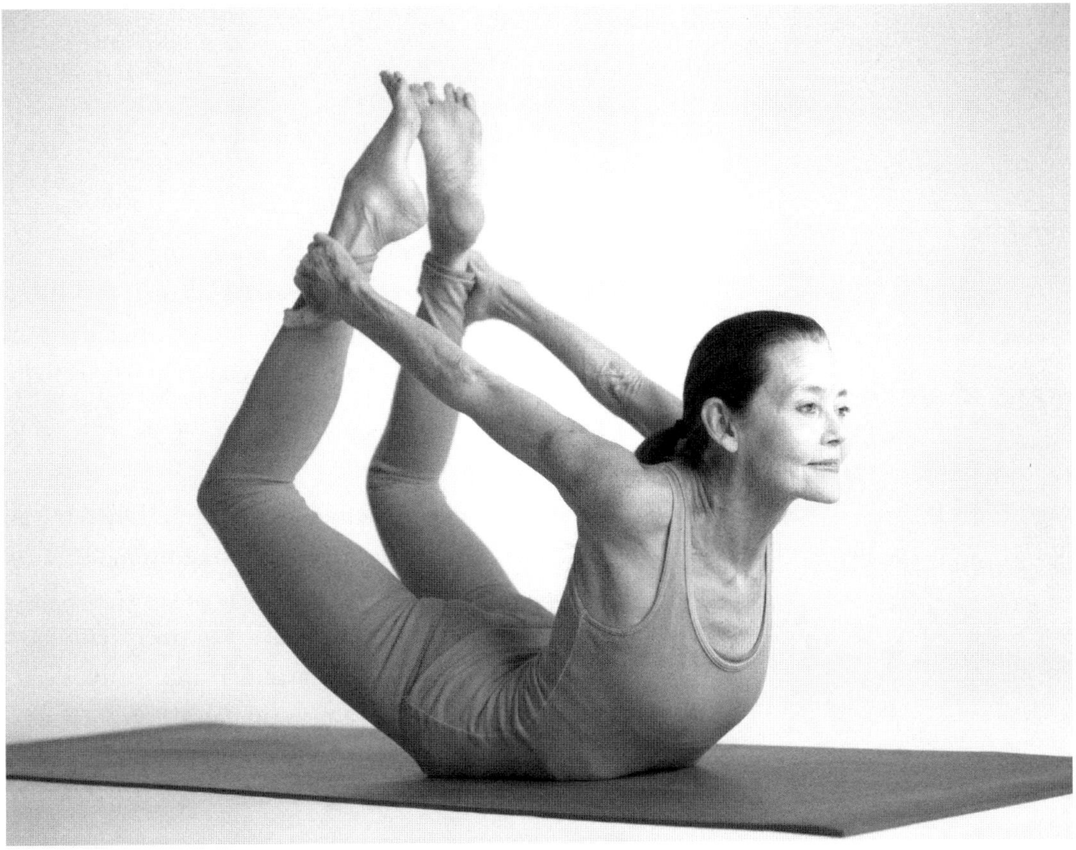

2. At the end of an exhalation, bring awareness to the coccyx, imagining it to be heavy and a ballast for the pelvic floor. Then, on an inhale lift the head, chest, and knees from the floor as you bend the knees and place the inner edges of the feet together. (This is technically a variation of Śalabhāsana.) Immediately clasp the ankles with the hands so that the feet are free to articulate. If you are flexible, you can clasp the legs with hands up higher on the shins toward the knees.
3. On an inhalation, lift the feet back and up, higher and higher as if you were a marionette and strings were drawing the inner edges straight up to the ceiling. Bend the elbows slightly to feel the small counter-inward or secondary rotation of the upper arms. Maintain an awareness of the coccyx, imagining it as a tail. Cultivate the sense of an empty palate to lengthen the front of the spine rather than compressing the back of the spine. Gaze along the line of the nose.
4. After five breaths, come down on an exhalation. Continuing with that same exhalation, enter Catvāri, and then inhale into Upward Facing Dog Pose. Exhale into Downward Facing Dog Pose to digest, study, and enjoy the residue of the pose. If you are practicing the Intermediate Series, instead of going immediately into Upward and Downward Facing Dog poses, do Pārśva Dhanurāsana on both sides before exiting.

Pārśva Dhanurāsana

Side-Angle Bridge Pose

Practice this pose immediately following Dhanurāsana, rocking from the Dhanurāsana over to the side and then returning to Dhanurāsana between sides. Of course this pose can be practiced on its own, but it is much easier and often more beneficial to practice after full Dhanurāsana.

1. Exhaling, lie down on your belly with the same alignment form as for Dhanurāsana.
2. If you are not working with Pārśva Dhanurāsana as part of the Intermediate Series, still incorporate some breaths in Dhanurāsana in preparation for this pose. As you inhale, lift the feet into full Dhanurāsana for five breaths. On an exhalation, rock over to the right, bringing the right arm and hip to the floor. Work the top of the arm back so you are resting as far to the front of the top of the humerus as possible. This action should feel good, and it helps to establish an openness in the heart.

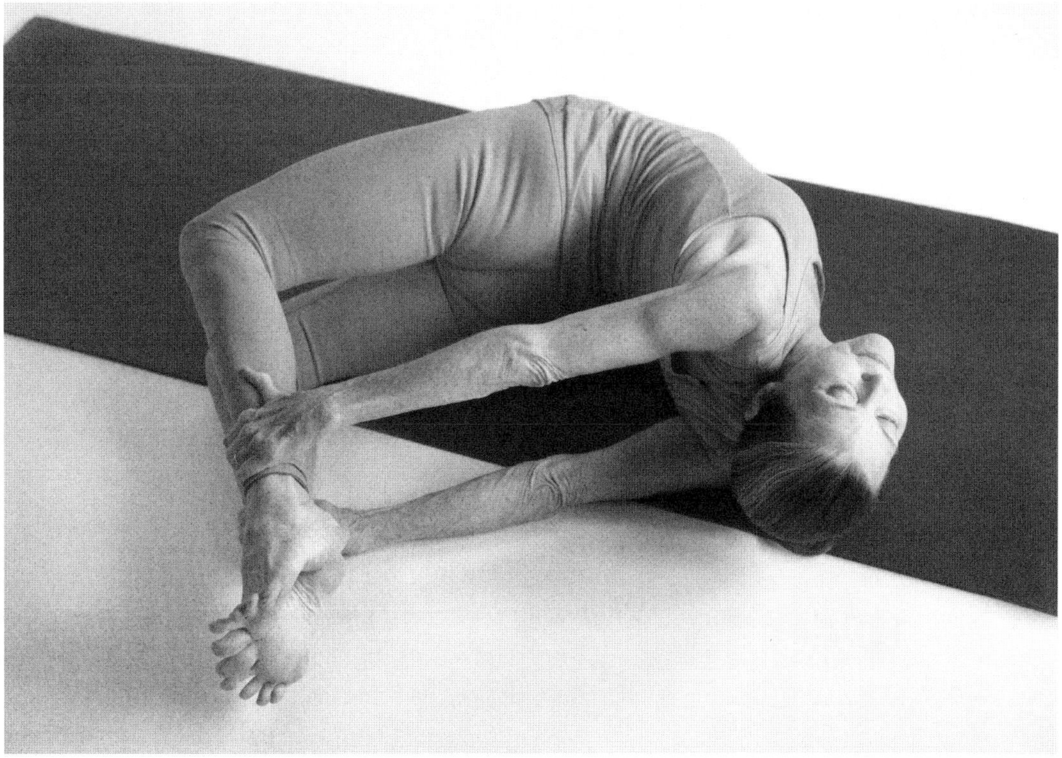

3. Inhaling, activate the pose by bring the sacrum up and into the body as you feel the coccyx moving down and in toward the pubic bone. Engage the quadriceps and reach out and back through both legs, keeping the feet even and thighs parallel to gradually move the legs to a straighter form.
4. When the posture feels fully expressed, turn the head back symmetrically as if looking at the toes. Then with the lower neck in full extension, turn the head to look up. Do *not* turn the head until the neck is first fully extended.
5. After five breaths, exhale and roll back onto the belly. As you inhale, lift back to full Dhanurāsana, then exhale and rock over to the left side and repeat the entire sequence of movements on that side.
6. After five breaths, exhale and roll back onto the belly. Inhale as you lift back to full Dhanurāsana, and hold for five breaths.
7. To exit the pose, lower the knees, release the feet, and straighten the legs down to the floor with the toes turned under. Place the hands in Catvāri position and immediately on an exhalation, lift your groins and belly into Catvāri. Inhale into Upward Facing Dog Pose, and exhale into Downward Facing Dog Pose. Again, take advantage of the open ears and the easy bandhas of this pose to digest the residue of Pārśva Dhanurāsana.

Ūṣṭrāsana

Camel Pose

Though this pose is found in the Intermediate Series, it can be beneficial and informative—and even accessible—to less seasoned practitioners. It is very instructional in terms of backbending basics: strong legs with an internal spin, and a connection to the pelvic floor so the spine elongates while entering backbends. The instructions that follow include a few extra breaths from the traditional sequence. These extra breaths allow the body to settle into the lines of the pose and move on the wave of the breath rather than from a place of muscular engagement. Once the pose has been practiced repeatedly and you are used to it, you can attempt it without these extra breaths.

1. From Downward Facing Dog Pose, at the end of an exhale hop forward to a kneeling position with the knees about hip-width apart. Keep the lower legs parallel and the tops of the feet against the floor. Place the hands on the hips.

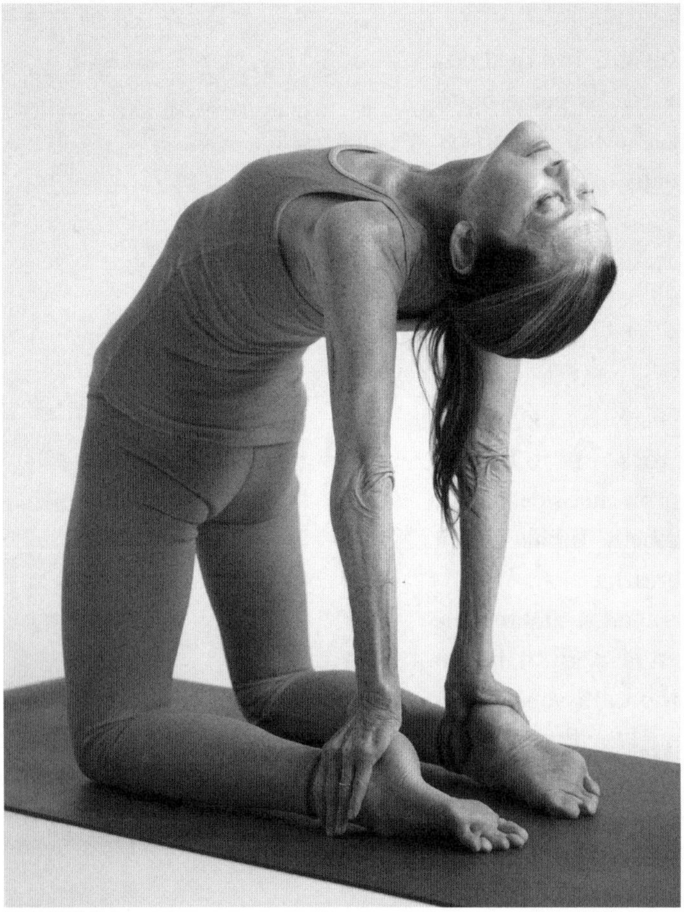

2. Exhale and drop the awareness into the base of the pose, grounding into the legs as they spiral down. Isometrically squeeze them together as you tone the PC muscle; drop the coccyx down and forward while keeping the internal action of the pubic bone moving down and back.
3. Inhaling, bring the awareness to subtle movements that straighten and elongate the spine along the plumb line of the body. Follow the wave of the breath as it arcs up through the central channel.
4. Gently push down on the hips with your hands and lift the heart, broaden the back of the body, and lengthen the spine from coccyx to crown. Keep the head lifted and gaze down the nose as you move into a subtle backbend. As in all backbends inhale with the gesture of lifting up and arching, and exhale with the sense of a heavy coccyx and dropping down through the legs into the earth.
5. Maintain the length in the spine and a sense of connection to the earth through the legs. Exhaling, place the hands on the ankles or

heels (if you are stiff, flex the feet with the toes turned under, or place the hands on blocks placed outside the ankles). Still gazing down the nose and keeping the jaw soft, tilt the head back by extending the neck and reaching out through the crown of the head. Do not allow the back of the head to fall back on the atlas and interrupt the smooth, even flow of the arc from the knees to the crown of the head.

6. The position of the hands on your ankles directs the shoulder action. As you become more flexible in the spine and shoulders, experiment with turning the hands so the thumbs are along the outsides of the ankles. If you are less flexible, place the hands on your heels, and when you can hold the ankles, place the thumbs along the insides.
7. Hold the pose for five smooth, full breaths, gazing down the nose and softening the jaw and tongue as you release the palate as if to drink nectar. To exit, ground down into the earth through the knees on an exhalation. Inhale, keeping the legs toned and in place, and gently squeeze the thighs together as you return to kneeling, bringing the head up last. Exhaling, place your hands beside the knees and jump back into Catvāri for a Half Vinyāsa.

Laghu Vajrāsana

Light Thunderbolt Pose

Ūṣṭrāsana and Laghu Vajrāsana are typically practiced in preparation for Kapotāsana. Laghu Vajrāsana is more difficult for many practitioners because the head is placed on the floor and the arms are kept straight. But moving slowly into the pose, working at it patiently over a period of weeks (or months), can eradicate—or at least tame—the fear, stiffness, and disorientation that are the usual obstacles to this āsana.

1. From Downward Facing Dog Pose, at the end of an exhale hop forward into a kneeling position with the thighs parallel and about hip-width apart. Exhaling, lean back to place the hands on the lower legs. Experiment with the position of the hands on the legs to fit with your proportions, level of practice, leg strength, and flexibility. The hands may be as far forward as the top of the calf and as far back as the ankles. Different hand positions change some dynamics of the pose, so adapt them to your circumstances.
2. Inhaling and keeping the legs strong with a sense of inward rotation, move the pelvis slightly forward to lift the sacrum in and up within the body, as you push down through the arms.

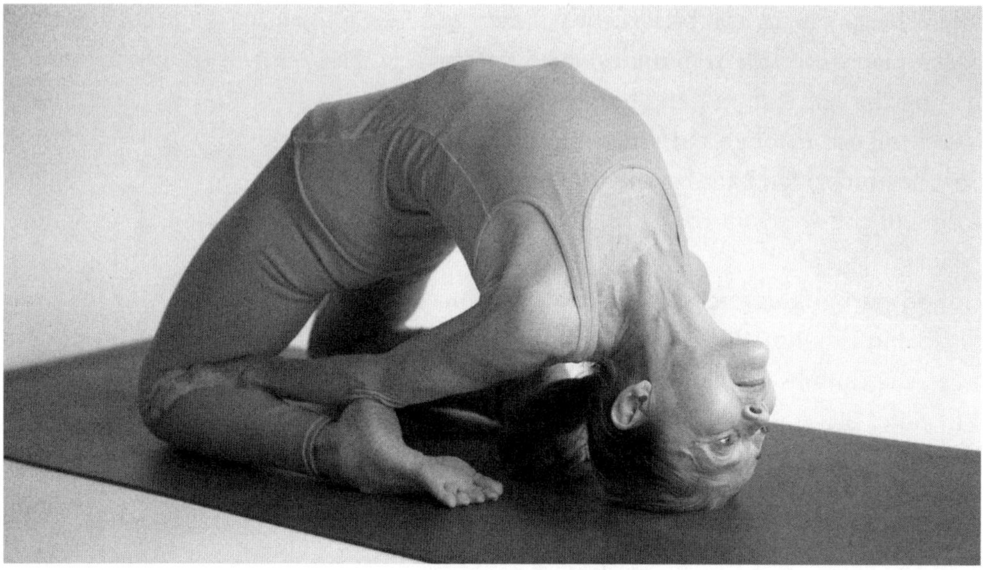

3. Keeping the arms and legs toned and strong, drop back until the head reaches the floor. Gaze down the nose as you descend and throughout the pose. Hold the position for five breaths, breathing smoothly and evenly.
4. At the end of an exhalation, engage and isometrically squeeze the legs together. From deep in the belly, on an inhalation, lift the pelvis to return the upper body to an upright position, bringing the head up last. Exhale into the legs and then, placing the hands on the floor next to the knees, hop back into Catvāri and move through a Half Vinyāsa.

Kapotāsana

Pigeon Pose

Imagining what it feels like to be a pigeon standing motionless on a city ledge with an enormous puffed chest and strong, straight legs can help as you move into Kapotāsana. It is a pose to work at slowly and with good form; for some practitioners, the full pose with the head resting on the feet may be a "next lifetime" event. Nonetheless, working the internal forms is accessible to everyone. Kapotāsana is a combination of flexibility and intelligent movement. Forcing the pose as if there is something to attain, or moving into a deep backbend by bending at the most flexible point in the spine, can have gratifying short-term results but usually ends in injury. Take time with this and other extreme poses.

1. Come to a kneeling position at the front of the mat with the legs about hip-width apart, the lower legs parallel, and the tops of the

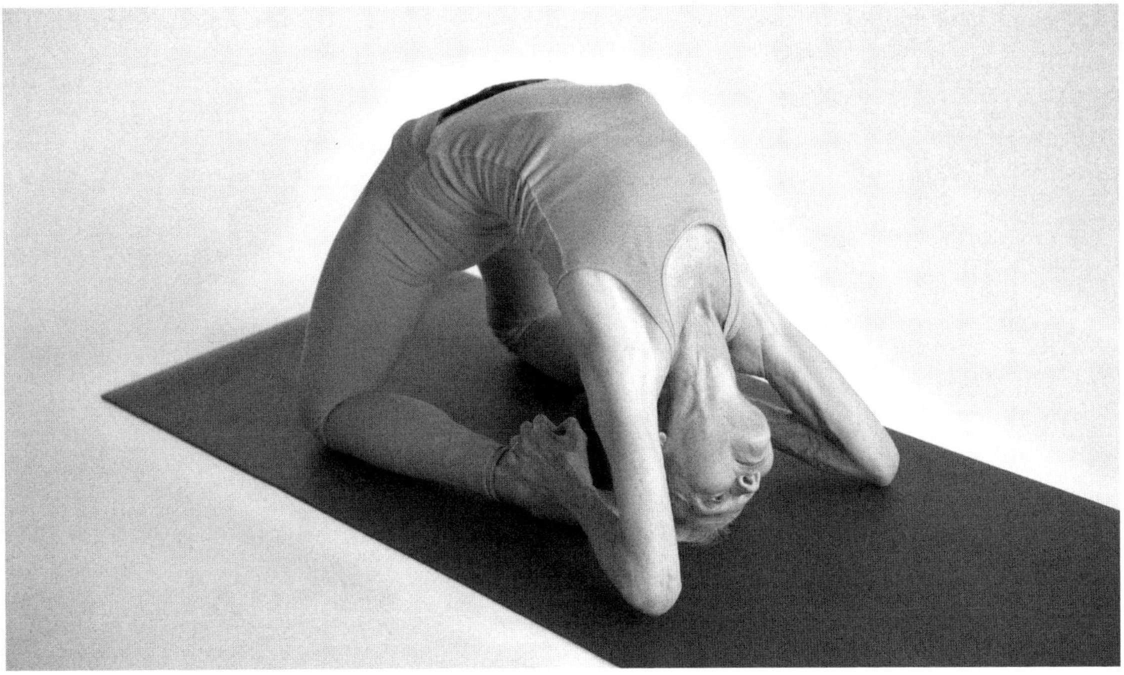

feet flat on the floor. Exhale to ground down through the legs and tone the pelvic floor.

2. Inhale, and begin to enter the pose as for Ūṣṭrāsana, extending through the core from the tip of the coccyx through the entire length of your upper body.
3. Inhaling, reach up through the torso, shoulders, and chest, then exhaling, lean back and begin to drop into a backbend with arms reaching up, back, and eventually toward the feet. Continue to follow in a smooth arc and extend through the spine from coccyx to crown. Gaze down the nose as you enter the pose. Soften the jaw, lift and broaden the kidney wings, and release the palate. Breathe smoothly.
4. Place the hands on the floor behind the toes or, eventually, on the heels. Bend the elbows and place the lower arms parallel to each other on the floor. Rest the top of the head on the soles of the feet as you continue gazing down the nose and breathing evenly. The smoother the breath in this pose—entering, exiting, and during—the more benefit you will get from the subtle internal actions.
5. After five breaths in the full form, move the hands toward the back of the mat, a few inches away from the toes and at shoulder width. Gradually straighten the arms, as if doing Ūrdhvā Dhanurāsana on your knees. Carefully protract the shoulder blades as the arms straighten. Continue to breathe smoothly, soften the tongue, and release the palate as you gaze down the nose. Hold this form for five breaths.

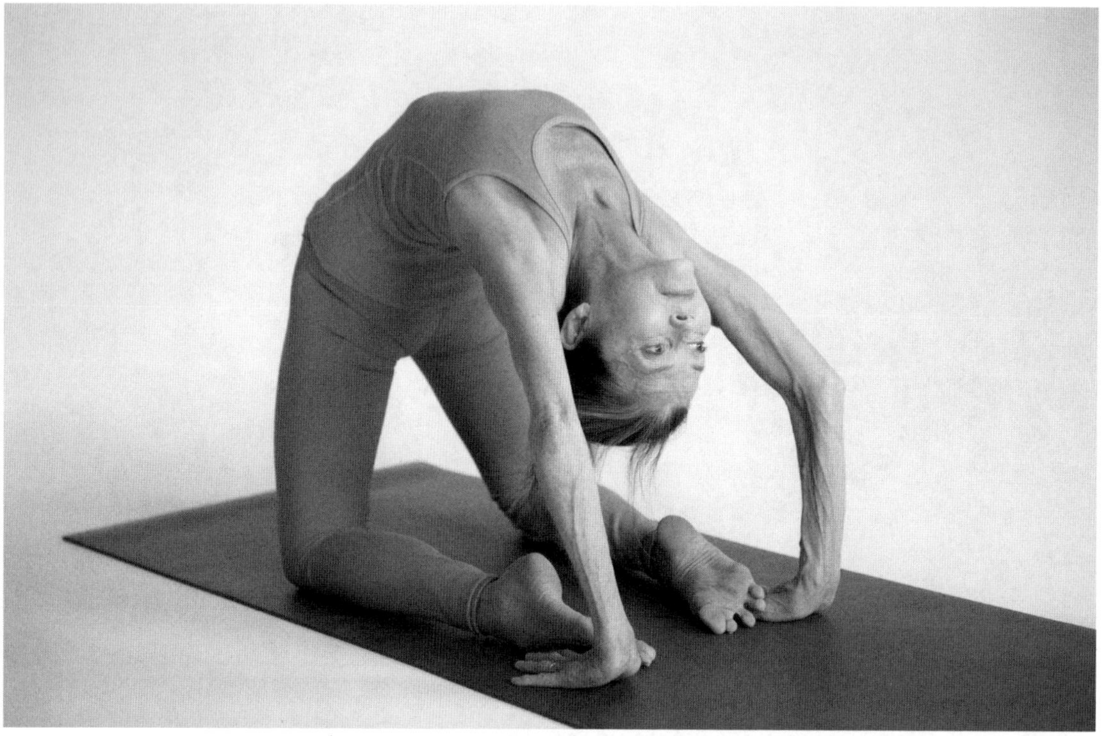

6. At the end of an exhalation, drop the awareness into the legs and pelvic floor by placing the hands on your hips. Inhaling, lift up out of the backbend to kneeling. Exhale, place your hands next to your knees, and jump back into Catvāri and a Half Vinyāsa.

Supta Vajrāsana

Reclining Lightning Bolt Pose

Though there are many ways to do this pose alone, it is helpful to have someone assisting to stabilize the legs. If you are practicing alone, you may try the advanced method by curling forward and then rocking back onto the elbows (place a blanket behind you where the elbows will fall), allowing the knees to lift away from the floor. Then extend back, lifting the heart as in Matsyāsana, the Fish Pose. To come up, reverse the process using a strong abdominal action to curl forward while still resting on the elbows. From there rock up to a seated position. If there is an assistant available and Padmāsana is not possible, sitting in Half Padmāsana or with the legs crossed is a viable option for completing the sequences (vinyāsas) of the pose.

1. From a seated position, come into Padmāsana with the left leg on top. Exhaling, reach behind the body leaning forward slightly to clasp the

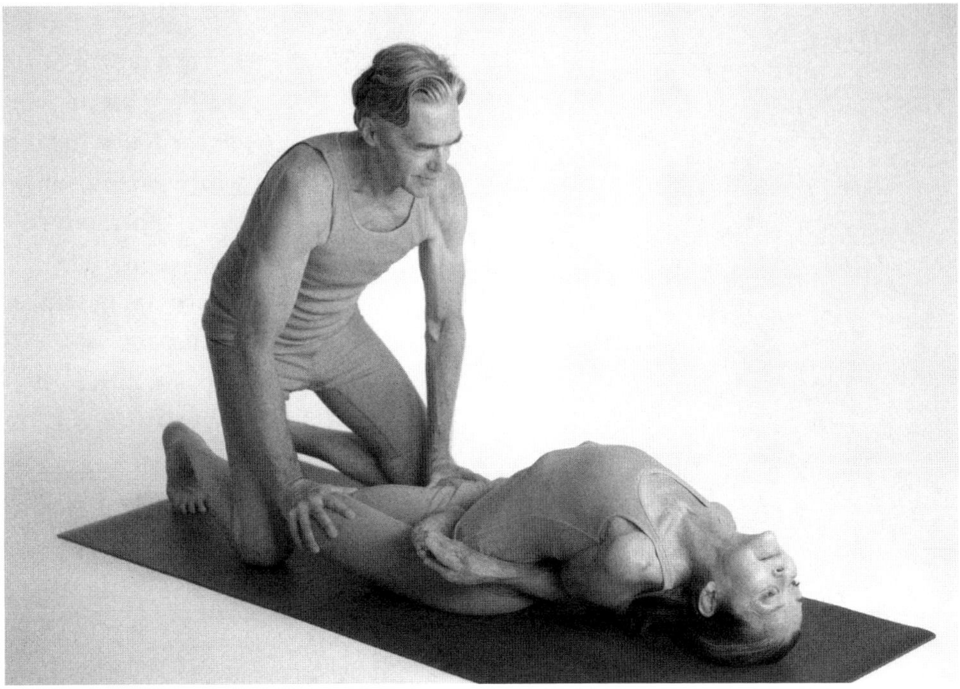

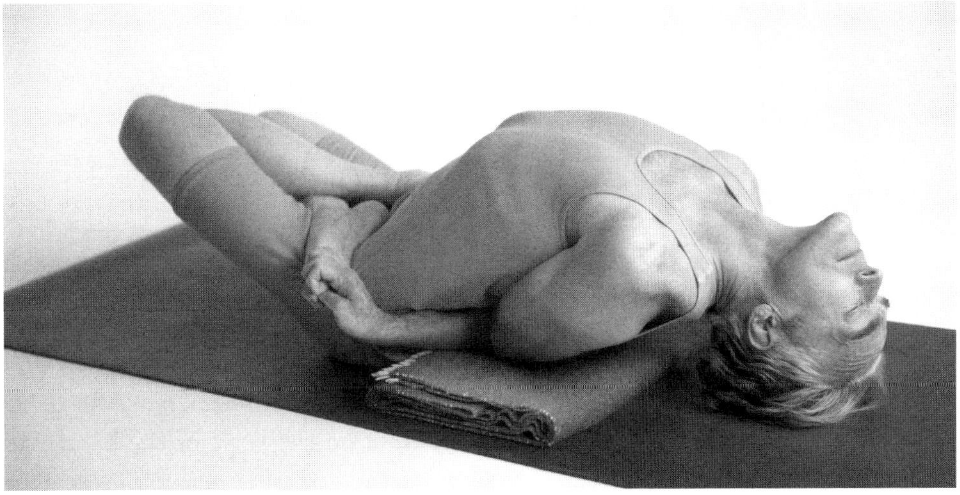

left big toe with the left hand. Inhale; on the next exhalation, again lean forward, wrap the right arm behind and under the left arm to grab the right big toe. Draw the shoulder blades down the back.

2. With an assistant to hold the thighs in and slightly down (allowing some room for movement in the lower body), inhale and lift the heart to form a backbend with deep lower neck extension. Exhale and drop the upper body back to place the top of the head on the floor as you gaze down the nose. Hold this position for five breaths. At the end of an exhalation, empty of breath, engage the pelvic floor and lower belly to initiate a lift in the upper body. Keep the head back and the chest puffed forward; return to a seated position on the inhalation.

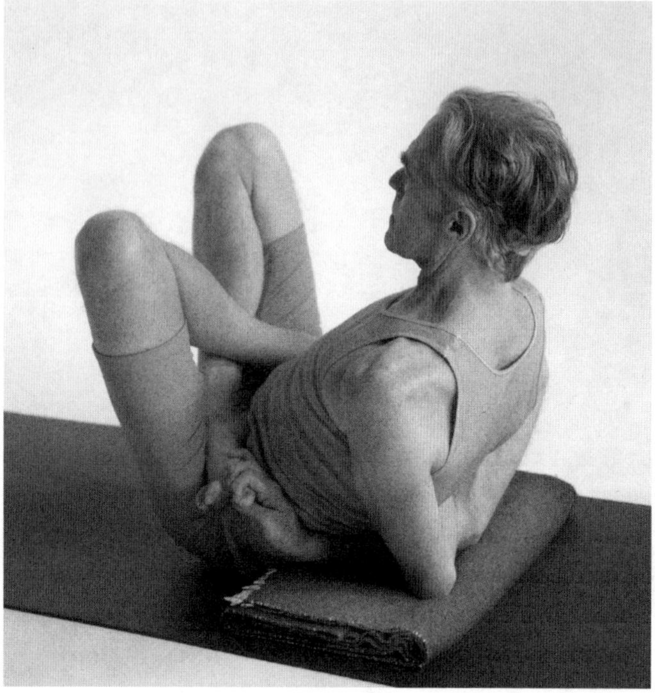

3. Keep the hands on the feet, and with the following five breaths, drop back to touch the head to the floor on the exhalation and return to sitting on the following inhalation; leave the head back while gazing softly down the nose the entire time. On the fifth exhalation having dropped back, remain with the head on floor for five breaths (as in step 2), then return to sitting on an inhalation.
4. To exit, place the hands on the floor beside the legs, lift up, and jump back, unlacing the Padmāsana position to land in Catvāri. If you cannot do this lift yet, unlace the legs from Padmāsana and lift up, which continues to train the apānic pattern of curling and lifting. This will eventually lead to swinging and jumping back through into Catvāri.

Setu Bandhāsana

Bridge Pose

Like Cakrāsana, Setu Bandhāsana can frighten the practitioner, who imagines the possibility of a broken neck for starters! But like in Cakrāsana, the neck is stable and safe when Setu Bandhāsana is practiced carefully and without excess tension in the neck and jaw. Using the legs intelligently and taking a certain amount of weight *forward* into the legs as you roll back is essential. Also, it is important to move into the pose on the wave of the breath while gazing down the nose. When practiced in this manner, Setu Bandhāsana can actually have not only a comfortable but brilliant opening effect in the palate.

1. Lie on the back with the legs stretched straight out. Place the heels together with the feet turned out with medial edges of feet touching the mat. The toes should be pointing to the sides.
2. Using the hands under the buttocks, come up onto the elbows briefly and tilt the pelvis up to place the sitting bones on the floor as you would for Matsyāsana (the Fish Pose). As you do this, the knees will automatically bend out to the sides in line with the feet, and the feet will be drawn closer to the pelvis. Depending on the length of your legs, your feet should be approximately 12 to 30 inches from your buttocks.

3. Holding the outer thighs with the hands, inhale and lift the chest and draw back the head. Roll the shoulders back, lengthening the throat as you gaze down your nose. Use your elbows, so that as you exhale, you can bring the top of the head to the floor (eventually bring the center of the crown of the head to the floor) as in full Matsyāsana. Sink the sitting bones as you open the center of the heart. Breathe freely and continue to gaze down the nose. This position should feel wonderful in the front of the neck.
4. Set and activate the coccyx on an exhale to begin the lifting of the pelvis, pulling it slightly toward the feet. Then with an inhalation, press the soles of the feet toward the floor. Lift the hips and slowly roll from the crown of the head back toward the forehead. Keep the heart open, the throat released, and the eyes looking down the nose. Cross the arms across the chest. Straighten the legs and contract the buttocks firmly. Hold the pose for five breaths.
5. Exit, on an exhalation, using the strength in the legs to bring the hips back down to the floor into a Fish Pose. Use the elbows on the next exhalation to lift the head from the floor and to roll the spine onto the floor from the sacrum on up, so that the head is the last to come back to the floor. If you feel discomfort in the full, extended form, the form is incorrect. Carefully follow the coiling and countercoiling vinyāsa when entering or exiting this pose.
6. If you are a beginner, you may try a training position with your legs and/or arms when moving into the pose. For one version, bend the legs with the feet flat on the floor as in Setu Bandha Sarvāṅgāsana

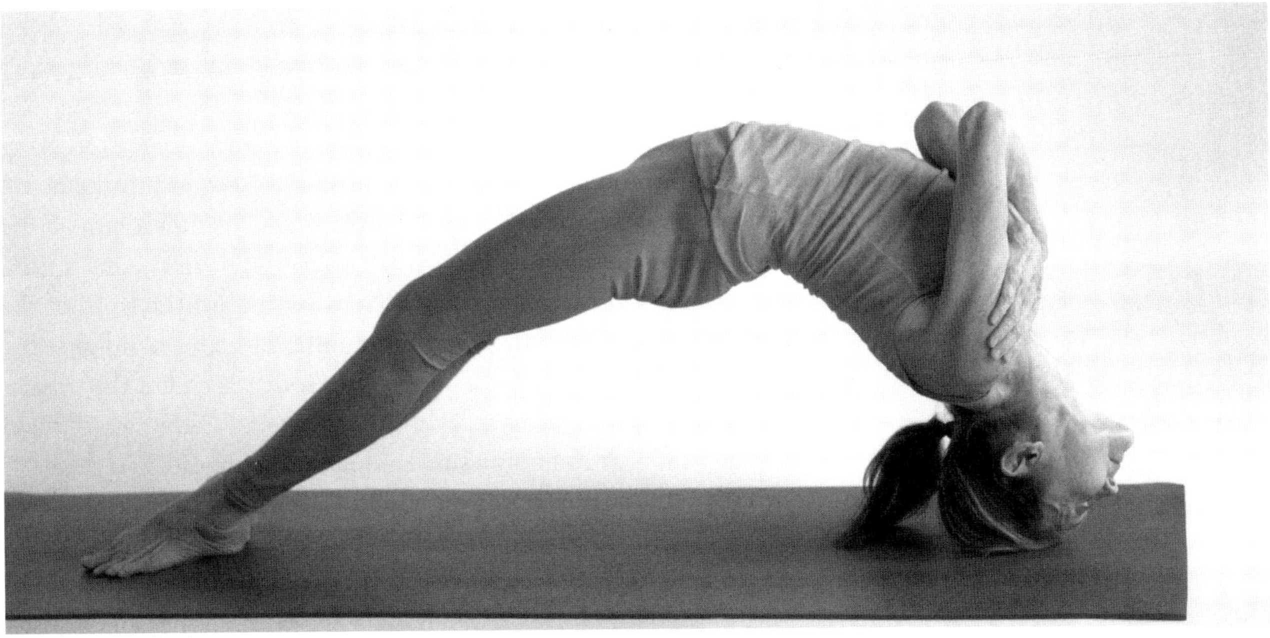

(Bridge Shoulderstand). Use the arms to position the head as for Matsyāsana (see Chapter 11), then straighten the arms along the sides and, inhaling, push through the legs to roll back on the head, gazing down the nose.

7. Alternatively, position the legs in the full form of Setu Bandhāsana with the arms along the sides of the body or reaching out to the sides as you initiate the roll. In this variation, you may eventually fold the arms over the chest, as in the full form, if the pose is strong and stable. Both variations use the arms as guides to draw the shoulders into their proper position and release the chest and throat. Note that the arms are rotated outward. If you have a neck injury or severe tension in the neck or shoulders, attempt only a Setu Bandhāsana variation.

Ūrdhvā Dhanurāsana

Upward Bow Pose

Ūrdhvā Dhanurāsana is the pose most frequently associated with the classic backbend and rightly so. Many of us played around with backbends as kids, and it's a form that seems more "normal" than many other contorted yoga āsanas. It is also the perfect ground for learning the internal and physical forms common to all backbends—from shoulder movement and strength in the legs to activation of the pelvic floor, stretching of the psoas line, and riding the wave of the breath.

1. Lie on your back with the feet parallel to each other and drawn up near the outer edges of the buttocks. The feet should be slightly wider than hip-width apart and are kept parallel throughout the pose.
2. Place the hands on the floor by the ears, with the fingers pointing toward the shoulders. Exhale to establish a connection to the pelvic floor and Mūlabandha. On another exhalation, lift the sacrum off the floor, moving the ring of the pelvis (coccyx, pubic bone, and sitting bones) toward the knees, which are moving toward the front of the mat as the heels lift. This tones the hamstrings, and highlights the coccyx and the entire apānic pattern. Pause at the end of the exhalation on the crown of the head, with most of your weight remaining in the arms and legs and only a small amount on the head. Lift the heels and observe the feeling of protracting the shoulder blades while keeping the arms parallel to one another.
3. On the inhalation, lift the hips toward the ceiling, straightening the arms as you spread the lower back. Lengthen the belly and move

the sacrum up and in toward the lower abdomen. Lower the heels to the floor if they are lifted. Take the head back completing the form only after everything else has rolled sequentially into place.

4. Spread the back surface of the body like a cobra's back. Relax the mouth and feel the skin on the back of the neck soften and then flow down the back as well as spreading up over the neck and forming a cobra hood over the head. Open, lift, and widen the fronts of the armpits and the shoulder blades, lengthening the psoas lines without limitation. Imagine that the coccyx is moving forward and slightly up as the pubic bone drops back and down as if to rest on the coccyx. Breathe freely.

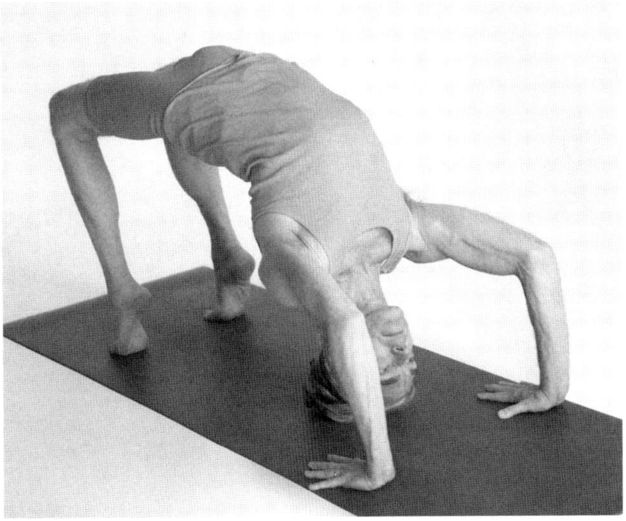

5. The buttocks muscles may be contracted while initially entering the pose, but after a time and with practice, they can soften and release. Maintain a feeling of the sacrum moving in and up toward the navel as the coccyx moves away from the sacrum toward the pubic bone. Draw the backs of the thighs up into the legs to encourage Mūlabandha.

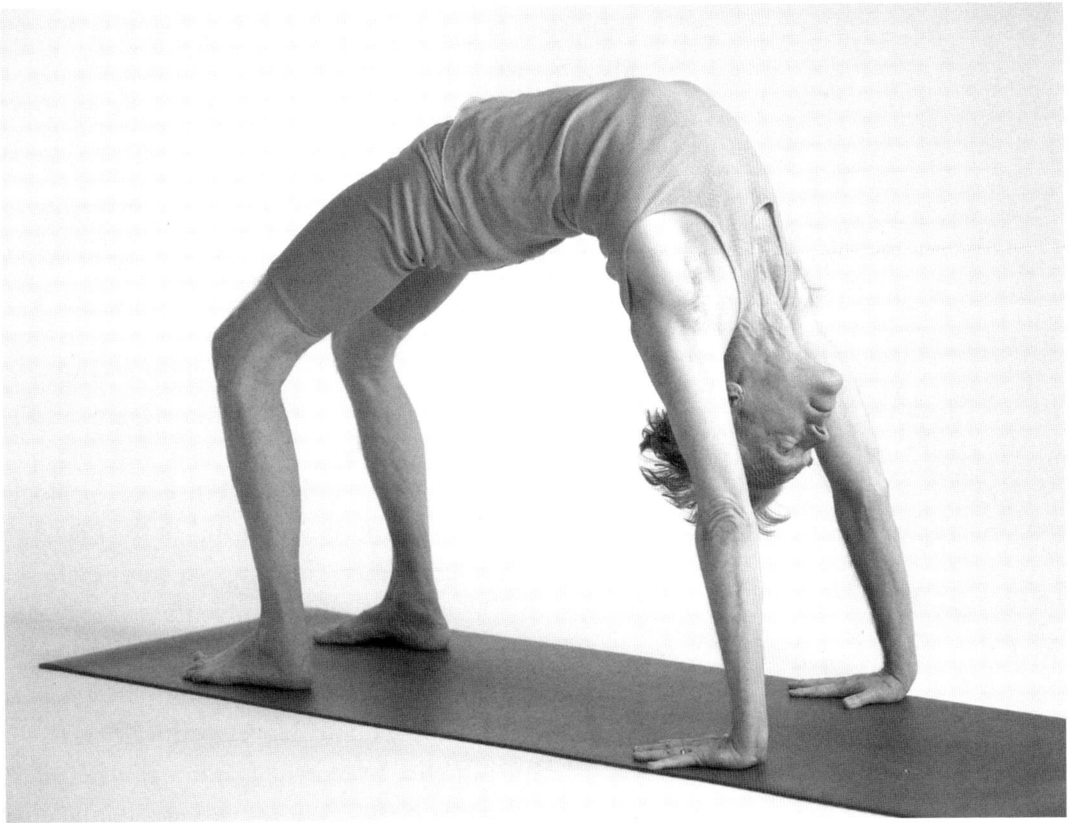

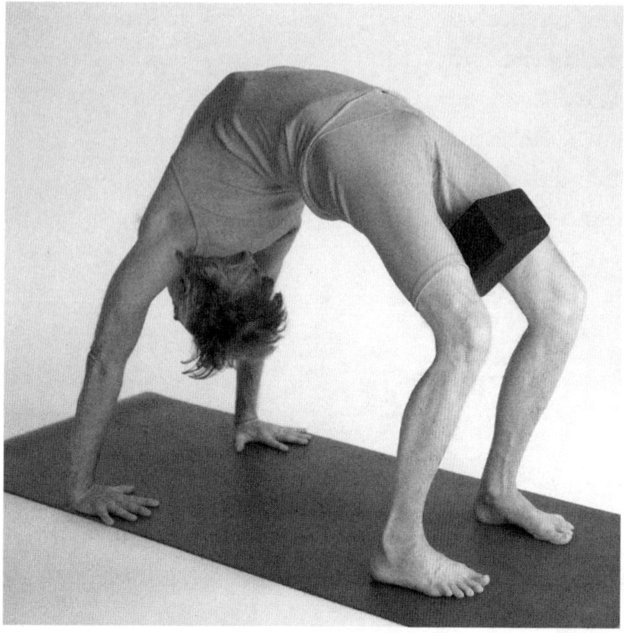

6. If you are a beginner and need motivation, gaze up between the eyebrows or at a point on the floor. When the pose is complete and easy, gaze down at the tip of or along the line of the nose.
7. Hold the full pose for at least five breaths. On an exhalation, lower carefully back down to the mat. To come down, first tuck the head, then place the shoulders down, unroll the spine flat on the floor, and finally inhale as you drop the sacrum to the floor. Rest briefly for one or two breaths and then repeat the pose. Each full Ūrdhvā Dhanurāsana in a series should become easier, more expressive, and more open.
8. After lowering to the floor on the final exhalation, placing the sacrum down last, rest in the residue of the pose for a few rounds of breath.

Dvi Pāda Viparīta Daṇḍāsana

Two-Footed Inverted Staff Pose

This and the following two poses are extreme backbends found in the Advanced A Series, but they are also informative for less advanced practitioners working to refine subtle movements and extensions of the spine in all backbends.

1. Begin in Baddha Hasta Śīrṣāsana A (see Chapter 10). On an exhalation, carefully bring the feet down to the floor and come into a backbend. Inhaling, spread the kidney wings and wrap the shoulders as you ground through the elbows to lengthen through the crown of the head as you would in a well-aligned headstand.
2. Move the feet so that the legs can straighten. Be sure to move the sacrum in and up to keep the back comfortable. If possible, place the inner edges of the feet together on the floor and hold for five breaths, gazing softly along the line of the nose.
3. If the primary form of this pose is comfortable you may increase the stretch. On an inhalation, pushing the sacrum up and in, lift the head off the floor and walk the feet in closer to the hands. Keep the feet parallel to each other and shoulder-width apart. If you are flexible, hold the ankles. Keep the shoulder blades distinctly protracted the entire time.
4. To exit, in either form exhale and place the top of the head on the floor. Then with the kidney wings spread and the elbows grounded,

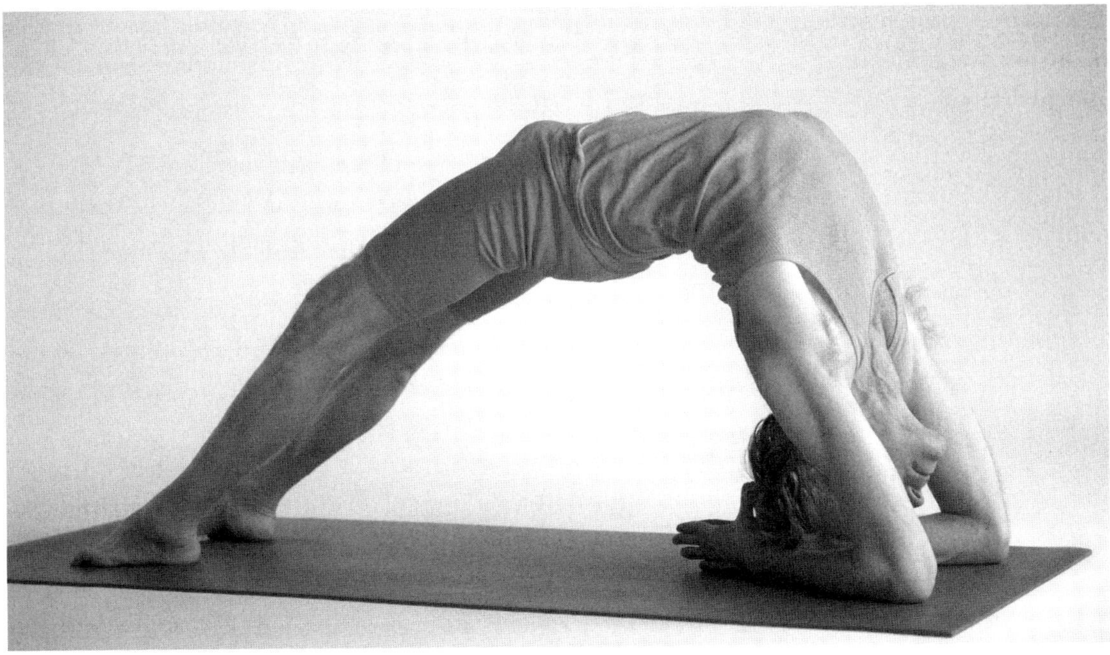

rock and inhaling come back up into Headstand, then drop down into Catvāri and move through a Half Vinyāsa. If this is not possible, simply lower onto the back and roll out of the pose into Cakrāsana to take a Half Vinyāsa.

EKA PĀDA VIPARĪTA DAṆḌĀSANA

One-Footed Inverted Staff Pose

1. Traditionally you come directly into this pose following step 2 of Dvi Pāda Viparīta Daṇḍāsana. Alternatively, you can drop into it as for step 1 of that pose.
2. In either case, leave the left foot on the floor and take the right leg up toward the ceiling, pointing the toes. Keep the hips level and the lower back wide. Eventually the left leg will remain straight with the mound of the big toe firmly grounded. Hold this pose for five breaths.
3. Lower the right leg and lift the left, holding this side for five breaths as well. Lower the left leg and exit the pose as for Dvi Pāda Viparīta Daṇḍāsana.
4. If flexibility allows you may walk the feet in close to the hands. Center one foot and, inhaling, lift the other leg straight up to the ceiling, pointing the toes. Hold for five breaths. Once you have completed the second side, walk both feet out away from the head and exit the pose as for Dvi Pāda Viparīta Daṇḍāsana.

Eka Pāda Rāja Kapotāsana

One-Footed King Pigeon Pose

Similar to Kapotāsana in feel, this more extreme version is an excellent method of exploring extension and flexion—without impingement—along the entire spine while working into backbends.

1. From Downward Facing Dog Pose, on an exhale jump forward bending the left leg to bring it forward and across the midline as you sit down, stretching the right leg out in back of you. Bring the right psoas button toward the left heel.
2. Pick up the right leg, and as you exhale, reach around with the right arm (palm up) and clasp the mound of your right big toe from the outside edge of the foot. On a deep, smooth inhalation, bring the right elbow and right kidney area forward and up as you drop the outer right hip toward the floor. This will rotate the right hand so the palm is turned down, and the chest will turn forward toward the front of the mat.
3. Lift the left arm and take the right foot (and eventually the right ankle) with both hands. Bring the right foot up, until eventually the sole meets the top of the head (or the heel may come to the eyebrows if

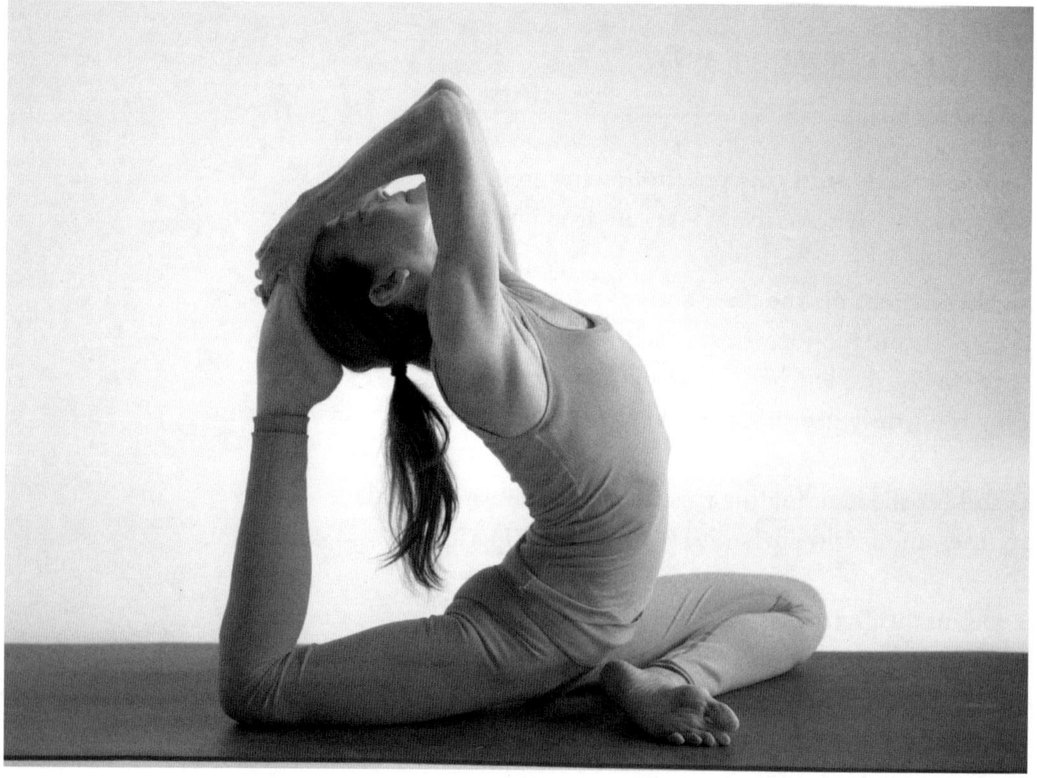

you are extraordinarily flexible). Bring the elbows toward each other. Spread and lift the kidney wings as the heart continues to float up. Hold this for five breaths. On an exhalation, release the foot, place the hands down next to the hips, step back into Catvāri, and move through a Half Vinyāsa for the other side.

4. When first clasping the foot, resist the action of the arms by using the quadriceps to push back through the foot into the hand. This will further lengthen the front of the body and will eliminate compression in the lower back, helping to open the thoracic spine.

9

Twists

COMPENSATING FOR OR BALANCING ASYMMETRIES in the body and breath comprises much of the work of yoga āsana and prāṇāyāma. With practice, we may begin to notice and track these imbalances as they relate to all poses, but twisting poses easily expose asymmetries in the legs, hip joints, SI joints, spine, rib cage, and neck. Twists also reveal a dramatic interplay of actions and counteractions throughout the body. Indeed, the appropriate use of counteractions and counterrotations is the key to the alignment, form, and benefit of twisting poses.

The basic movement and breathing patterns entering, exiting, and during all twists is similar. Before you even begin, you exhale to tone the pelvic floor creating a sense of being grounded—usually through the feet or, in seated twists, through the sitting bones. This grounding contact with the foundation of the pose gives space within the body, mind, and nervous system to pause for an instant and then really feel the full movement pattern on the inhalation that follows. These first two breathing patterns are vital "setup steps" to the actual pose.

Exhaling establishes evenness, stability, and full lines of the apāna pattern of the twist, often using the abdominal wall. Inhaling brings in counteractions: extension of the torso and spine as well as a lifting of the heart and more awareness of the palate and pelvic floor connection. The inhalation wakes up the seeds in the nervous system of all the counterspins, rotations, pushes, and pulls for the primary actions of the particular twist. Having set up these two important patterns, we move into the actual twisting pose on the next exhalation. The following inhalation switches on or "lights up" the full pose and in theory pulls the central thread of the pelvic floor up into the body. This introduces all of the counteractions to the primary actions without the primary actions disappearing. Then they work together, churning out the nectar of integrated prāṇa and apāna.

In many twists, there are important counteractions to level the hips or minimize lateral flexion/extension (depending on the twist). These counteractions are an important means of identifying, balancing, and correcting bad postural habits. In the fine-tuning of twists, the side-to-side work across the midline is asymmetrical and creates rotations in opposite directions—like unscrewing two halves of a sphere or moving as if opposite ends of the body were opposing wheels in a system of gears that rotate in complementary yet opposite directions.

Most twisting occurs in the upper lumbar and lower thoracic sections of the spine (the junction of T12 and L1) and in the neck at the atlanto-axial joint (the junction of C1 and C2). There is very little twisting in the upper thoracic spine and the lower part of the neck. The SI joint may be injured by improperly aligned twisting, although micro-twisting in the SI joint *is* allowed with good communication of complementary rotations side to side and through the pelvic floor.

The most common forms of twists are flexion twists, like Paśāsana (Noose Pose). Others, like Trikoṇāsana (Triangle Pose), are referred to as extension twists. Less common are spiraling extension twists, such as Parighāsana (Hinge Pose). We initiate movement into flexion twists on the exhalation, working the abdominal muscles to keep the lumbar spine slightly flexed and the coccyx curled. This is the apāna pattern. After initially getting into any flexion twist, the next inhalation brings in a slight amount of counterextension through the spine. This can be complemented on the following exhalation with a bit more flexion and on the next inhalation with additional extension.

As in flexion twists, extension twists are entered on the exhalation. The PC muscle is toned, the coccyx is awakened, and the spine is relatively straight when entering the pose. Extension twists allow for more length in the whole spine, particularly in the lumbar region and the neck. They do not involve as strong an initial compression of the abdominal muscles as in flexion twists, and they allow for more space between the vertebral bodies along the spine.

A flexion twist has more of a compressive effect on abdominal organs because it shortens the abdominal muscles, which may distort the positioning of the stomach, liver, and intestines in the abdominal cavity. Therefore it is easier and advisable to practice twists, especially flexion twists, when the bowels and bladder are not full. An extension twist has a more dramatic effect on the relationship of the diaphragm and the abdominal organs. The ribs and abdomen are less compressed and allow fuller motion in the diaphragm. It is usually easier to breathe in extension twists, and they are often pleasant to hold for longer periods of time or to use in more therapeutic contexts.

In all twists, there should be a feeling of dignity in the final pose—as though you are growing longer up through the center of the spine and out through the crown of the head. Whatever form the final twist takes, it is really important not to lock the pelvis and sitting bones in place either when entering the pose or when continuing to make subtle microadjustments while pausing in it. Also important is a strong awareness of the hips and pelvic floor. When you are first learning some new and "gnarly" twists, such as Marīchyāsana D, there may be a certain amount of strain getting into the pose, but this should be minimized by smoothing out the ends of the breath and not pushing or pulling yourself into the pose from an external perspective. It is sometimes difficult for beginners to breathe fully in extreme twists, so a feeling of anxiety may arise. In this case, it is important to soften the gaze and the tongue and sometimes even to back out of the twist a tiny bit in order to calm the mind. Grimacing, clenching the teeth, and grunting are usually methods of forcing a situation and ignoring an awareness of pain, but they don't help the pose unfold.

A general benefit of twists is that they can aid the "fire of digestion," helping the movement of the gastrointestinal track and possibly the function of the liver and stomach. This is mostly mechanics—the organs in the abdomen are moved around as you twist your torso, and this can help to get things moving! Another benefit of twisting is that you can distinctly feel the side-to-side imbalances around the hip joints, pelvic floor, abdominal wall, shoulders, and neck. Consequently, twisting can give you a real handle on how to work with and lessen these individual imbalances.

Commonsense contraindications for twists are herniated disks (especially those that have been recently herniated); a fractured spine; broken ribs; and swelling, such as with abdominal tumors. Spinal irregularities such as scoliosis require the practitioner to work slowly and carefully so as not to exacerbate the problem. Those with inguinal and other hernias should use caution with or avoid twisting in certain dimensions as well. It is also contraindicated to practice extreme twists during pregnancy (though open twists in which the belly is not compressed are usually alright). In all of these cases, or if you experience difficulty or pain when twisting, you should seek the advice of a highly experienced yoga teacher.

Marīchyāsana C

This simple twist from the Primary Series is wonderful in that it can be done to some degree by almost everyone. It is easy to discover the main actions that underlie all twists and to really *feel* counteractions deep in the body that are reminiscent of churning butter.

1. From Downward Facing Dog Pose, at the end of an exhale jump through to a seated position inhaling as you land. You may land with the right foot in place on the floor or with both legs stretched straight out in front. In the latter case, bend the right knee and place the right heel near the right hip and buttock, about a hand-width from the inner left thigh.
2. With the spine straight, place the right hand on the floor behind you and lean back to turn the belly to the right. This will initially turn the pelvis to the right, giving the feeling that the left leg is lengthening in an inward spiral.

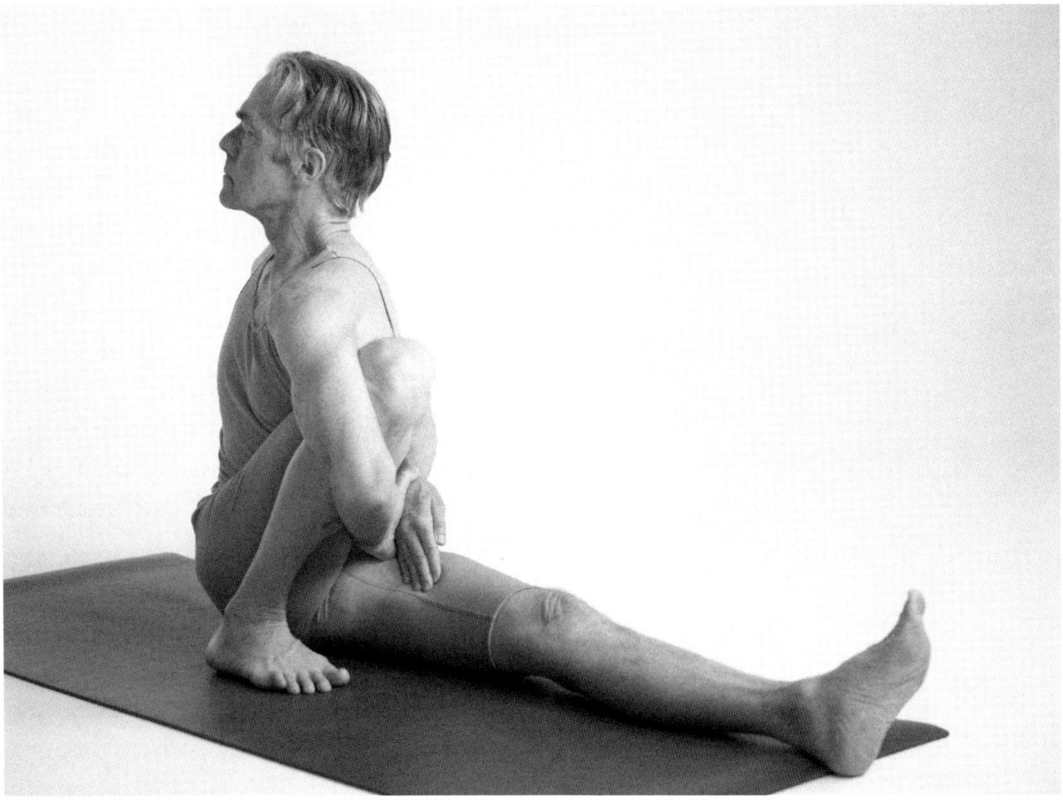

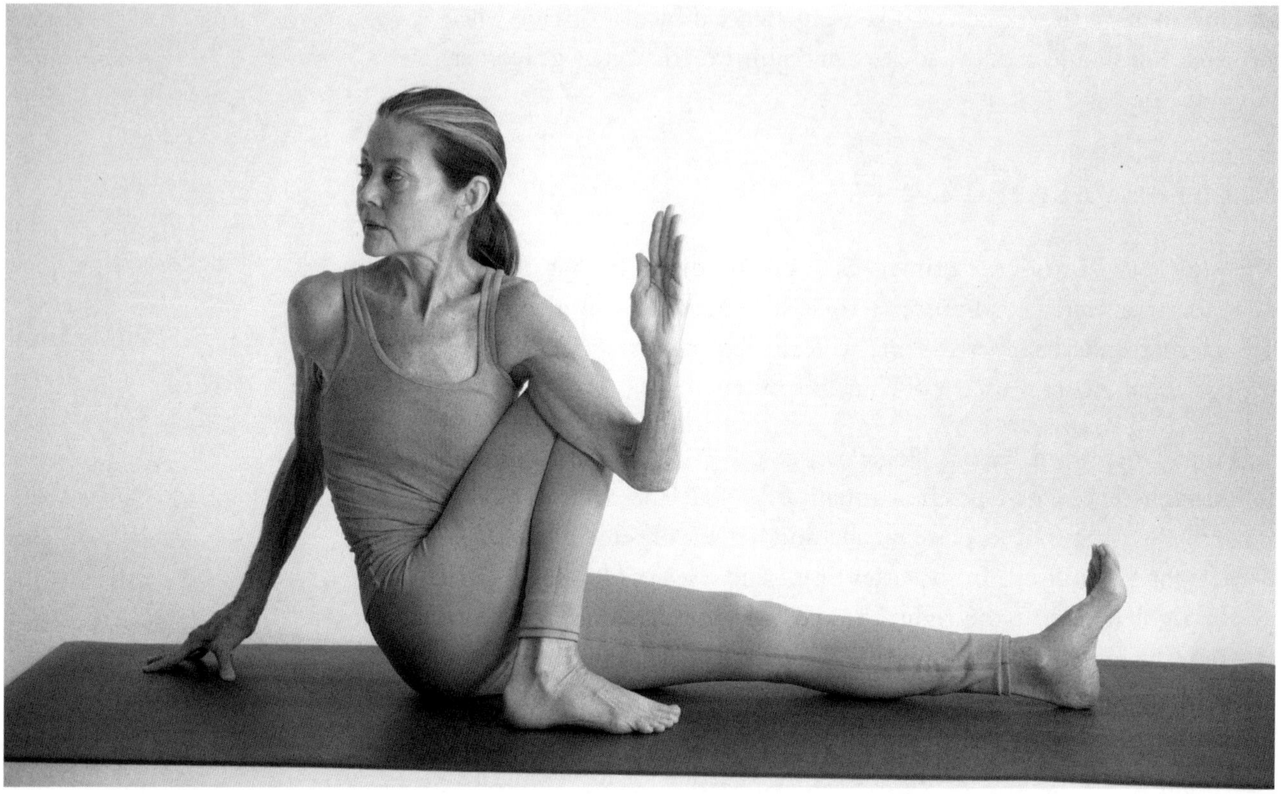

3. Reach up with the left arm while inhaling, then exhale and wrap the arm around the outside of the right leg or simply hook the left elbow or hand on the outer right knee. If the arm is wrapped, reach behind the back with the right arm and clasp the left wrist.
4. The next inhalation "activates" the pose, bringing in all of the movement components and counteractions. The outer right hip and right sitting bone come back down toward the floor and slightly forward. This brings the pelvis somewhat back into a countertwist, which seems to shorten the left leg with a subtle outward rotation. Here it is possible to play with and listen to the dialogue between prāṇa and apāna while toning the pelvic floor.
5. Turn the head in the direction of the twist (over the right shoulder), and select an easy gazing point on the horizon. Notice transformations that occur in the body, mind, and breath over the course of five breaths.
6. To exit the pose, first exhale fully to deposit some tone in the pelvic floor. Inhale releasing the arms and turn the upper body toward the front. Exhale to settle the pelvis steadily onto the mat and square the body to the front, then proceed through the appropriate vinyāsa to repeat the same pattern on the other side.

MARĪCHYĀSANA D

This is just like Marīchyāsana C, except that one of the legs is in Padmāsana. One small detail like that can make a seemingly accessible pose impossible! But even if the pose is difficult, don't give up. Work steadily and carefully just to the edge of your ability, and over time the pose will evolve.

1. From a seated position with the legs out in front of you, bend the left leg into a deep Half Padmāsana position with the heel near the psoas button area of the right lower belly and the ankle at the crease in the right groin.
2. Bend the right knee, placing the foot flat on the floor up toward the right sitting bone. Rotate the hips to the right as in Marīchyāsana C, pressing forward and down with the left knee.
3. Inhale as you lean back and slightly to the right to move the belly up out of the way and to the right. It is helpful on the next exhalation to rest the upper body on the right arm as you do this. On the following inhalation, reach up high with the left arm. Then with the top of the arm bone moving forward, exhale, flex the lumbar spine slightly as if lengthening the coccyx along the floor. Continue to wrap the arm as low around the right leg as possible. Reach behind the back with the right hand. Clasp the right wrist with the left hand and, if possible, hold the left ankle with the fingers of the right hand.
4. To activate the pose, inhale and pull in opposite directions with the arms so there is a sense of the heart spreading and lifting and a feeling of spiraling up through the crown of the head as you sink into the pose. Play with the counteraction, which brings the right sitting bone back down and forward toward the floor. Find a steady gazing point on the horizon, and keep the tongue silent and still.
5. Hold the twist for five breaths. At the end of an exhalation, ground into the base of the pose, and on the next inhalation, release the arms and turn the upper body to the front.

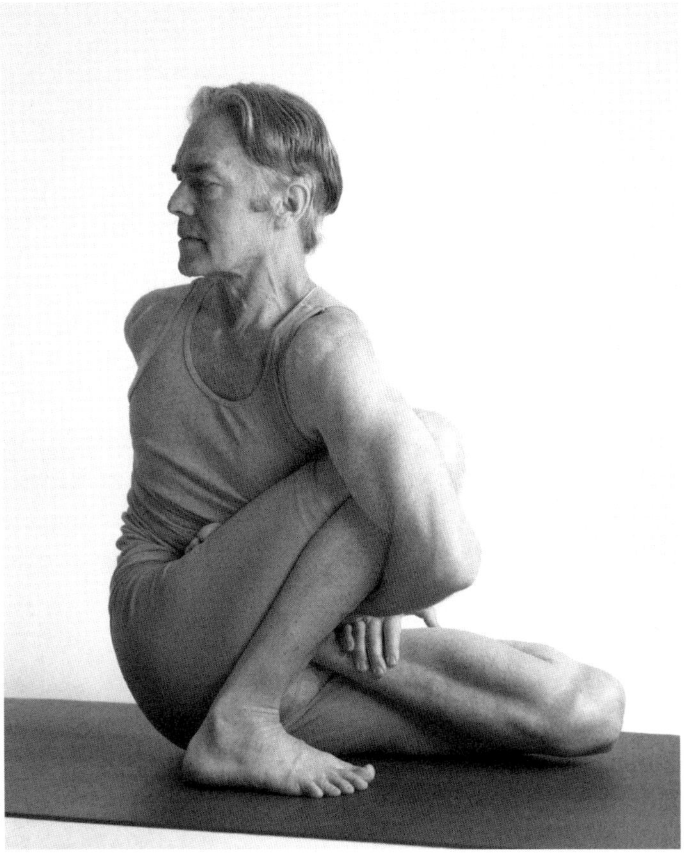

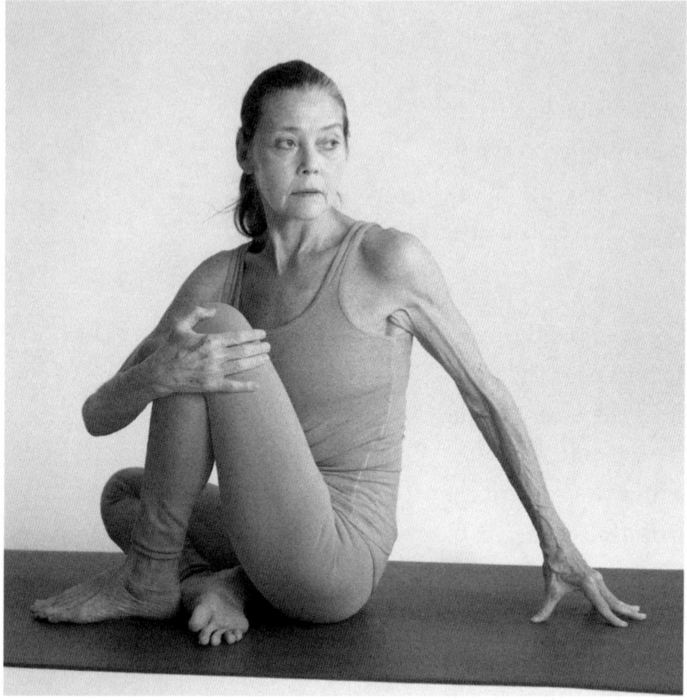

Continue to release the arms, grounding into the pelvic floor on the exhale. After going through the appropriate vinyāsas, practice the posture on the second side.

6. If you cannot bind the arms, catch the right knee with the left elbow or hold the knee with the palm of the left hand. Press the elbow/hand against the knee, and push back into the elbow/hand with the knee. You may also use a strap to connect the hands behind you. In form D, if Padmāsana is not possible, you may fold the left foot in front of the body and place it on the floor with the heel in front of the right sitting bone. You can then put the right foot in front of the left ankle to work the pose from there.

PARIGHĀSANA

Hinge Pose

This twist from the end of the Intermediate Series allows a radical lateral spinning, spiraling movement in the lower spine and pelvis. It profoundly impacts the hip joints, SI joints, abdominal wall, and diaphragm.

1. Begin by floating through from Downward Facing Dog Pose or simply sitting and folding the right leg into Half Vīrāsana. Open the left leg out to the side so the thighs form a little more than a 90-degree angle. Sit with the pelvis and upper body turned out to face the folded leg.
2. Inhaling, reach up high with the left arm, releasing the left psoas line. Exhaling, reach straight out and forward with the left arm on the floor, palm up. Next slide the left arm and shoulder down along the floor to create the initial twist and lateral flexion.
3. Inhaling, reach up toward the ceiling with the right arm, then bend the elbow as you continue to stretch the arm and the right side in order to take the outer edge of the left foot with the right hand (or secure a connection between the hand and foot using a strap) with the elbow pointing up toward the ceiling. Then, if possible, bring the left hand to the left foot. Eventually the back of the head can rest on the left shin.

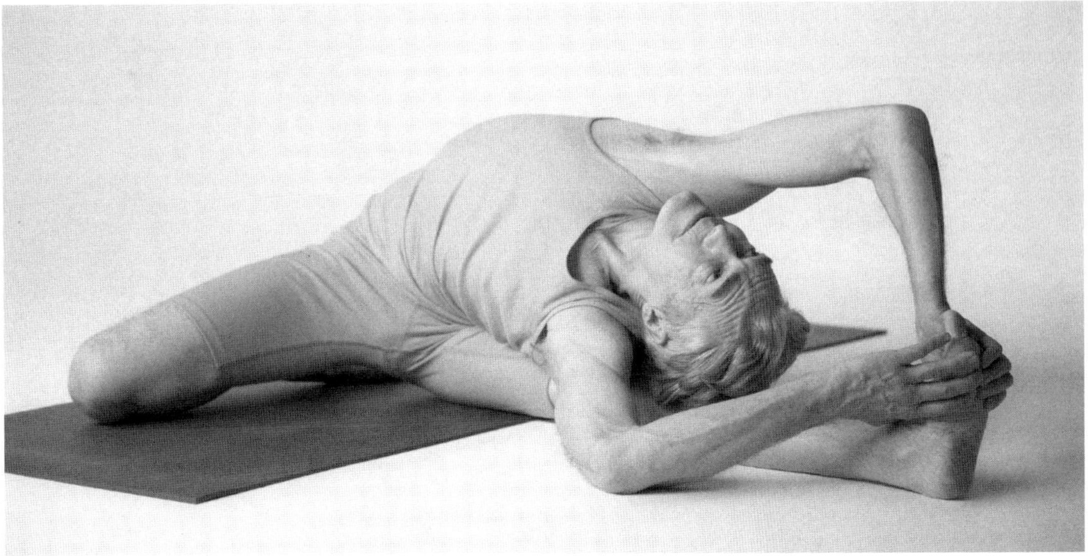

4. Gradually introduce a slight outward rotation to the right femur. This will bring the right sitting bone back toward the floor. Do this just the right amount to create Mūlabandha, remembering that the inward rotation of the right femur is the primary, leading action that takes your torso out over the straightened leg and that deeply and correctly lengthens the left hamstrings and adductors.
5. If you are flexible, the gazing point is the left big toe as the back of the head rests on the left shin. If you are stiffer, gaze along the line of the nose while smiling and breathing kindness into the whole-body patterns as they manifest. Hold the pose for five breaths.
6. Come out of the pose by releasing the hands on an exhalation and sitting up on an inhalation, then place the hands on the upper rims of the pelvis to ground the sitting bones equally for one breath. This provides a unique space for digesting the residue of this radical pose.
7. Move through a Half Vinyāsa to get back into the central axis, then float through to begin the pose on the other side.

Paśāsana

Noose Pose

In Indian mythology, Gaṇeśa's vehicle was once Krauñcha (literally "crane"), a celestial musician who was cursed and turned into a huge mouse or rat. He was tamed when Gaṇeśa sat on him after throwing a noose around his neck. (Krauñcha really *wanted* to be tamed, so he was delighted.) Paśāsana is the embodiment of this story; while squatting, the folded legs feel a like huge mouse or rat. Summoning the combination of

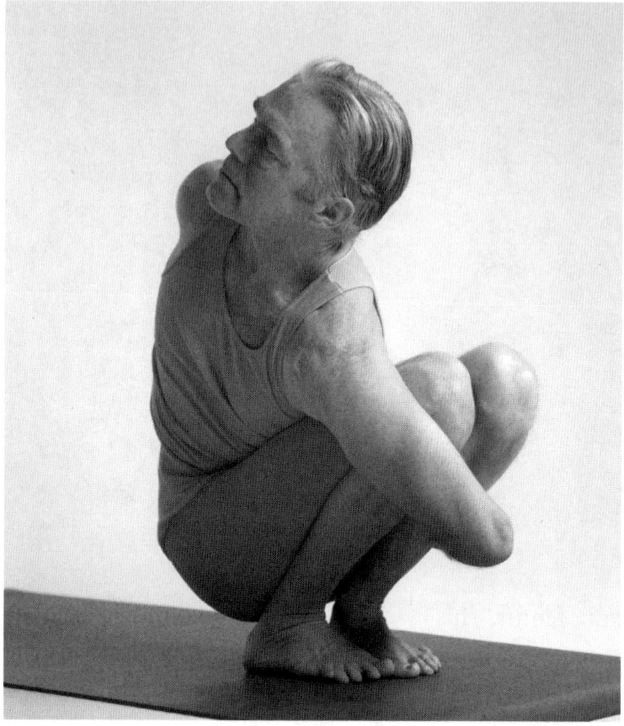 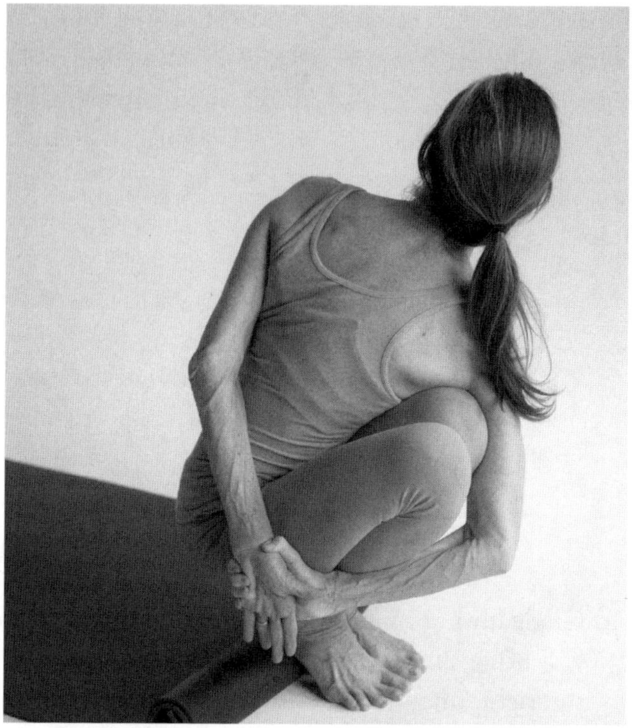

forward bending with the action of an oblique stretch, we can throw our arms around and "lasso" our own legs, summarizing the Primary Series, to bring both the image of the mouse and the apānic residue from the series together.

1. From Downward Facing Dog Pose, at the end of an exhalation, hop to the front of the mat, landing with the feet together and sitting down in a squatting position. If it is difficult to squat with the heels flat on the floor, you may roll the mat slightly to provide support.
2. On an inhalation, lean back onto the left hand and reach up with the right arm as you turn the upper body to the left. Exhaling deeply, reach around the outside of the left thigh with the upper right arm, bending the elbow to bring the lower part of the arm near the left shin and up behind the back. Reach behind you with the left arm to clasp the hands together or hold the left wrist with the right hand.
3. Now turn on the juice in the pose. Inhaling, push down through the feet as if to stand up, but at the same time, keep a sense of the sitting bones being heavy, so you do not actually stand but instead activate the legs. Move the left sitting bone back down toward the left ankle to create a countertwisting of the pelvis.
4. Roll the top of the left arm back, sliding the shoulder blade down the back as the sternum lifts. Turn the head to the left, keeping the chin neutral, and gaze at a point on the wall over the left shoulder.

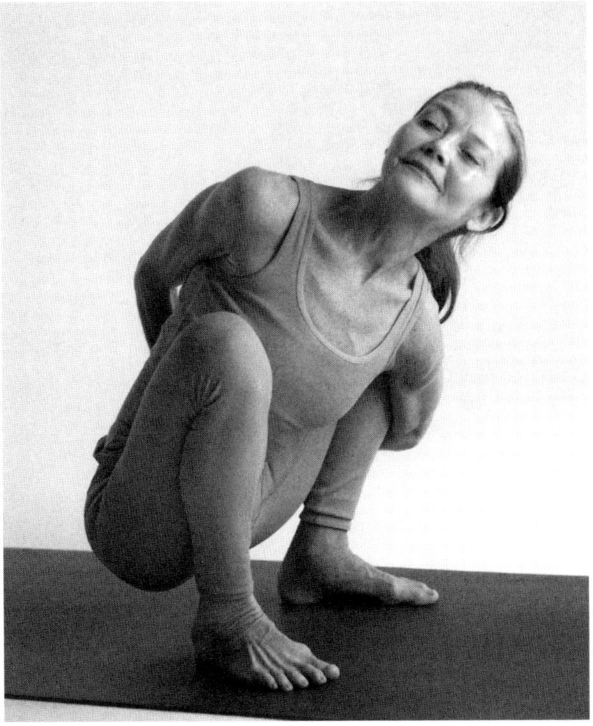

5. Pull the arms in opposite directions, as if to break the clasp of the hands, but keep them clasped so the pose comes to life. Pull the hands up the back as if to squeeze the rat. Keep the gaze steady and the breath smooth and even. Hold this for five breaths.
6. At the end of an exhalation, bring the awareness to the tone in the pelvic floor. Keeping this awareness, release the hands and return the upper body to center on the inhalation. Exhale to reawaken the feet and pelvic floor, then switch sides twisting to the right. After five breaths on the second side, exit the pose by setting the tone in the pelvic floor on an exhale before jumping back into Catvāri.
7. Two variations on full Paśāsana can be used when you are learning the pose or are using it therapeutically. If squatting is not possible, sit on the heels as in Vajrāsana. Inhale and reach up with the right arm to release the psoas line. Then exhaling deeply, reach across the thighs, bringing the right shoulder to the outer left knee and the right elbow to the floor near the left shin or ankle. Inhaling, reach up toward the ceiling with the left arm, then bend it at the elbow to drop the left hand behind the back to take the inner right thigh with the left fingers. This is a flexion twist. Work with the counteractions of pushing the right elbow into the left thigh and pulling the left hand back and up keeping the head away from the floor, extending and spiraling long through the spine.
8. If you are pregnant or for a variation that works for most, squat with the feet and knees about hip-width apart. Inhale and reach up with the right arm, then exhale and reach forward to wrap the right arm back around only the right leg. Clasp the hands behind the back, and work the pose intelligently as you would in the full form. Release after five breaths and repeat on the second side.

Bharadvājāsana

Bharadhvāja's Pose

This pose, named after the sage Bharadhvāja, appears in two similar forms within the Intermediate Series. The first Bharadvājāsana appears midway through the series, just before beginning poses with the legs behind the head. The second form appears at the very end of the series and is called Supta Ūrdhvā Pāda Vajrāsana.

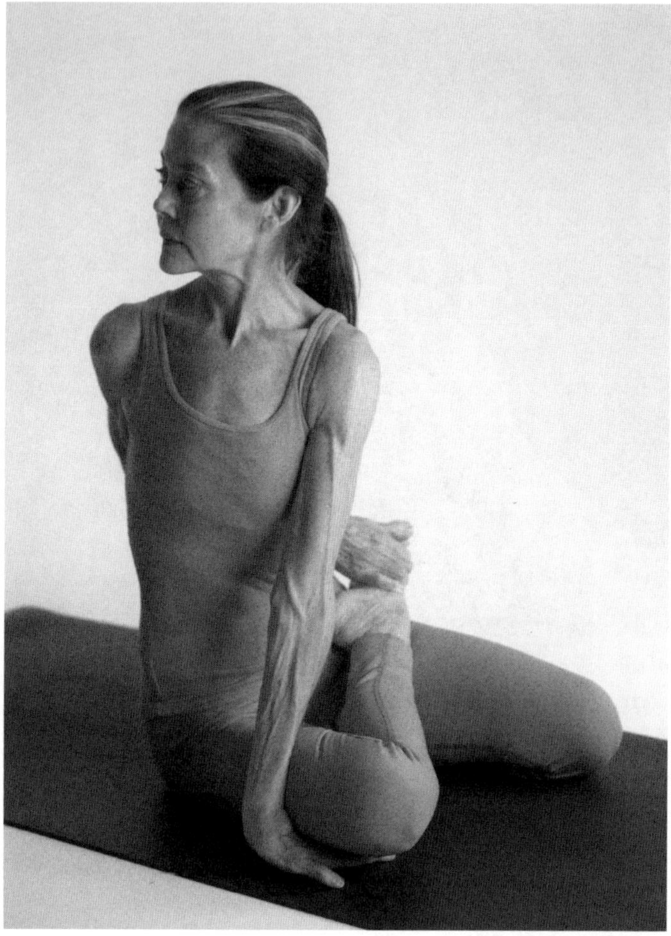

1. From Downward Facing Dog Pose after an exit, slide through to a seated position and inhale with the left leg folded in Vīrāsana and the right leg stretched straight out in front. Angle the left knee out to the side and draw the right foot back toward the lower belly to put the right leg in Padmāsana as you exhale.
2. Spin the torso to the right, elongating the spine as you reach up through the left arm and fingertips, rotating the arm and protracting the shoulder blades. Exhaling, place the left palm on the floor under the right knee, with the fingers pointing toward the midline of the body. Wrap the right arm behind the back to clasp the right big toe or foot.
3. Activate the twist by engaging the arms, pushing down and forward through the left arm and hand and bending the right elbow to pull the right foot as the top of the right arm rolls back. Turn the head to the right, keeping the tops of the shoulders broad and dropping away from the ears as you find a steady gazing point on the horizon over the right shoulder.
4. Bring the awareness into the midline of the body and the sense of the sternum lifting, the kidney wings broadening and lifting, and the palate releasing. Experiment with the countertwist of the pelvis by bringing the left sitting bone back down toward the floor. The rotations of the femurs at the hip joints shift with different degrees of counteraction. Notice the effect of this on the pelvic floor. Hold this position for five breaths.
5. At the end of an exhalation, tone the pelvic floor, release the arms, and as you inhale, turn back to center. Cross the legs, place the hands next to the hips, lift up and jump back to Catvāri for a Half Vinyāsa. Then glide through and do the pose on the other side.

Supta Ūrdhvā Pāda Vajrāsana

Reclining Feet Up Thunderbolt Pose

Similar in final form to Bharadvājāsana, the entrance to this pose is quite different as is the effect of the final form on the pelvic floor. It's an interesting exercise to practice the form with wide knees (Bharadvājāsana) and then immediately after with the knees close together (Supta Ūrdhvā Pāda Vajrāsana) to tune in to the subtle differences.

1. Lie on the back with the legs stretched out straight along the floor arms along the sides of the body, palms down as in Tāḍāgī Mudrā. At the end of an exhalation, begin to lift the legs and hips and at about a 30-degree lift from the floor inhale to continue the lift, until feet are straight overhead, then exhale to place the feet on the floor above your head as in Halāsana.
2. Still in Halāsana position, fold the right leg into Padmāsana and wrap the right arm behind the back to clasp the right big toe. Gaze down the line of your nose, and hold this position for five breaths.
3. On a well-defined exhalation, still in Halāsana position, fold the left leg into Vīrāsana, grabbing the left big toe or the side of the foot with your left hand. On the next inhalation, rock up to a seated position, keeping the hold on the feet as you roll up. The knees should be about 4 to 6 inches apart, and you should still be holding both feet with the hands.
4. Exhaling, release the left hand from the foot and place the left palm on the floor under the right knee, with the fingers pointing toward the midline of the body. Wrap the right arm behind your back to clasp the right big toe or foot.
5. Activate the twisting action by engaging the arms, pushing down and forward through the heel of the left hand and bending the right elbow

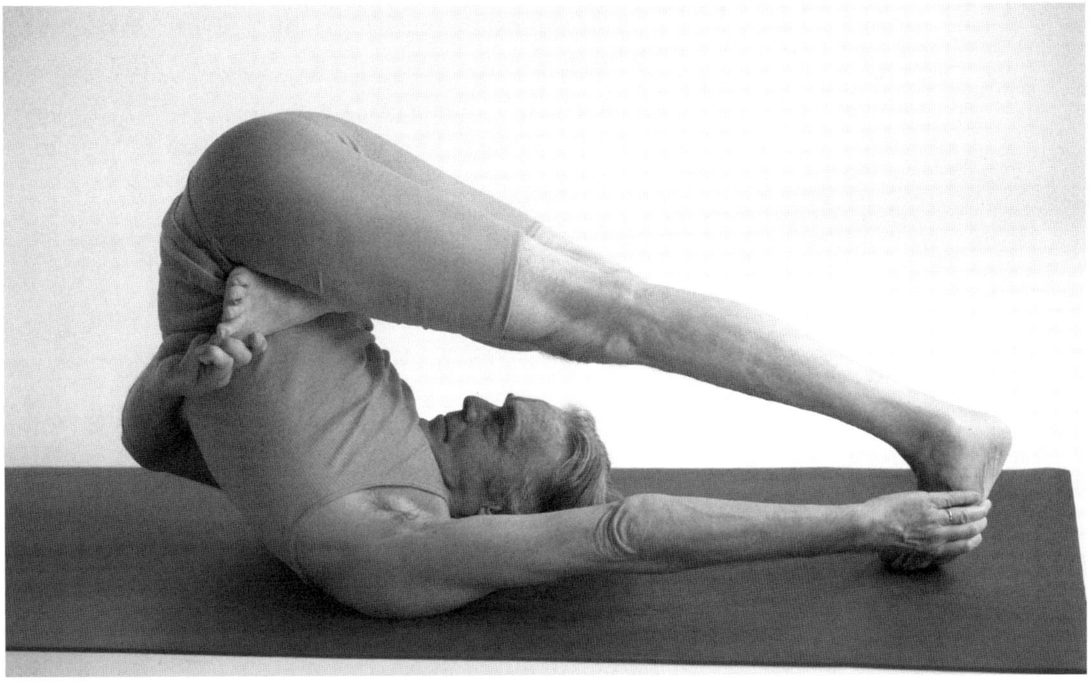

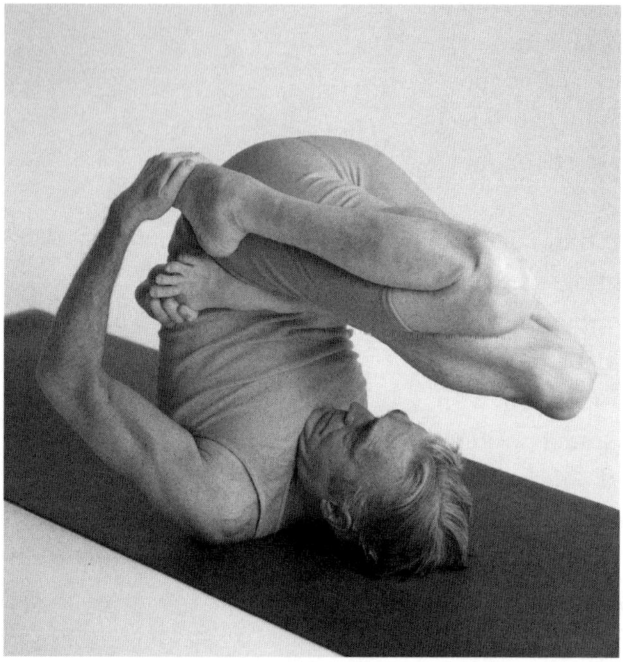

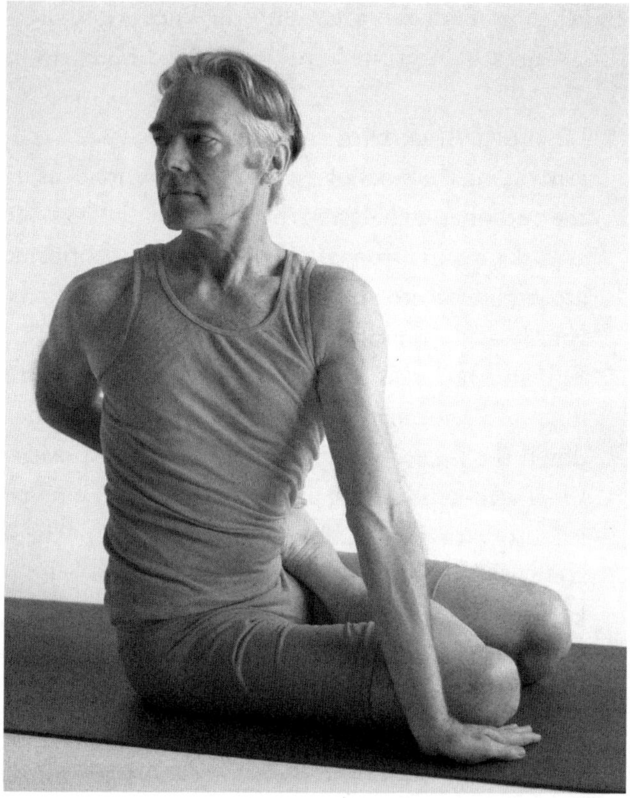

to pull the right foot as the top of the right arm rolls back. It is similar to shooting a bow and arrow behind your back. Turn the head to the right, and gaze at a point on the horizon over the right shoulder. Hold this position for five breaths.

6. To exit, bring tone back to the pelvic floor, release the arms, and turn back to center. Place the hands next to the knees and jump back, or unravel the legs, cross them, lift up, and jump back to Catvāri for a Half Vinyāsa. Next jump through and lie down to repeat the pose on the other side.

Ardha Matsyendrāsana

Half Spinal Twist Pose

This extended spine twist appears in two forms within the Intermediate and Advanced A series. The half twist, in the Intermediate Series, is accessible and informative as an exploratory pose, even for those who do not practice Aṣṭāṅga Vinyāsa. It can teach us how, when breathing fully, the pose is refined as an endless subtle conversation between prāṇic and apānic patterns, and between our different theories and techniques. Close attentiveness to these conversations can give us insight into the nature of reality as well as our biases, beliefs, and emotional conditioning.

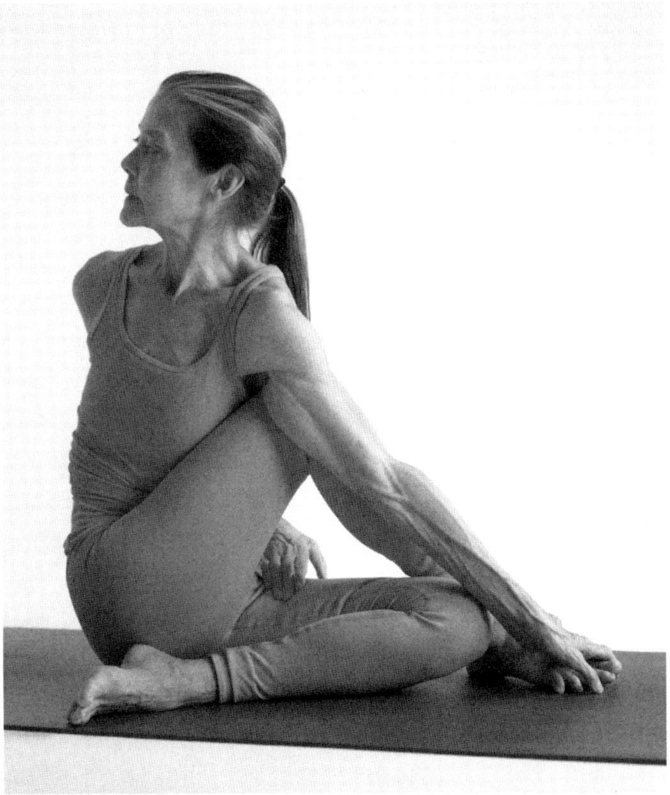

1. From Downward Facing Dog Pose, at the end of an exhalation, jump forward and inhale just as you land in a seated position. As you exhale, turn the pelvis to the right and bring the left heel back toward the sitting bones, pointing the left knee toward the front of the mat. Place the right foot on the floor just inside the left knee, with the toes pointing forward and the entire sole on the floor.
2. Inhaling, reach up with the left hand, rotating the arm and protracting the shoulder blade to stretch and open the psoas line. Exhaling completely, reach around the right leg, catching the upper part of the arm on the outer knee. Take the inner edge of the right foot with the left hand. If you are a beginner, you might need to exhale again to move fully into the twist. Wrap the right arm behind the body and clasp the inner left thigh.
3. Inhaling, turn on the pose by feeling the coccyx wake up to flow in toward the pubic bone. Bring the outer right hip and sitting bone back down and in toward the floor, moving them gently toward the front of the mat in a slight countertwist. Push the right leg back against the left arm and resist this push through the upper arm.
4. The arms stretch and pull in opposite directions both to open the heart and to extend the tail (as in holding the tail of a serpent). The back-and-forth conversation frees the head of any extraneous tension so that it floats and can inspire a feeling of nobility. (Any and all of the Internal Forms practices and visualizations can be used as we align the āsanas.) Find a steady gazing point over the right shoulder, and breathing smoothly, hold the pose for five breaths.
5. Before exiting, exhale to consolidate the actions, counteractions, thoughts, feelings, sensations, and the overall effect of the pose that can be sensed into at the root in the center of the pelvic floor. Then on an inhalation, release, and unwrap the form to return to a symmetrical seated position.
6. Cross the legs and place the hands beside the hips. Inhale as you lift up, and exhale back into Catvāri and complete a Half Vinyāsa to do the other side or simply switch sides.

Pūrṇa Matsyendrāsana

Full Spinal Twist Pose

This pose is similar to Ardha Matsyendrāsana, except the bottom leg is in Padmāsana rather than on the floor.

1. From Downward Facing Dog Pose, at the end of an exhalation, jump forward and inhale just as you land in a seated position. Inhale again as you draw the left leg into Padmāsana, dropping the knee to the floor and toward the middle of the mat with a slight internal spin of the left femur. Place the left heel down in the area of the right psoas button.
2. Place the right foot on the floor just inside the left knee, with the toes pointing toward the front of the mat and the entire sole on the floor.
3. Inhaling, reach up with the left hand, rotating the arm and protracting the shoulder blade to stretch and open the psoas line. Exhaling, curl the spine and slide the left arm outside the right thigh, wrapping the lower arm along the edge of the right shin so you can take the right foot at the inner edge of the mound of the big toe with the fingers of the left hand. Exhaling again, wrap the right arm behind the body and clasp the inner left thigh.
4. Inhaling, resist the hold with each hand so that the spine is invited to twist and extend as you lift the core of your heart.
5. Keeping the head and neck neutral, turn the head to the right and gaze softly at a point on the horizon beyond the right shoulder. Hold the pose for five breaths.
6. Exhale and bring the awareness to the toning of the pelvic floor. Maintaining that awareness, return to center on an inhalation.
7. Cross the legs and place the hands on the floor next to the hips. Inhale as you lift up, and exhale back into Catvāri for a Half Vinyāsa before repeating the pose on the other side.

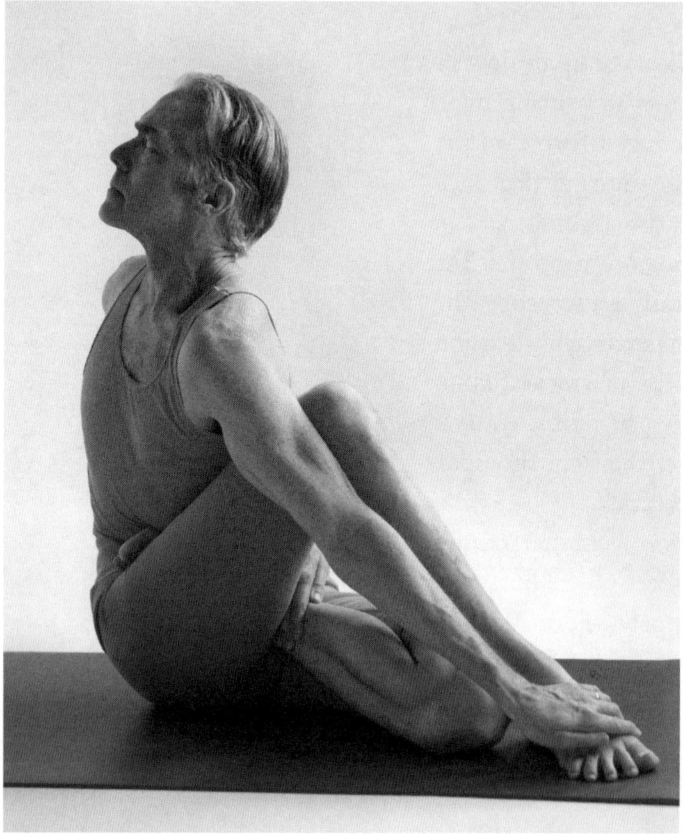

10

Balancing Poses

IMAGINE YOU'RE STANDING IN SAMASTHITIḤ ON TOP of a flagpole, finding whatever it takes within your body and mind to keep you upright and stable—even when the wind picks up. That's the feeling we're after in all balancing poses, from simple standing poses like Samasthitiḥ with the feet together (which is challenging enough and could be considered the quintessential balancing pose) to more complicated poses such as Utthita Hasta Pādāṅguṣṭhāsana.

Balance is mostly unconscious and automatic, the result of a fine dialogue between opposing patterns of movement, alignment, and thought within the body and mind. Balancing embodies the awakening of a focused and refined intelligence. In successful balancing poses, the mind is open to a whole background of sensations, yet it is intensely focused on a seed pattern of sensation within the body that is a synthesis of kinesthetic relationships. It is never just smooth breathing, a steady gaze, or intelligent legs that are required for balance; it's always an open, focused, multifaceted, and adaptive conversation between many aspects of body and mind. If we concentrate too strongly on lower levels of technique, like a particular muscular line in the body, then balance becomes difficult and usually fails. If the mind is scattered, balancing is impossible! In balancing, the attention is focused, but it is difficult to say exactly on what the attention is focused.

In yoga, when we think of balancing poses, extreme forms such as a one-armed handstand may come to mind. Yet even these more demanding types of poses function in the same way as Samasthitiḥ, requiring deep and open focus. Of course, they usually also involve a specialized and intense awareness of particular patterns within the body, but their foundation is the same. Even in Samasthitiḥ, which could be considered the "beginner's" balancing pose, there is a constant flowing of synthesized techniques into the plumb line. When practiced in this way, Samasthitiḥ comes to life as vividly as any of the more intense balancing poses; it practically becomes an adoration of the plumb line by countless subsystems. Sri K. Pattabhi Jois used to say, "Correct Samasthitiḥ is very difficult." Perhaps this subtle level of awareness is what he was referring to.

The logical next step in understanding balancing poses is to turn Samasthitiḥ over into a headstand. The basic requirements are more demanding, and the attention needed is more intense, as is the necessity of integrating the opposing actions of prāṇa and apāna for a successful and useful headstand. However, the basics of open-mindedness and clear focus are the same. As we increase the difficulty of the balance in even more complex poses, we work toward āsana in which legs veer off in opposite directions or in which we balance on just one limb; all of the same integrating principles and patterns apply, just with increasing difficulty. Good balance is the perfection of the whole mental process of finding a pattern on which to focus and then opening the background of that pattern. This ability is of particular significance in yoga.

Daṇḍāsana

Staff Pose

Daṇḍāsana seems almost like a "nonpose," one that is difficult to put into a family because it's just sitting, not doing much of anything. Looked at closely, however, it is revealed to be a pose in which we are doing a great deal and becomes the epitome of what is meant by joining together opposite patterns of form, breath, movement, and mind—a tribute to balancing on the plumb line.

1. From Downward Facing Dog Pose, at the end of an exhalation jump through to a seated position at the front of the mat. Stretch the legs straight out, with the feet together and the sides of the big toes touching. Square the feet and press the inner edges of the feet forward and out. Draw the upper, inner backs of the knees and the skin of the

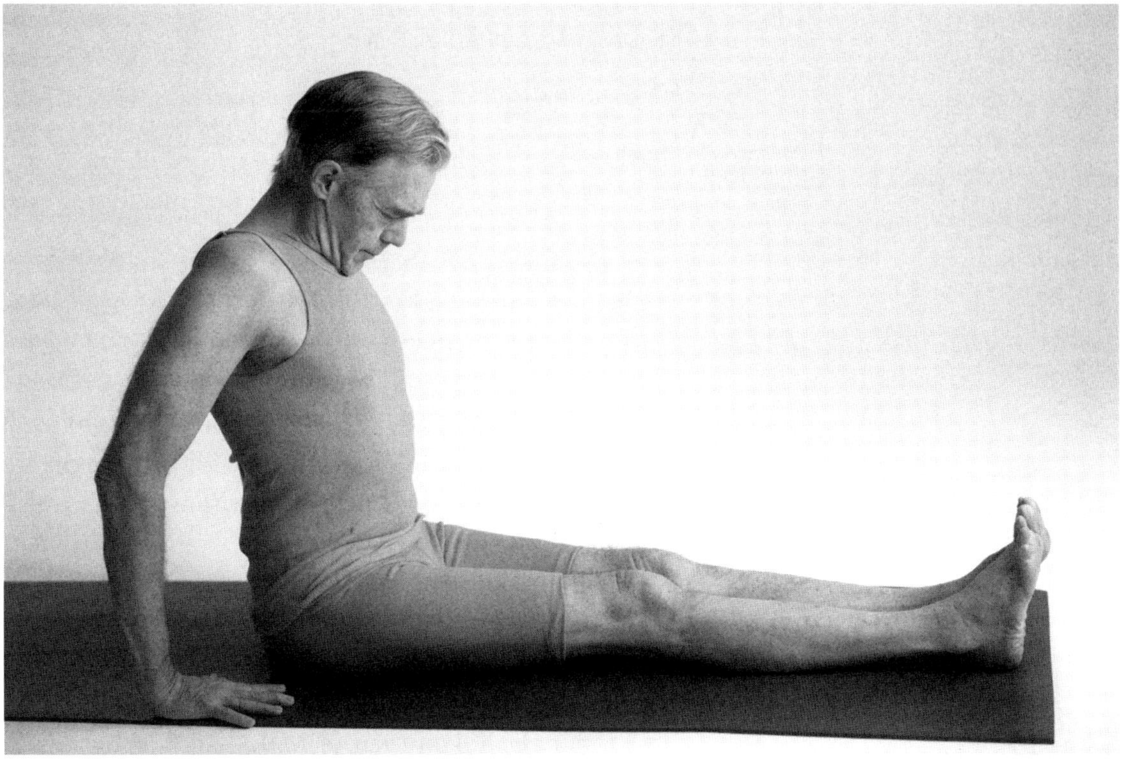

inner thighs toward the floor. The heels may come up off the floor slightly, but do not hyperextend the knees to achieve this.

2. Place the hands behind the back at the outer edges of the buttocks, with the fingers pointing toward the front of the mat. The elbows should not be locked; you may come up onto your fingertips to bend the elbows and rotate the tops of the arms up, back, and down while spreading the shoulder blades, as if shrugging.
3. On an inhalation, begin to place the chin in Jālandhara Bandha position (see Chapter 1), extending through the neck, spreading the skin on the back of the neck, and releasing the tongue and palate as you reach up through the center of the head. Exhale and nestle the chin down into the sternum.
4. Pull the sitting bones back and then ground them by imagining the kidney wings broadening and spreading up the back. Draw the lower belly, about two inches below the navel, into Uḍḍīyāna Bandha. Lift the front of the spine and broaden the back of the head, neck, and entire body as you hold the pose.
5. Lift the heart, as if that entire area is light and buoyant. It may be helpful to imagine that the chest is that of a swan, rounded and puffed, so the chin can settle easily into the core of the heart. Gaze along the line of the nose with a soft smile that opens the back of the palate. Hold this position for five breaths.

HANUMANĀSANA

Hanuman's Pose

Like Daṇḍāsana , this classic split is a refined internalized pose that epitomizes the process of making tiny adjustments to stay balanced.

1. From Downward Facing Dog Pose, step the right leg forward between the arms and as you exhale slide the heel along the floor out in front of you, squaring the foot and reaching long through the leg. Breathe smoothly and over the course of one or several breaths, lower down so the right sitting bone rests on or close to the floor, reaching out and back through the left leg, with the toes pointed. Keep both legs activated. Do not collapse into the hip joints, and do not attempt to square the hips to the front.
2. Keep the upper body straight, the heart lifted, and the pelvic floor awake. If you cannot come into a full split, keep the hands along the side and support the weight, gradually, over several weeks or months, gently working the pose to eventually be able to sit fully down into it. When in the full position, place the hands on the hips for five breaths, gazing along the line of the nose.

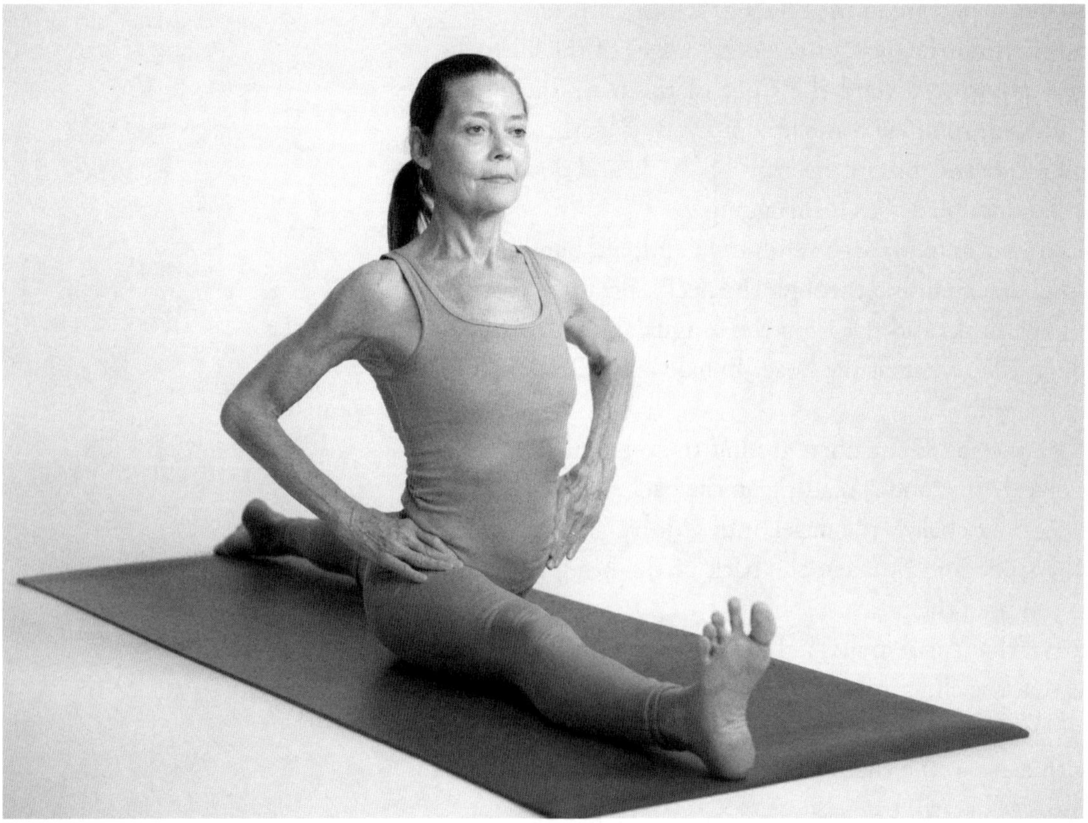

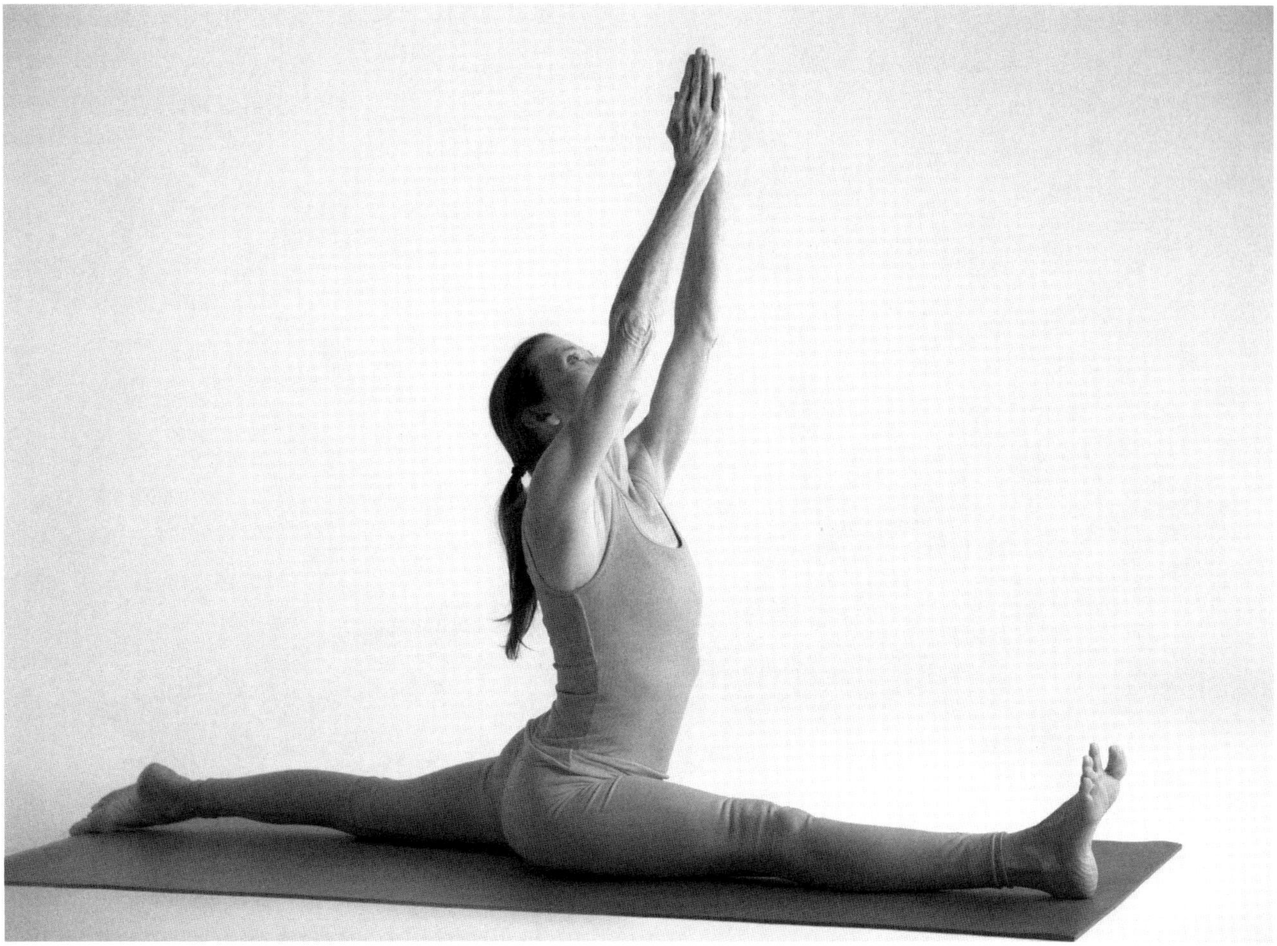

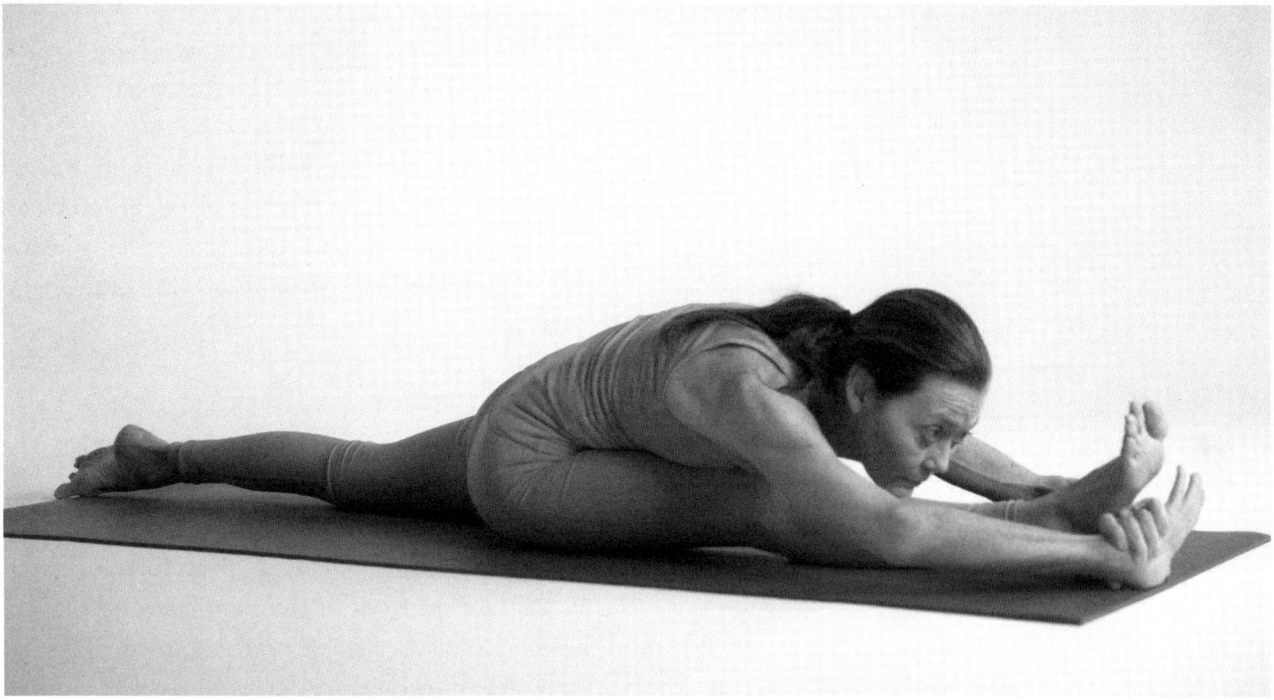

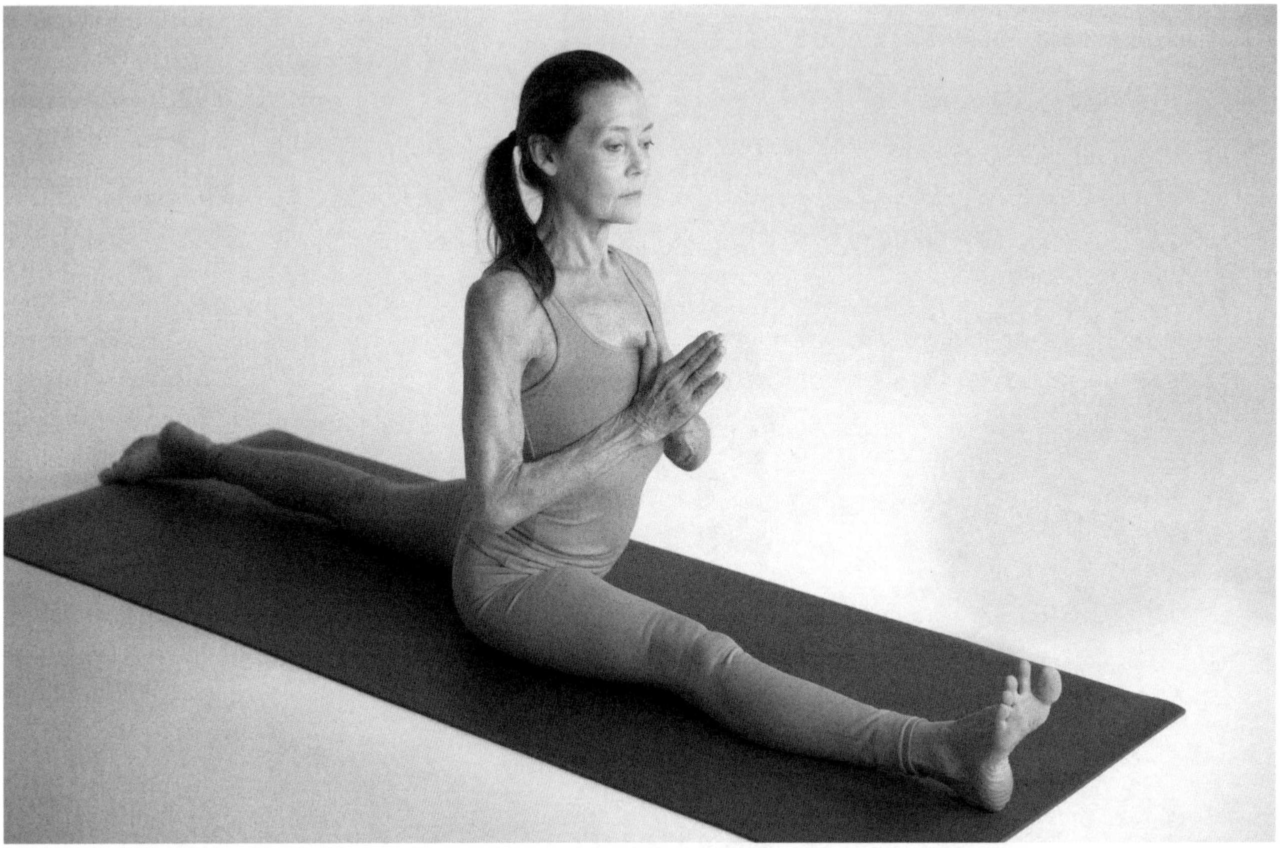

3. Inhaling, reach the arms above the head, palms together, as in Ekam, and gaze at the thumbs for five breaths before releasing the hands down to the sides.
4. On an exhalation, fold forward over the right leg, and clasp the left wrist with the right hand beyond the sole of the foot, again holding for five breaths and gazing at the toes.
5. Inhaling, return to an upright position and fold the palms in front of the heart in Añjali Mudrā for five more breaths. Place the hands on the floor by the hips, lift up and step back into Catvāri, then move through a Half Vinyāsa before repeating the pose with all of the hand positions on the other side.

Bhujapīḍāsana

Arm Squeezing Pose

1. From Downward Facing Dog Pose, exhale and hop forward, landing with the feet on the floor in front of the shoulders and the legs wrapped around the outsides of the arms. Breathing smoothly, work the inner knees up as high as possible on the arms and, while bending

the knees and leaning back slightly, inhale and lift the feet off the ground.

2. Cross the right ankle over the left and squeeze the heels in toward the sitting bones. Lift the core of the heart toward the ceiling, lift the chin slightly, and gaze between the eyebrows or at the horizon. Hold the pose for five breaths.
3. An alternative is to hook the inner knees around the upper arms and lean back to balance without crossing the feet. This is a way of working toward the full form of the pose and is still effective. Do not expect to do poses like this without a lot of practice!
4. On an exhalation, pull back the sitting bones and heels to curl as you slowly rock forward. Place the top of the head on the floor. Alternatively, you may bend the elbows deeply to place the chin on the floor. In this case, your spine is not as flexed, but the center of gravity is farther back. Both variations of this stage of the pose are beneficial. In both forms the hands and the crown of your head or your chin should form an equilateral triangle.
5. In this form pull the shoulders high and wide. Make the arms parallel to each other. Draw the feet off the floor, squeezing them

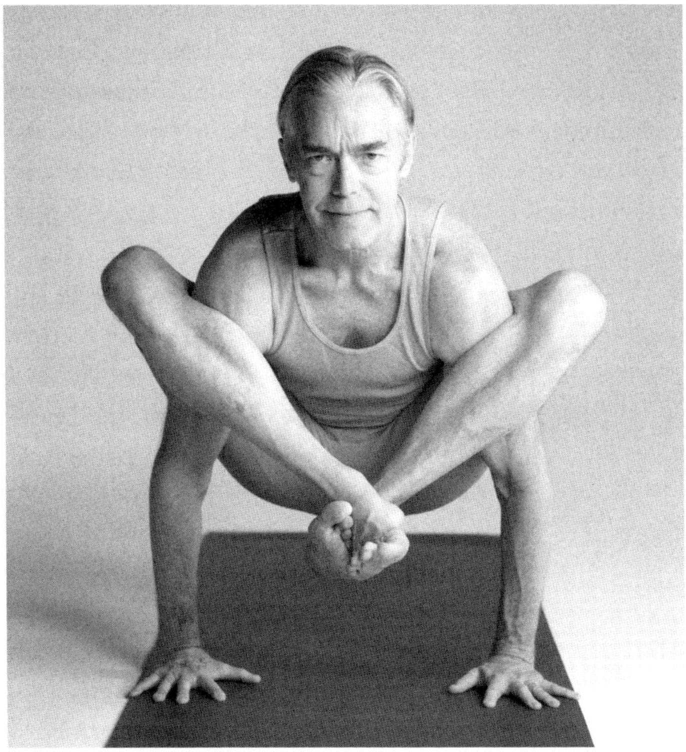

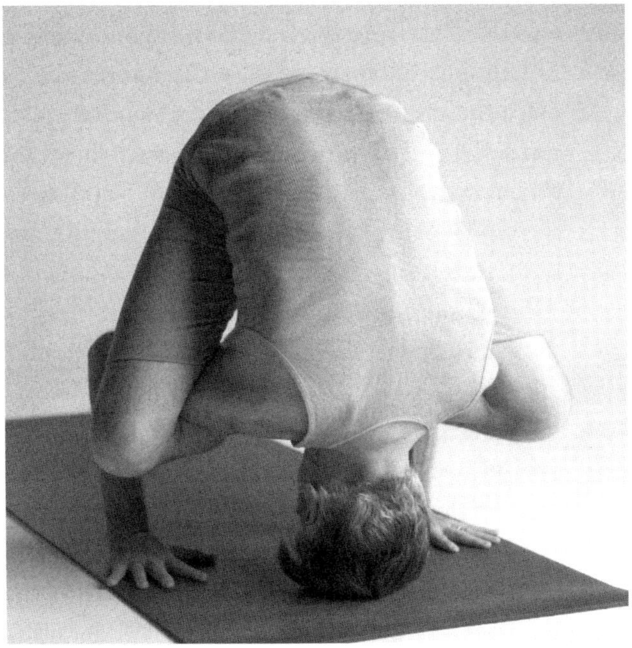

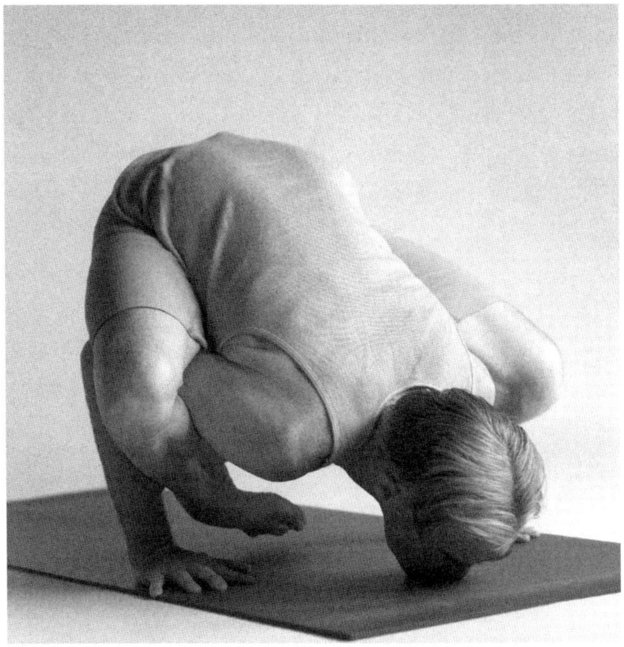

up and in toward the sitting bones. Gaze at the tip of the nose. Hold for five breaths.

6. Exhale and, empty of breath, carefully lean back to lift the head. As the head ascends, inhale and gaze up between the eyebrows. Exit by separating the feet and straightening the legs out to the sides in Ṭiṭṭibhāsana (see pages 258–60) for one breath. On the exhalation, draw the knees back and straighten the arms in Bakāsana and jump back into Catvāri. You may also jump back into Catvāri directly from Ṭiṭṭibhāsana.

BAKĀSANA (CRANE POSE) A AND B

This pose is the embodiment of the apāna pattern. Like other poses named after animals, imagining yourself to be a crane with long, straight legs and a broad, round upper body can be helpful here. In the full form, the knees rest on the outer edges of the straightened arms, the feet are together and flexed, and the heels are drawn up toward the sitting bones.

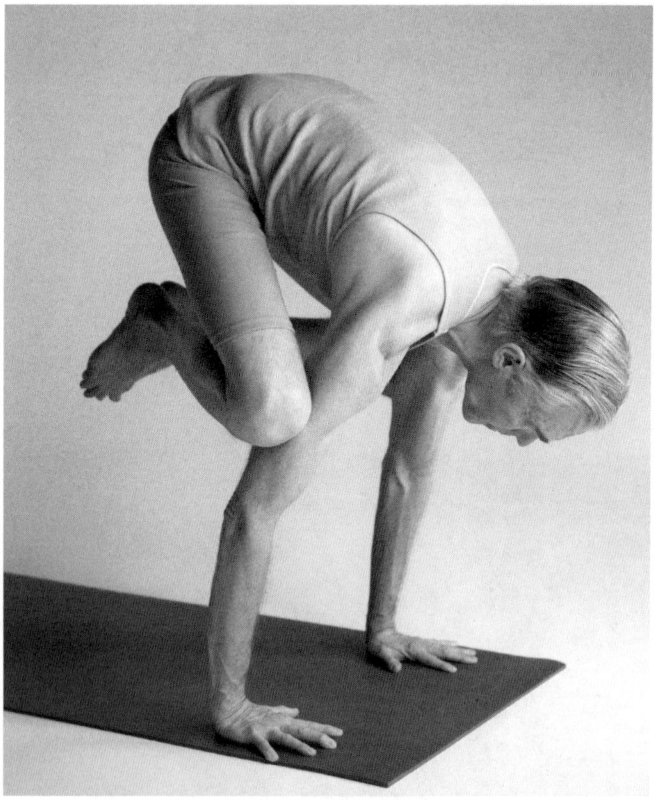

BAKĀSANA A

1. From Downward Facing Dog Pose, hop forward at the end of an exhalation, then inhale as you land in a squatting position with the feet about 6 or 8 inches from the wrists.
2. Exhaling, lean forward over the hands as you place the knees on the outer edges of the upper arms. Drop the hips and push into the floor through the arms to connect them strongly to the sides of the body; puff out the area of the kidneys by toning the pelvic floor, curling the coccyx, and broadening the low back. Push your shoulders down away from the ears and let your feet begin to lift up away from the floor.
3. Inhaling, lift the head, heart, hips, and feet working the arms to eventually straighten them. Keep the feet flexed and square, with the inner edges touching as you squeeze the heels up toward the sitting bones. Squeeze the knees into the

arms and simultaneously push out through the arms to resist the squeeze, drawing strength and awareness into the lower belly and pelvic floor.

4. Gaze along the line of the nose to a point out in front of you on the floor, and hold the pose for five breaths. Take a full inhalation, then on the next exhale jump back into Catvāri. Move through a Half Vinyāsa and on to form B.

Bakāsana B

1. From Downward Facing Dog Pose, hop forward on an exhalation as for Bakāsana A, but instead of landing in a squat, bend the knees midflight and land (on the arms) lightly with the knees on the outer edges of the upper arms. Having landed in the full form of the posture at the end of an exhalation, you can then inhale to pull the heels even closer to the sitting bones. Imagining yourself to be a small bird landing in a tree (the tree being your arms) and looking forward optimistically can help when learning to float into this form.
2. Once in the pose, follow steps 3 and 4 for form Bakāsana A, holding the pose for five breaths as for form A, before jumping back into Catvāri and moving through a Half Vinyāsa into the next pose.

Piñcha Mayūrāsana

Peacock Feather Pose

This pose is excellent training for the important shoulder action of connecting to the serratus anterior muscles while protracting and stabilizing the shoulders. This action supports many poses, from Piñcha Mayūrāsana itself to Śirṣāsana and even Catvāri.

1. From Downward Facing Dog Pose, step forward and bend the elbows to bring your forearms down on the mat, with the elbows directly beneath the shoulders and the palms facing down. The upper arms should be parallel to each other as should the lower arms, so they form a square or box that can support the body evenly. Roll the shoulders back and around to activate the serratus anterior muscles to spread the kidney wings. Lift the hips away from the floor so you are supporting the pose with the arms and slowly step forward bringing the hips closer to the hands. The wrists, elbows, forearms, and the

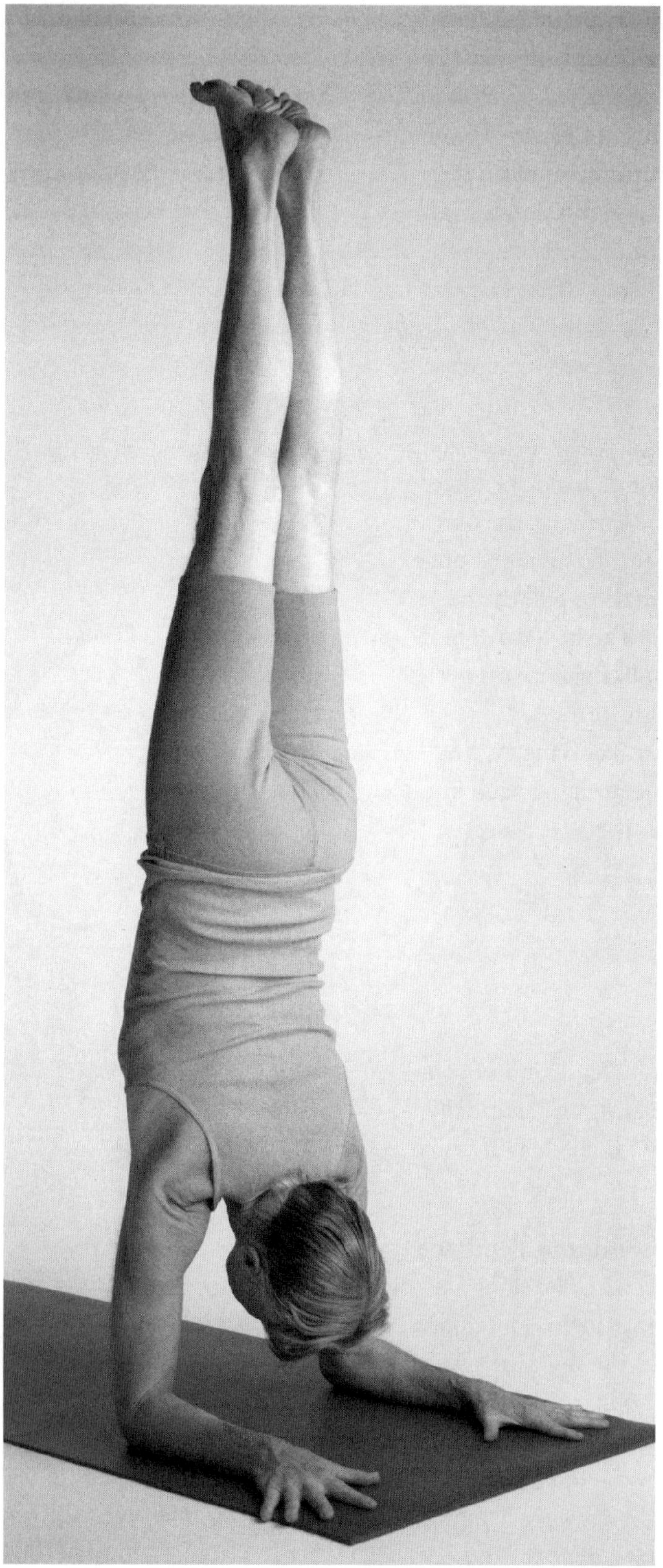

inner edges of the hands (the heel of the thumb and the index finger) root into the earth. Lowering the hips slightly and bending the knees can facilitate the stepping forward movement, especially while you are learning the pose.

2. As you move closer to the hands with the upper body, keep the 90-degree angle (or just a little past that) in the elbows. Lift the hips toward the ceiling and root again into the sense in the outer shoulder blades of protracting (wrapping around the sides of the body) as you ground thoroughly through the elbows and wrists. Feel the kidney wing power in the elbows.
3. Exhale to set the base of the pose, then inhale to step or kick up one leg at a time. Keep the serratus muscles and protraction of the shoulders engaged and pressed back, maintaining the 90-degree bend in the elbows. If the elbows bend less than 90 degrees, the posture is more difficult and unstable. Engage the legs, squeezing them together and reaching up toward the ceiling through the inner edges of the half-flexed feet. Feel the coccyx lifting up toward the ceiling, as the arms work to press against the floor. Imagine that you are holding the central axis between the legs as if it were a long, thin straw. Lift the head slightly to gaze at a point between the wrists or thumbs. Keep the tongue soft and the palate released. Hold the position for five breaths.
4. To exit, on an exhalation, step back down and move into Catvāri. Alternatively, after completing the breath cycle, inhale and quickly, with a small push upward, move the hands next to the heart as you snap down into Catvāri. This quick exit takes practice. Move through a Half Vinyāsa into the next pose.

Karandavāsana

Crane Pose

This pose is not easy (which is a major understatement). For many practitioners, it is one that may not be part of the menu this go-round. But even if dropping into the full form and then lifting back up doesn't quite happen, the actions we work on to prepare for and eventually do these movements are very informative and integrating.

1. From Downward Facing Dog Pose, step forward and place the elbows on the floor and follow steps 1 through 3 as if to set up and move into Piñcha Mayūrāsana. Once balanced in the pose, you may take a few extra breaths or immediately move into Karandavāsana.
2. On an exhalation, cross the legs in Padmāsana. The key to this is that once the right leg is in Padmāsana position, extend that hip joint by reaching up toward the ceiling and slightly back through the right knee. This way, the folded right leg is not in the way of the left as it moves into Padmāsana.
3. With a firm and complete exhalation, curl the legs and lower torso to bring the tops of the shins in to rest on the middle back portion of the upper arms. This exhalation must be smooth and audible to go with the careful, firm contraction of the rectus abdominis and a strong sense of puffing the kidney area while strongly protracting the shoulders and maintaining a sense of pushing down through the elbows and wrists. At no point while in the pose should you release the abdominal contraction. If you do, you will not be able to return to Piñcha Mayūrāsana.
4. In the pose, push the shoulders back to minimize the flexion at the elbows. Do not allow the nose to go forward past the line between the thumbs. This rolling and pushing back of the shoulders makes it feel as if the heart is open, even though the spine (from the lower thoracic area down through the coccyx) feels

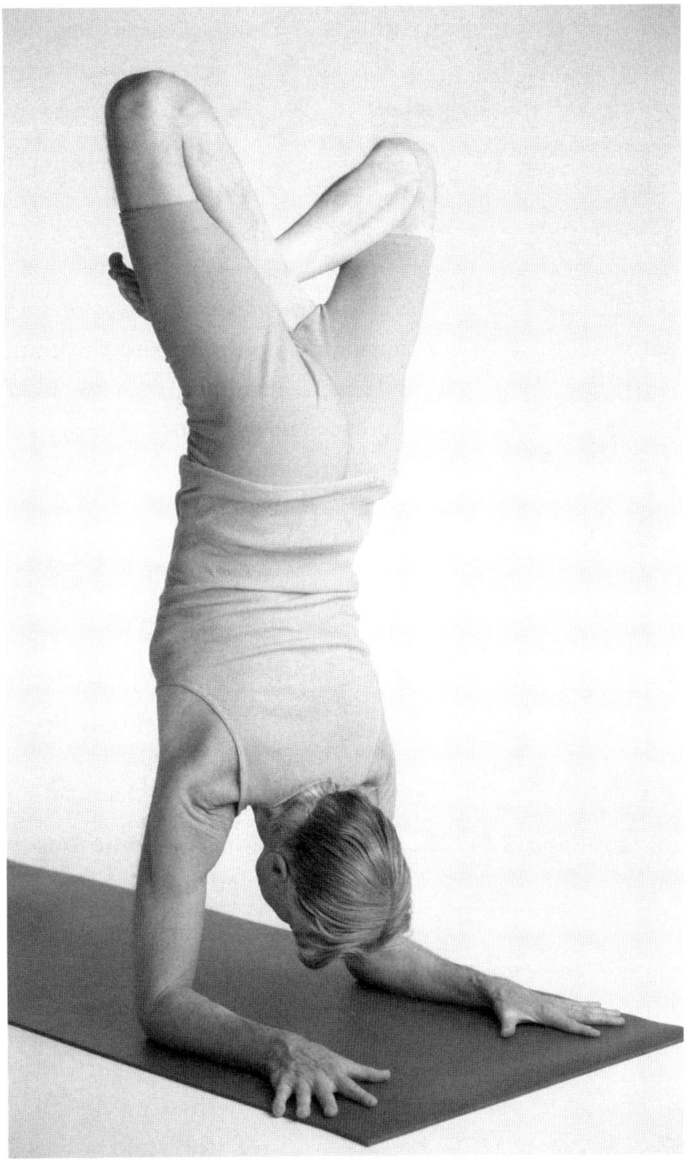

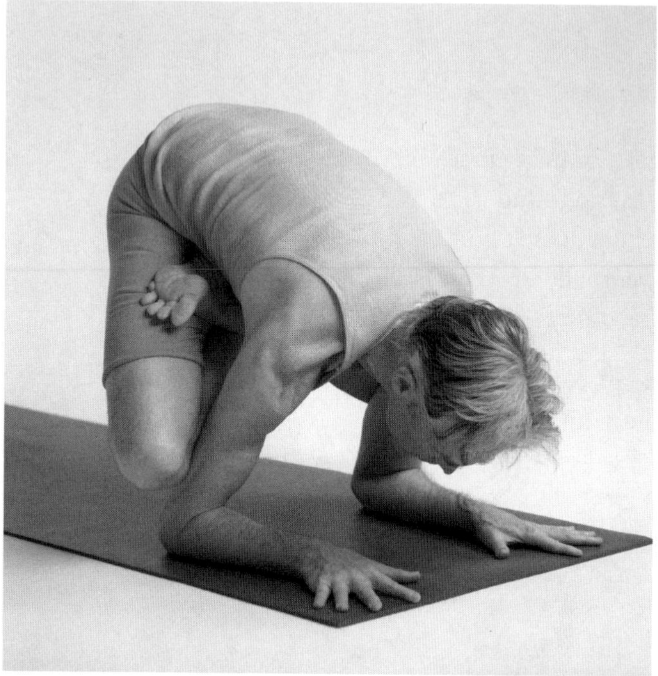

as if it is coiled tightly. Strong apāna is held with strong prāṇa. Hold this position for five breaths.

5. To come out of the pose, exhale and redouble on the apānic coil the sense of curling deeply through the spine, dropping the coccyx and maintaining the tone in the abdominal muscles. Before you inhale, start bringing the legs, still in Padmāsana, back up toward the ceiling. Do not inhale until you clear the tight point halfway up. Then unfold the legs into Piñcha Mayūrāsana and exit as for Piñcha Mayūrāsana.
6. One way to train that may allow you to feel the pattern of the movement is to place the legs in Bakāsana position instead of Padmāsana as you bring them down and to then place the upper shins on the backs of the upper arms.
7. Another training trick is to sit in Padmāsana on the floor. Stand up on the knees and place the elbows on the floor just in front of the tops of the shins as if you were setting up for Piñcha Mayūrāsana. Exhale and pull the shins to the elbows and then up a few inches onto the backs of the upper arms. Notice the patterns that need to be strengthened and coordinated.

Mayūrāsana

Peacock Pose

This pose requires that the engagement and use of the abdominal muscles be differentiated correctly to provide both a strong surface on which the elbows can rest and the ability to continue breathing while doing so. It can be considered an arm balance not only because we literally balance the body on the arms, but also because it requires strong core awareness and toning in coordination with a sense of release. In the Intermediate Series, Mayūrāsana comes after Karandavāsana, and there is a Full Vinyāsa—with Mayūrāsana hand placement—between the two poses.

1. From Samasthitiḥ, on an exhalation, hop the feet approximately hip-width apart, placing the hands on the hips. Inhaling, extend long through the spine and upper body. Exhale and fold forward to place the hands on the floor between the feet, with your fingers pointing toward the back of the mat and the outer sides of the hands almost

touching. Inhale and straighten the arms, lifting the head and the heart while gazing along the line of the nose.

2. Exhale and jump back into a transitional version of Catvāri, with the elbows only slightly bent and the hands in this preliminary position. Flex the lower spine and slide forward on the feet to place the elbows close to one another and against the abdomen, slightly above and near the navel, keeping the legs strong and the feet flexed with the toes on the floor.
3. Keep the rectus abdominis muscle toned and the core of the body engaged as you move your center of gravity forward, reaching forward through the sternum and lifting the head to look at the floor just in front of the body. Remember this initial setup is done as a complete exhalation.
4. As you glide forward with the heart on an inhalation and reach the balance point, the feet will automatically lift off the floor. Hold this position for five breaths, then roll back slightly until the toes touch the floor.
5. Leaving the hands as they are inhale and move directly into Upward Facing Dog Pose with hands close together and fingers pointing toward the back of your mat. Exhaling, back into Downward Facing Dog Pose with hands reversed, and then jump forward to Sapta (seventh form of the Sun Salutation). Inhaling, release the hand position and stand up, placing the hands on the hips. Exhale and hop to bring the feet together for Samasthitiḥ.

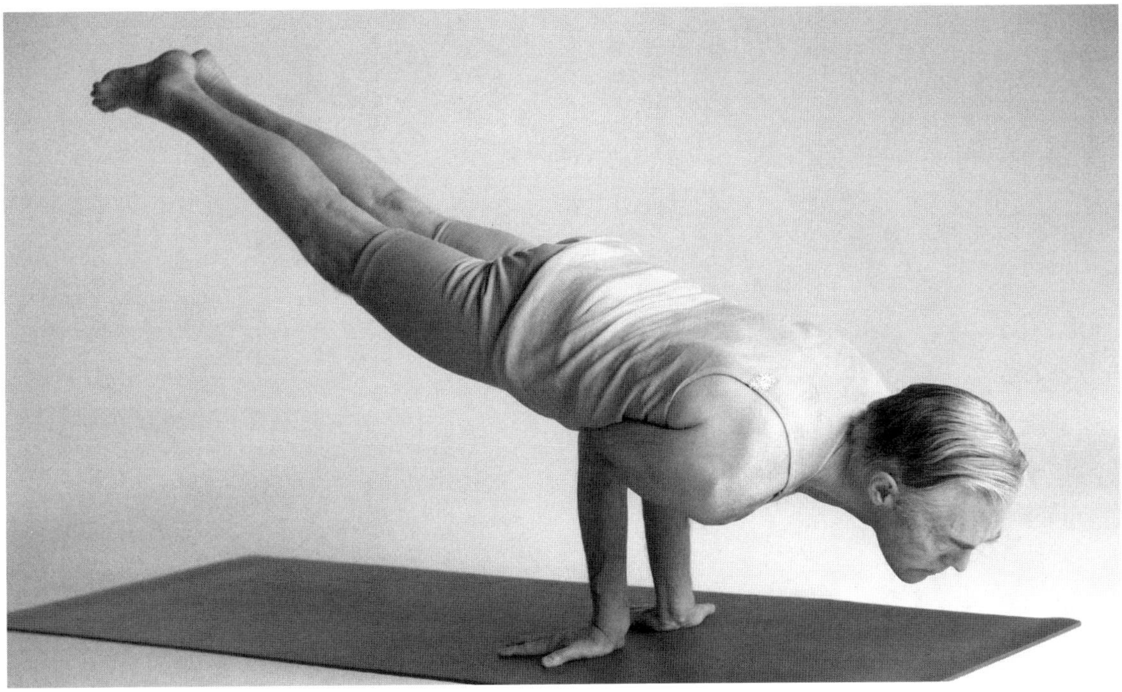

Ṭiṭṭibhāsana (Small Water Bird Pose) A, B, and C

Watching the small birds that fly between prime spots and then hop along on an open stretch of beach, moving side to side while pecking at the sand for delicacies that lie beneath the surface, is an image that can be helpful to keep in mind when you're working on this pose. When practicing Ṭiṭṭibhāsana in its various forms, there *is* a sense of being that small creature with sea-soaked, sandy feet moving along the shore. The first form of the pose is an arm balance, which is used as a transition form in vinyāsas out of other arm balances such as Bhujapīḍāsana, while the second and third forms are extreme forward bends similar to balanced upright variations of Kūrmāsana.

Ṭiṭṭibhāsana A

1. From Downward Facing Dog Pose, at the end of an exhalation, jump forward and wrap the legs around the outside of your arms, keeping your feet flat on the floor and knees bent. Work the inner knees up the arms to the area of the deltoid muscles.

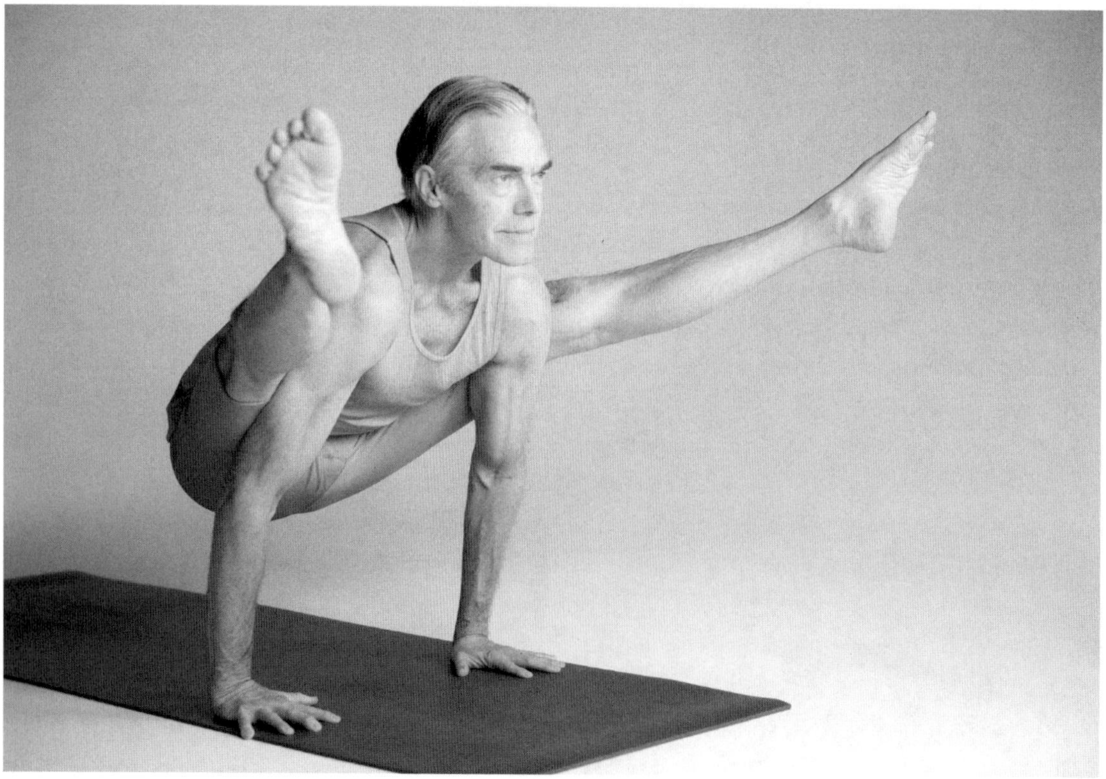

2. Finishing the exhalation, drop the sitting bones toward the floor and lean back, while reaching forward through the sternum and spreading the collarbones to lift up and balance on your hands. Finally inhale to reach out through the legs and straighten the arms.
3. Hold this position for five breaths. As you exhale, drop the head forward and puff out the kidneys. On an inhalation, bend the knees and draw them up the outer edges of the arms to rest for one breath in Bakāsana. Jump back into Catvāri on an exhalation and move through a Half Vinyāsa to the next pose.

Ṭiṭṭibhāsana B, C, and D

These three forms of Ṭiṭṭibhāsana are practiced one immediately after the next so even though they are distinct forms, they are included in one continuous instruction because that is how they are best practiced.

1. Follow step 1 for Ṭiṭṭibhāsana A to position the feet flat on the floor beyond the arms. If you are a beginner, you should place your feet wider than in the previous form.
2. Exhaling and leaving the legs slightly bent, curl the spine and move the upper body more deeply through the groins into a strong forward bend. Work the upper arms, head, and shoulders through and behind the legs. Reach up to clasp the hands behind the back. Straighten the legs as much as possible, and lift the head slightly to look at a point on the floor just in front of the head. This is Ṭiṭṭibhāsana B and can be held for five breaths. Without exiting form B, move immediately into form C.

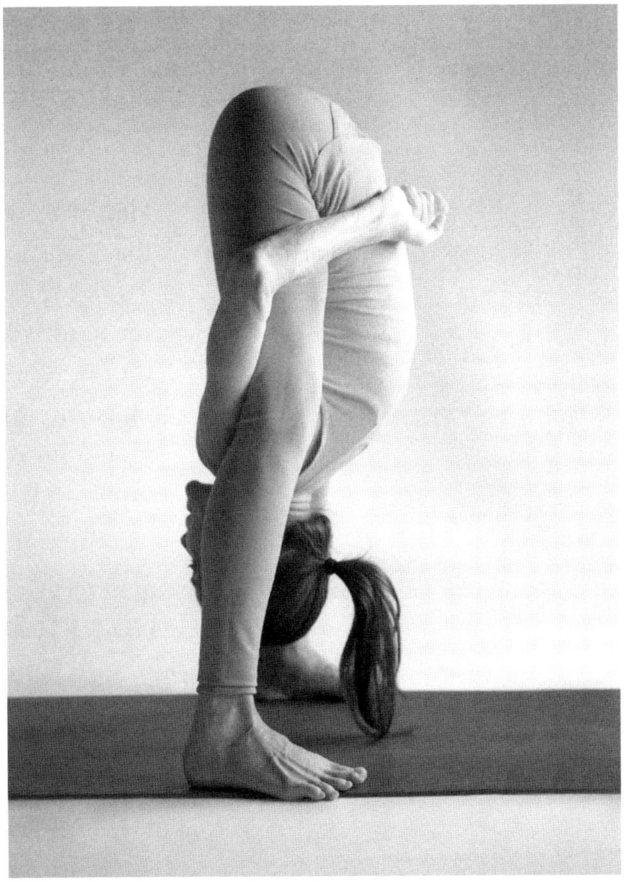

3. On the inhalation, lean to the left, putting more weight in the left leg. Exhaling, step forward with the right foot. Then lean to the right as you inhale, and step forward with the left foot as you exhale. Repeat this walking motion, forward and then back, for five breaths in each direction to complete Ṭiṭṭibhāsana C.
4. When you are back to the starting point at the front of the mat, immediately move into form D. Release the hands, but keep your arms wrapped behind the legs. Inhaling, move the feet closer

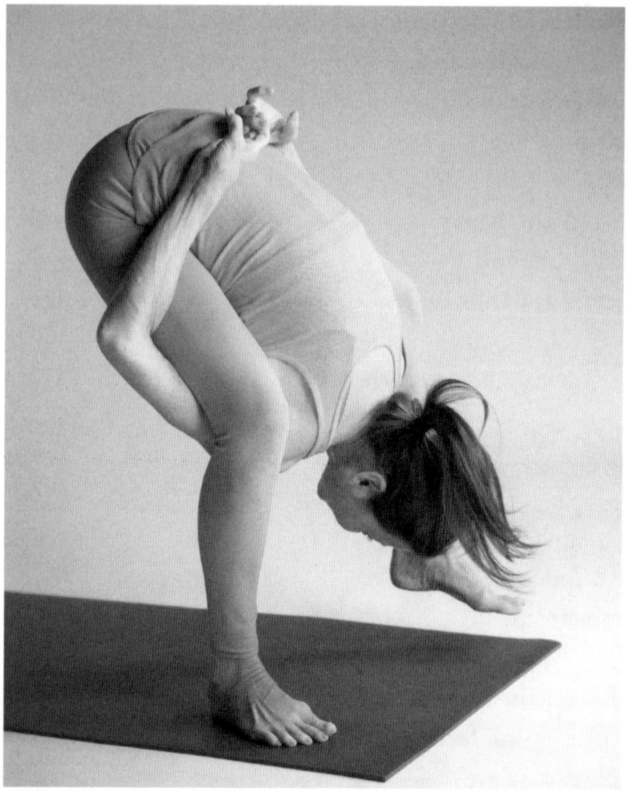

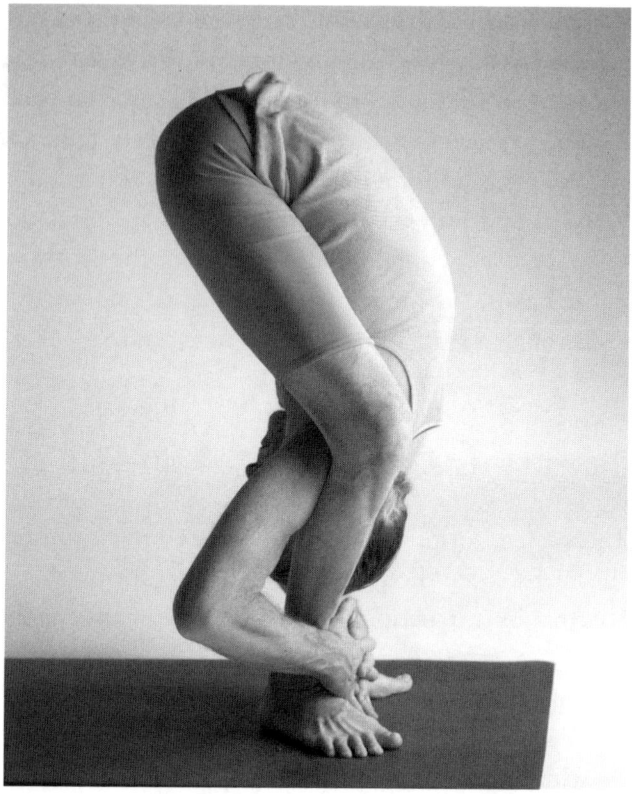

together, with the toes pointing out to the side and the heels touching. Exhaling, work the upper arms even more deeply through the legs and lace the arms around the lower legs, clasping the hands in front of the ankles. Spread and push the elbows back to move the lumbar spine farther through the legs. Gaze softly along the line of the nose and hold this position for five breaths.

5. To exit the pose, release the hands and, exhaling, place them flat on the floor as you move the feet apart to lower the sitting bones toward the floor. Inhaling, lift and engage the legs and point your toes as you move into form A, then move through Bakāsana into Catvāri and a Half Vinyāsa. Jumping back into Catvāri directly without pausing briefly in Bakāsana is a matter of style, but it is also effective.

Vāsiṣṭhāsana

Vāsiṣṭha's Pose

This advanced balancing pose is beautiful in its expression of the central axis and is named after Vāsiṣṭha, a legendary sage who carried a magical staff that is represented by the raised arm in this pose.

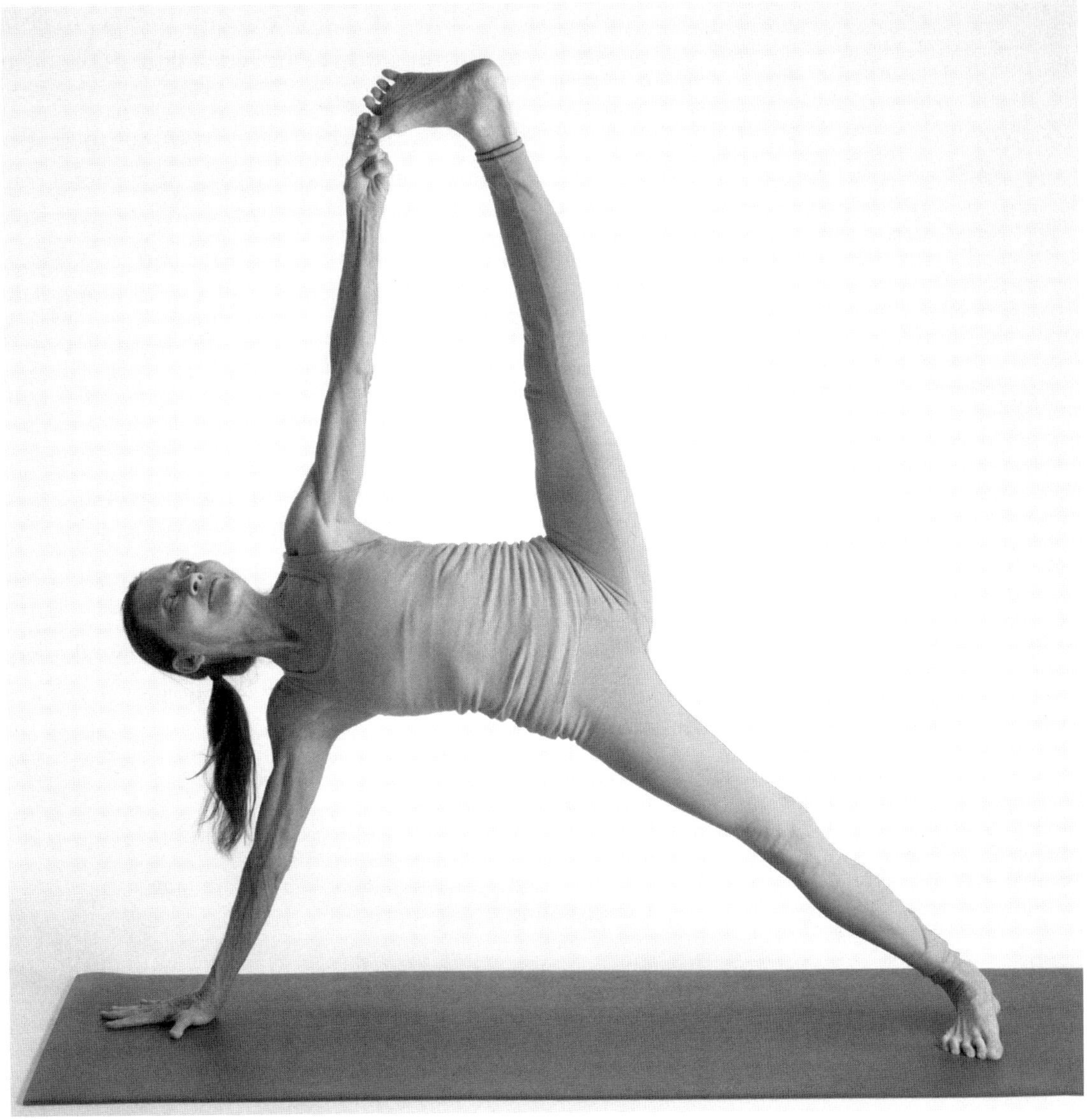

1. From a well-aligned Downward Facing Dog Pose, exhale and turn the feet so the toes point to your left. This will place the outer edge of the right foot on the mat. The left leg will rest on the right leg as you turn the belly to the left while swinging the left arm up off the floor. In the first position of this pose the right arm and outer right foot support the straightened torso. The left arm is straight up, and your head is turned so that you gaze at your left thumb.
2. On an exhalation, ground through the right arm and right foot to stabilize the pose. Inhale and straighten the left leg up toward the ceiling and take the left big toe with the middle and index fingers of the left hand. Keep an emphasis on the external rotation of the femur at the left hip joint. If lifting the left leg while straight is not possible,

you may bend the leg in order to take the toe. In either case, press the left big toe firmly into the fingers holding it and lift the right outer thigh away from the floor.

3. Established with full complements of counteractions and counter-rotations on the inhalation, this pose expands radiantly out. The head, heart, shoulder, and kidney wing actions spread both the front and the back of the torso. The unique patterns of force around the hip joints are organized by Mūlabandha.
4. After five breaths with the left leg up, exhale, release the toe, and bring the left leg down to join the right leg. Leave the left arm up and continue to gaze at the left thumb.
5. On the next exhalation, bring the left arm down to your side. Turn the torso toward the floor, spreading the feet apart slightly as you step onto the toes and place the left hand down so you are in a high plank position like Catvāri, but the arms are only slightly bent.
6. Rolling from the cave of the sacrum, drop the coccyx and, inhaling, unroll into Upward Facing Dog Pose. Then ride that same wave back into Downward Facing Dog Pose on the exhale. Repeat the pose on the other side.

Nakrāsana

Crocodile Pose

There is something both entertaining and confounding about this pose. It can be helpful to imagine yourself as a crocodile, with strong, short legs and a deft ability to hop forward and back on the floor.

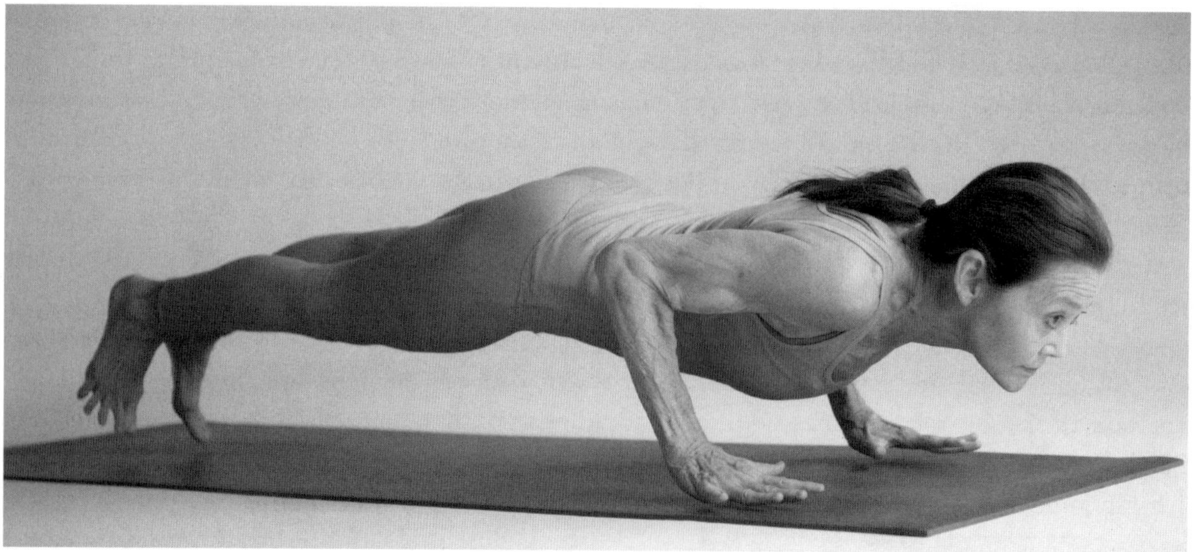

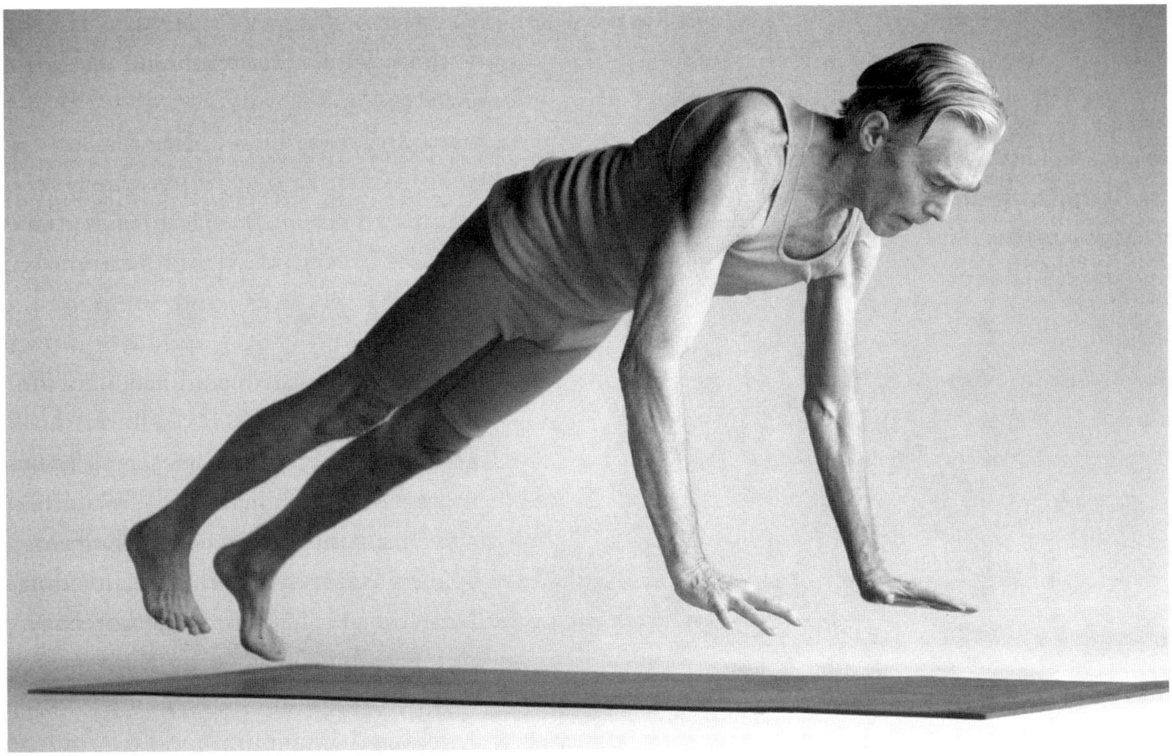

1. From Downward Facing Dog Pose, lower down into Catvāri on an exhalation. Keep the core of the body and the abdominal muscles toned, the legs and arms strong, and the shoulders set properly for Catvāri.
2. As you inhale, hop up off the floor in the plank position, moving forward by working the hands and feet almost as if walking on all fours, then land as you exhale. This pattern is triggered by engaging the psoas muscles just as you are preparing to leave the floor, which pulls back the groins allowing you to hop. Repeat this five times, hopping forward.
3. Reverse the pattern in the hands and feet to hop backward five times, again lifting on the inhalation and landing on the exhalation. From Catvāri, move directly into Upward Facing Dog Pose on the inhalation, then a Half Vinyāsa and into the next pose.

Vatayanāsana

Air Vehicle Pose

This interesting pose appears near the end of the Intermediate Series and, although it doesn't *look* terribly difficult, it is surprisingly hard to balance in the final form.

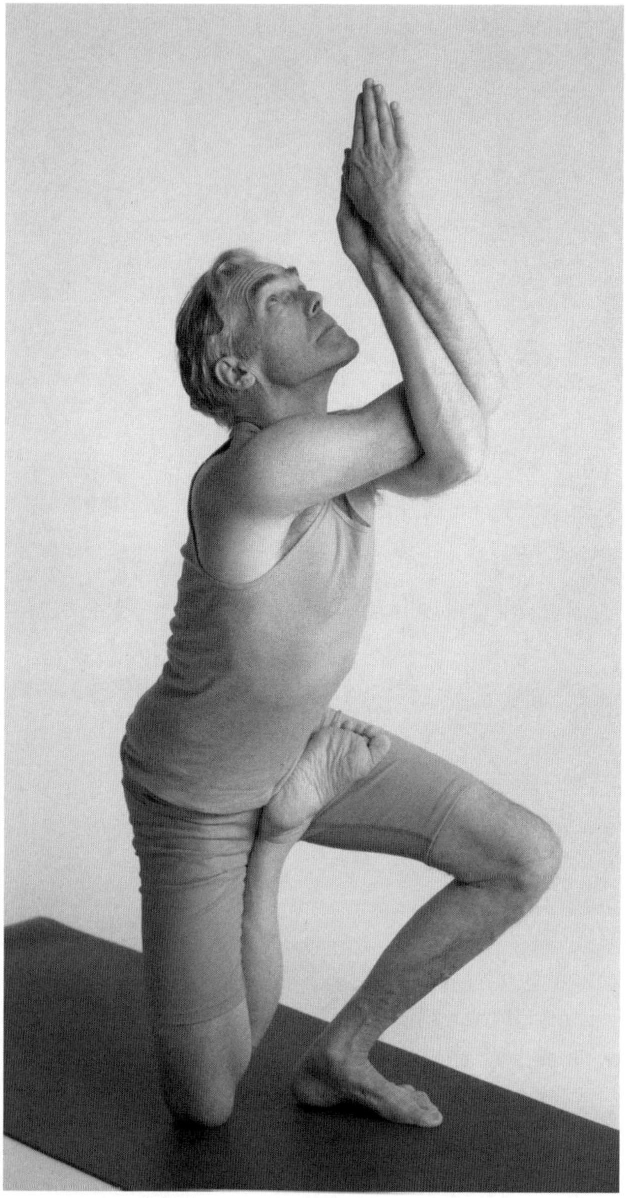

1. Begin in Samasthitiḥ. Fold the right leg into Half Padmāsana and reach behind you with the right arm to clasp the right big toe.
2. Inhaling, reach up with the left arm, protracting the shoulder blade and stretching the psoas line on the left side of the body. At the peak of the inhalation, release the right foot and, exhaling, fold forward to put both hands on the floor beside the left foot.
3. Inhale and come to a modified Trīṇi position, with the right leg still in Half Padmāsana. On the next exhalation, jump back into Catvāri, then inhaling move through a one-legged Upward Facing Dog, and exhale into Downward Facing Dog Pose, with your right leg remaining in Half Padmāsana.
4. Next, on an exhalation, bend the left leg. Inhale as you jump forward, placing the right knee and left foot on the ground. The left heel should be near or touching the right knee, and the toes should point out to the side at about a 45- to 90-degree angle, depending on your flexibility.
5. Inhaling, begin squaring the hips toward the front and lift the upper body out of the pose, pushing down into the earth through the right knee and the left foot to maintain balance. If it is impossible to balance, you may move the left foot away from the right knee slightly until the pose is accessible.
6. Draw the arms to the front of the body. Bend your elbows and place the right upper arm on top of the left, then wrap the right lower arm around the left so the palms of the hands are together.
7. Inhaling, gradually lift the hands and arms straight up toward the ceiling, and gaze at the tips of the thumbs. Hold this for five breaths.
8. Exhale and release the arms, placing the hands on the floor by the knees with the right leg still in Padmāsana. Jump back into Catvāri on an exhalation, then keeping the Half Padmāsana form, move through a Half Vinyāsa to Downward Facing Dog Pose.
9. Take the right leg out of Half Padmāsana to place the foot in full Downward Facing Dog Pose position for one breath. Inhaling, draw the left leg up into Half Padmāsana, using your hand to help position

the foot if necessary. Jump forward as in step 4, this time with the left knee on the ground and the right foot flat on the floor. Wrap the arms with the left one on top and inhaling reach up through the arms, gazing at the ceiling. Hold the pose for five breaths.

10. To exit the pose, work through a Half Vinyāsa to Downward Facing Dog Pose with the left leg in Half Padmāsana. Jump forward to land on the right foot and inhaling, lift the head and heart into a modified Trīṇi position. Reach behind the back, take the left foot with the left hand on the wave of the breath, then fold forward, exhaling. Inhaling, come back up to standing, and exhaling, bring the left foot down from Half Padmāsana into Samasthitiḥ.

Gomukhāsana

Calf Face Pose

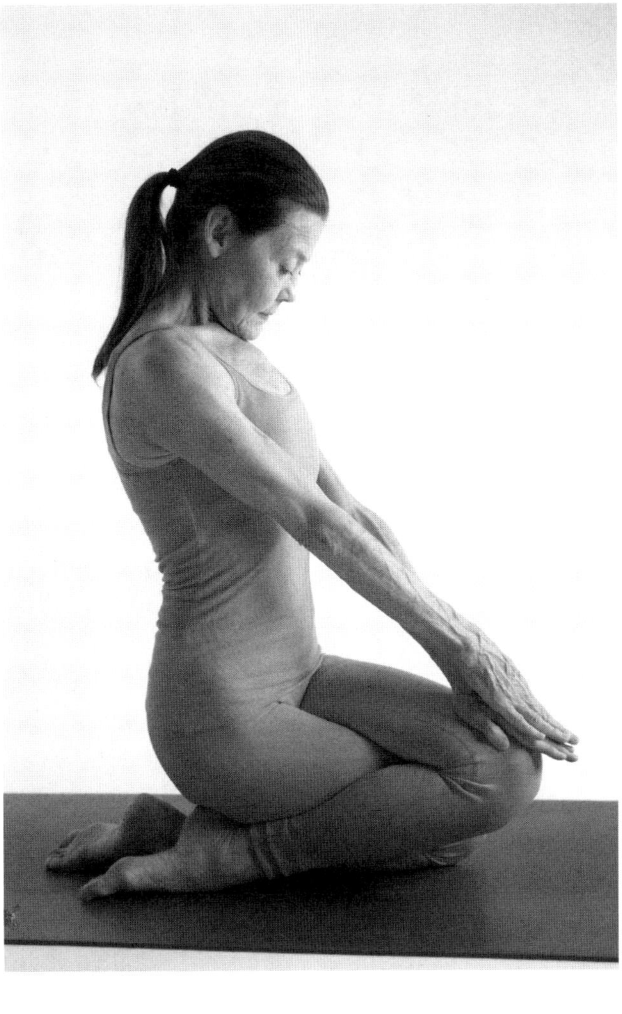

Gomukhāsana in the Aṣṭāṅga tradition is slightly different from the form practiced by many other traditions in that the feet are very close and one almost hovers to balance above the legs while sitting. Finding the plumb line and pelvic floor in this version makes the pose possible, and it is representational of the skills needed to find balance in any pose. There are two phases to this pose that affect the throat and lower neck at the home of the Udāna Vāyu. It grounds and integrates the intensity that can arise within the nervous system, emotions, and the physical body.

1. From Downward Facing Dog Pose, at the end of an exhalation hop through and land on your knees with the right thigh in front of the left, feet slightly out to the side. Sit down, and as you do so, move the lower legs and the sides of the feet so they are touching, if possible.
2. Drop the awareness into the sitting bones, making them heavy in order to stabilize the interplay of the pelvic floor muscles. Place the hands on the left knee, palms down, with the left hand under the right. Roll the shoulders back and down, spread the collarbones, and drop the chin into Jālandhara Bandha position.

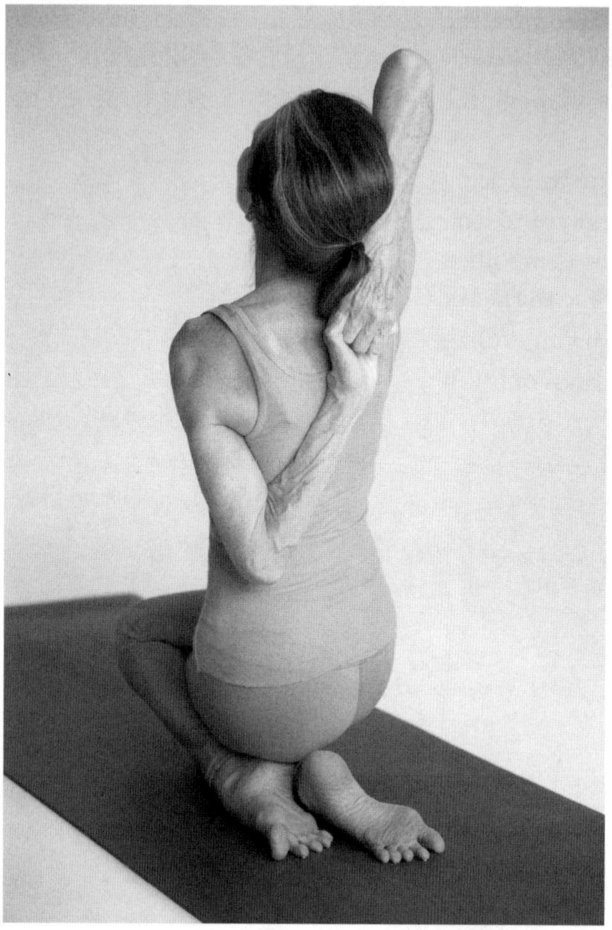

3. Gaze softly inward with the eyes half open and downcast. Hold this position for five breaths.
4. Release the hands. Bend the left elbow and wrap the left arm up the back of your body with the back of the hand on your back. Reach up with the right arm, then bend the elbow to reach down the back with the palm facing the back and clasp the fingers or hands together. Reach up and slightly forward through the right elbow, which will protract the shoulder blade. Tilt the head back and gaze down the nose, holding this position for five breaths.
5. To exit the pose, release the arms, move through a Half Vinyāsa, and do the pose on the other side.

Dikāsana

Compass Pose

Dikāsana appears at the end of the Advanced A Series in the Aṣṭāṅga Vinyāsa system, and even though it isn't as showy as some of the others within that series, it is possibly one of the more difficult poses for many. It is a fine example of the subtleties of working into balancing poses by finding actions and counteractions, maintaining a strong yet soft wave pattern of the breath, and of incorporating the plumb line even when the body is not in a straight or upright form.

1. From Trīṇi, exhale and ground well through the left leg, toning the PC muscle. While inhaling, lift the right leg straight back and up so it is parallel to the floor. Lift the arms and bring them forward with palms of hands together if possible and head behind the arms, closer to the ceiling. Gaze at a point on the floor out in front, balancing for five breaths.
2. Be sure to stretch back through the inner edge of the right foot and use the pelvic floor and scooping up of the lower belly as a strong base for the pose. Do not collapse into the left hip, which can be avoided by micro-bending the left knee and fully articulating the left foot while following the breath. This keeps the hip joint comfortable and keeps the pelvis level.
3. After five breaths, on an inhale take the arms out to the sides angled slightly back behind you, but still parallel to the floor. The arms will be like wings of a bird in flight. Hold this form five more

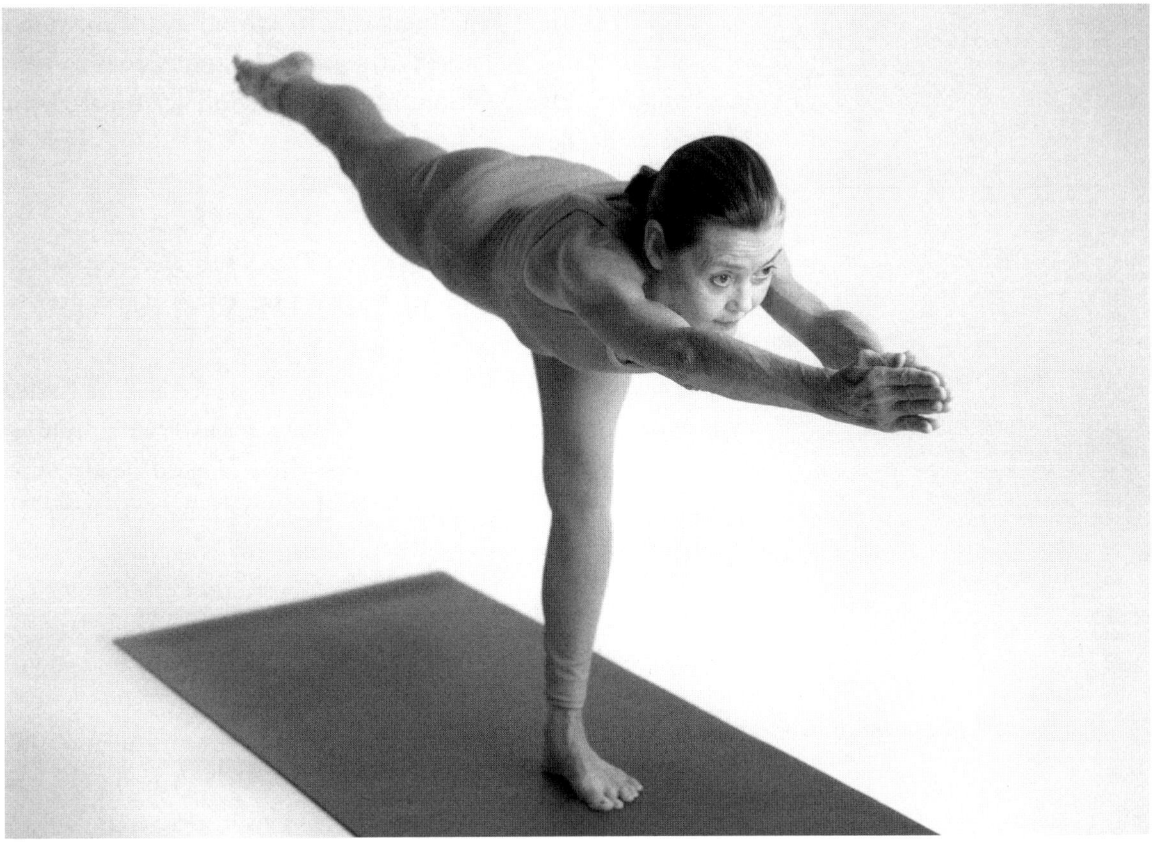

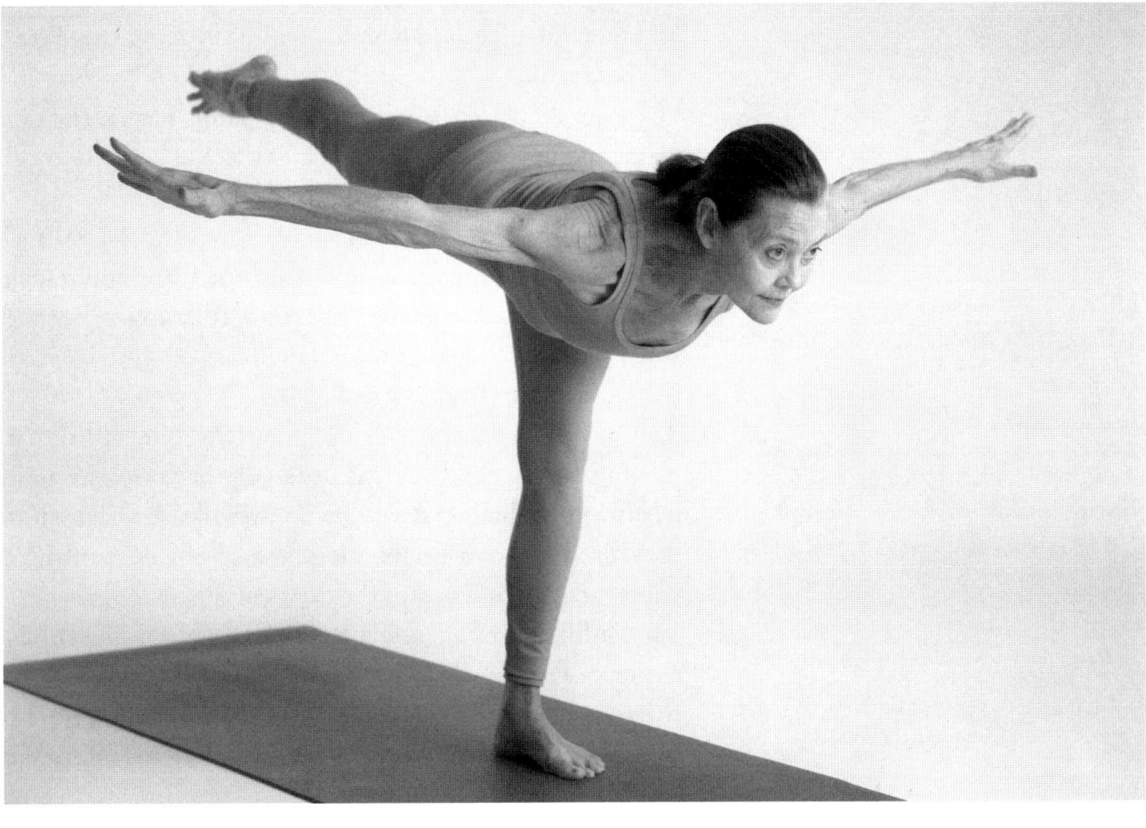

breaths. Then inhaling, reach overhead again for just one breath and on an exhale bring the leg and hands down to the floor coming into Dve position. On the next inhale repeat the pose on the second side.

MUKTA HASTA ŚĪRṢĀSANA (UNBOUND HAND HEADSTAND POSE)

The final sequence of poses within the Intermediate Series comprises seven headstands practiced one following the other, dropping down into Catvāri between poses. In the first three of these headstands, the hands are not clasped together, and in the remaining variations, they are (see Chapter 11).

Mukta Hasta Śīrṣāsana A, B, and C

1. From Downward Facing Dog Pose, on an exhalation, hop forward to place the head on the mat in front of the hands, with the hips raised and the feet on the floor. If you are a more advanced practitioner, you may position the hands for the variation being practiced and then float forward from Downward Facing Dog Pose, landing in the headstand.
2. For form A, place the palms of the hands flat on the floor with the fingers pointing toward the back of the mat, at a distance that allows the arms to be parallel to one another.
3. Exhale fully to establish the base of the pose as you protract the shoulder blades, drawing them up toward the waist and out slightly away from the ears and away from the floor. Inhaling, tone the legs and lift them together, keeping them straight, as you lift into Śīrṣāsana. Hold this position for five breaths.
4. At the end of the final exhalation, take one additional in-breath, moving the hands back into the original position as for a tripod headstand. Exhaling, drop down into full Catvāri, then immediately move into Upward Facing Dog Pose on the next inhale and Downward Facing Dog Pose on the exhale. Prepare for form B.
5. For Mukta Hasta Śīrṣāsana B, from Downward Facing Dog Pose, at the end of an exhalation, position the head as for form A, but place the arms straight out along the floor so you are looking at them, keeping the arms parallel with the palms facing up. Exhale to establish

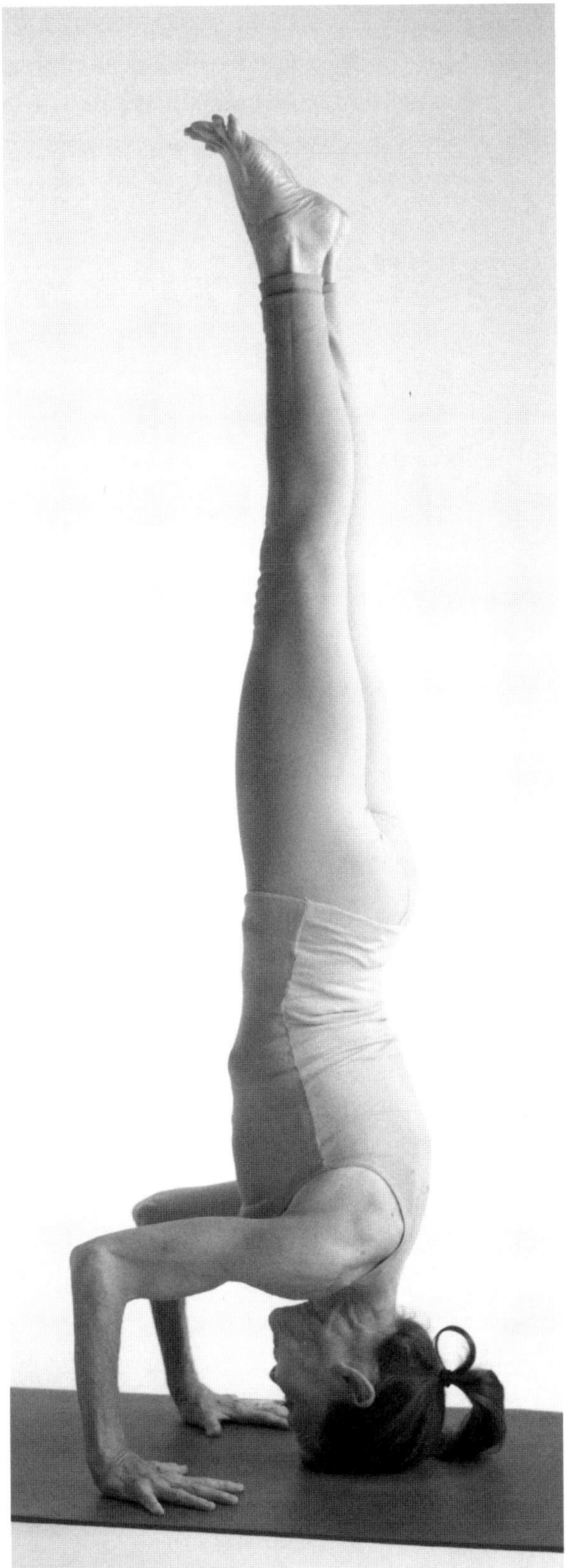

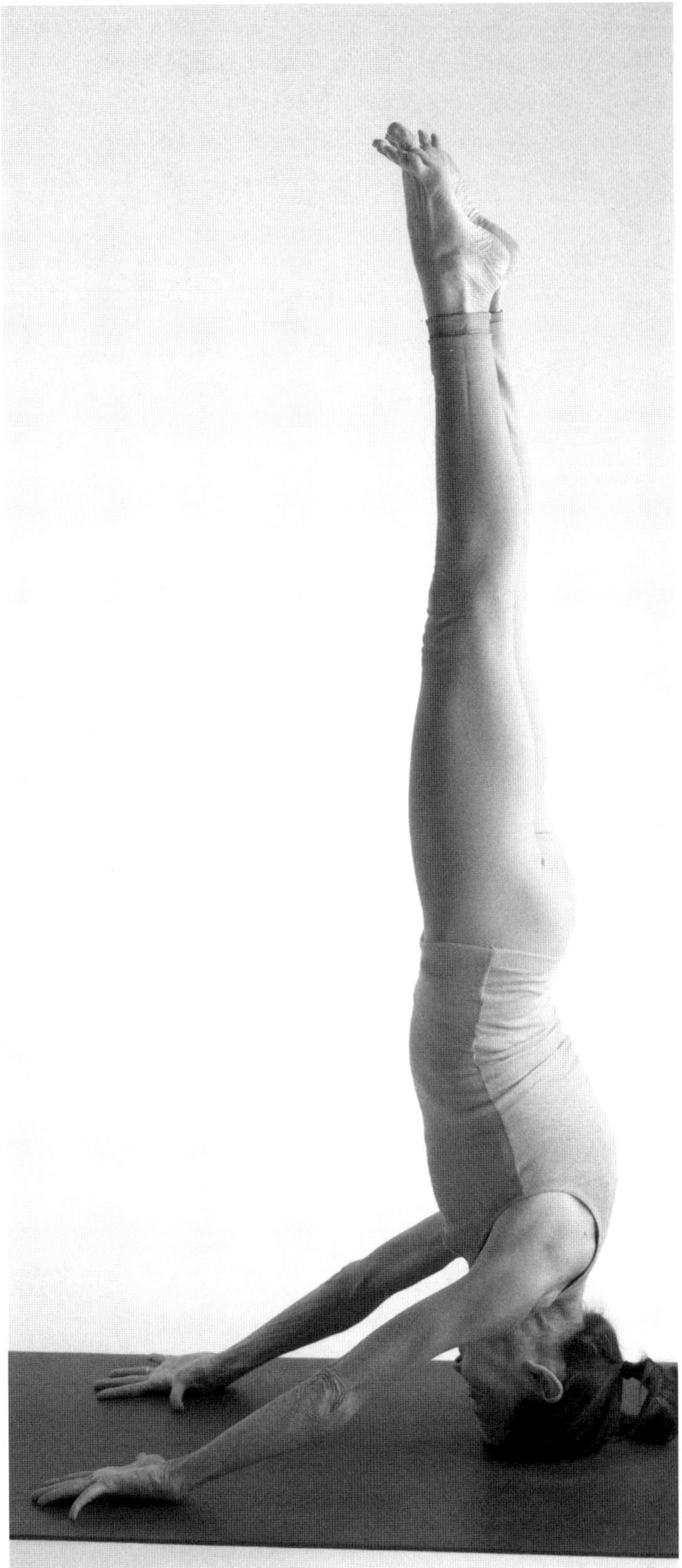

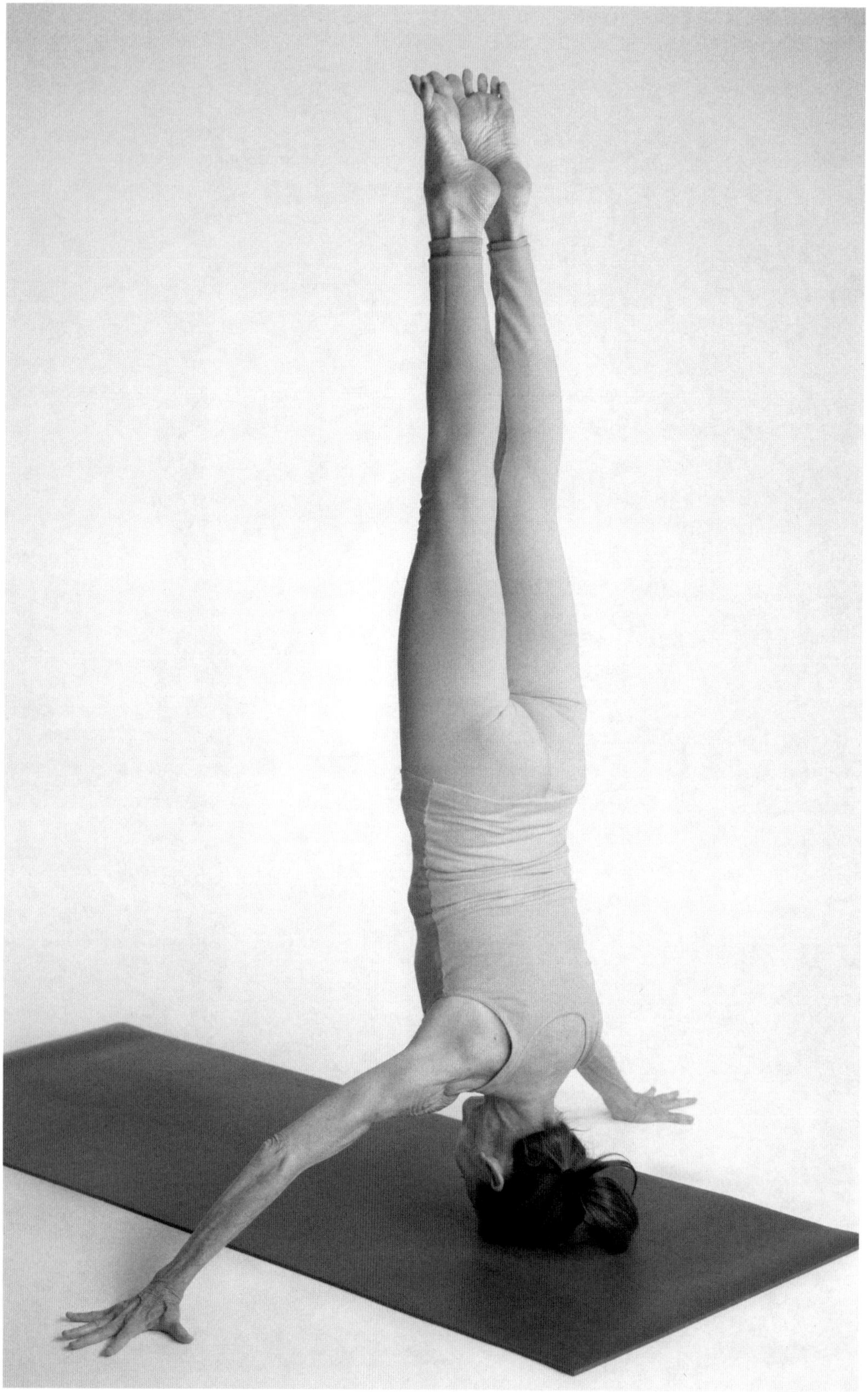

the base of the pose, then, keeping the arms firmly in place, lift the legs into Śīrṣāsana. Adjust the pressure in the backs of the hands, and make subtle adjustments in your shoulders and arms to find strength and balance. Hold this form for five breaths, then, as in step 4, move the hands back to a tripod position and drop into Catvāri and move through a Half Vinyāsa.

6. For Mukta Hasta Śīrṣāsana C, enter the pose as for form B, except place the palms down and reach the arms out to the sides of the body. Your hands may be angled slightly forward toward the end of the mat you are looking at in order to allow for easier balance. Lift the legs into Śīrṣāsana, keeping the arms straight and using subtle adjustments in the arms and hands to facilitate balance. Hold the posture for five breaths.
7. Exit the pose by placing the hands flat on the floor in front of your face on an inhalation. As in step 4, drop into Catvāri and move into a Half Vinyāsa ending in Downward Facing Dog Pose.

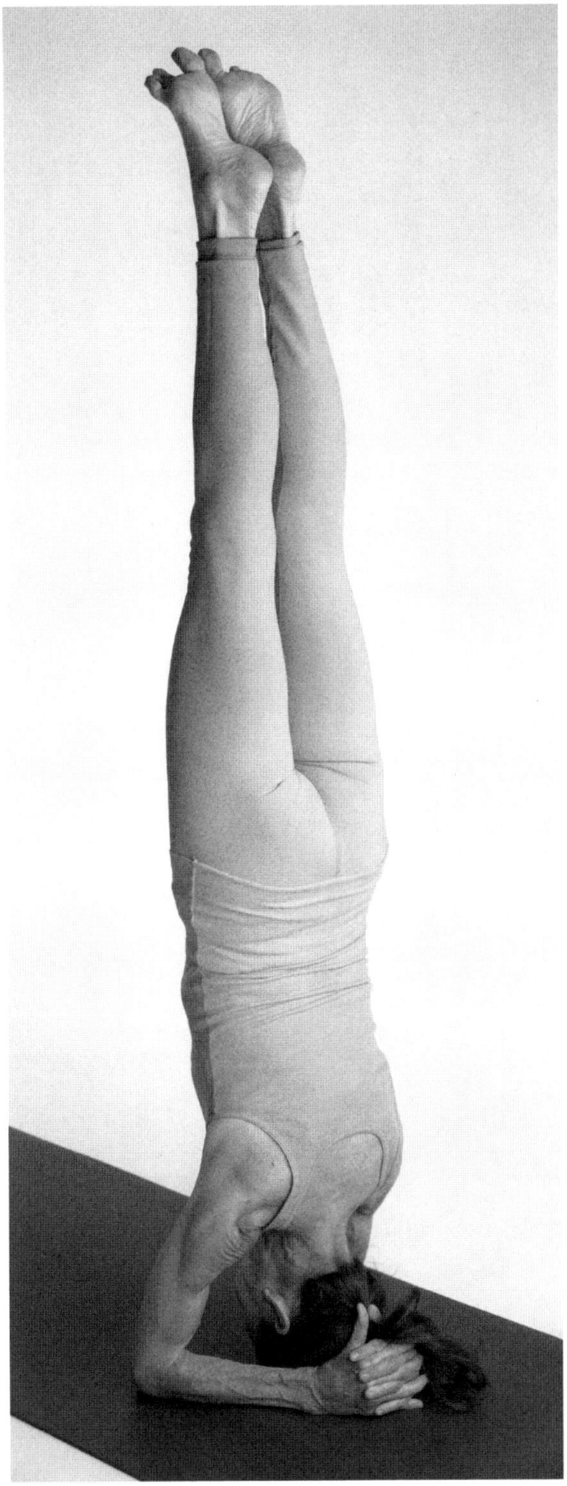

Baddha Hasta Śīrṣāsana A, B, C, and D

In all of these variations of Śīrṣāsana, the hands are bound, touching each other or another part of the body.

1. For form A, from Downward Facing Dog Pose, on an exhalation, place the head on the mat in front of the arms. Position the arms in the classic Śīrṣāsana position with the hands clasped and cupped and the head placed in the nest of the hands.
2. Establish a strong base in the pose, then on an inhalation, lift the legs straight into Śīrṣāsana. Hold this pose for five breaths. As in step 4 for Mukta Hasta Śīrṣāsana, on an inhalation, move the hands so they are flat on the floor to prepare for Catvāri. Drop down on the exhalation and move through a Half Vinyāsa before coming into the next form.
3. For Baddha Hasta Śīrṣāsana B, position the arms in front of your face with the elbows bent and hands holding opposite elbows. Again, lift the legs into Śīrṣāsana

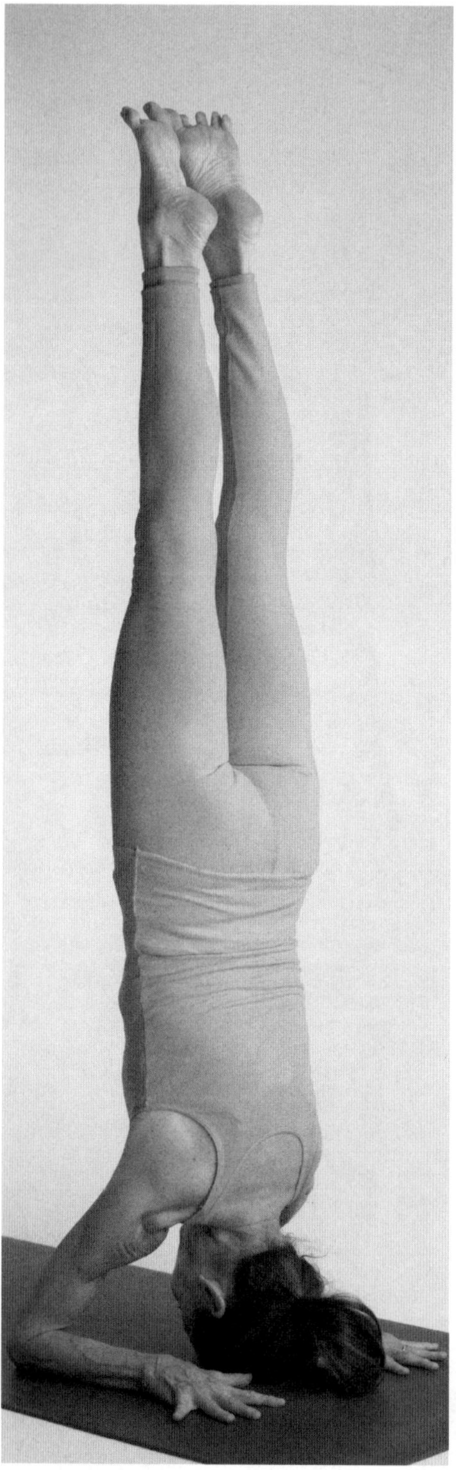

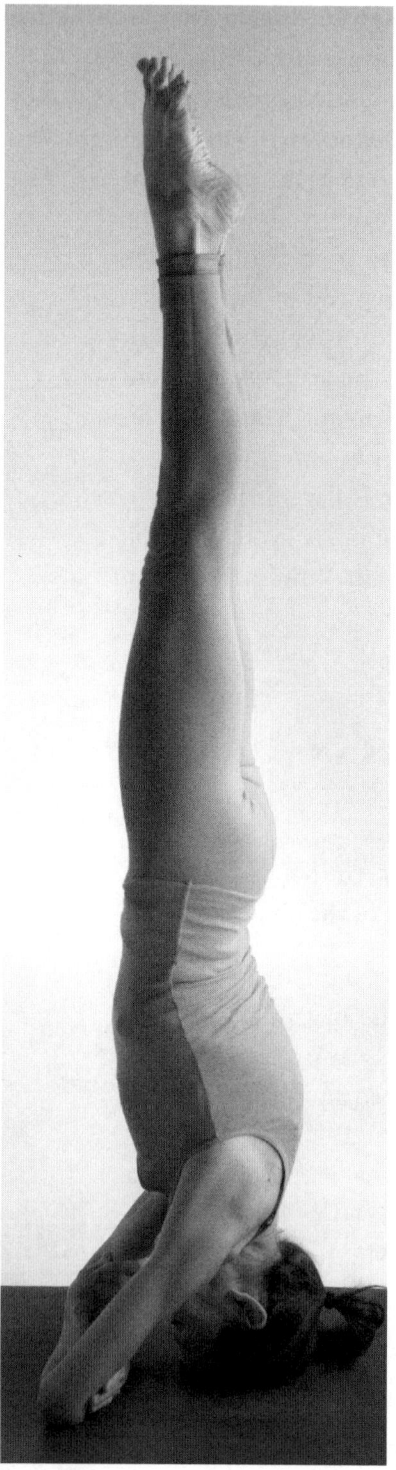

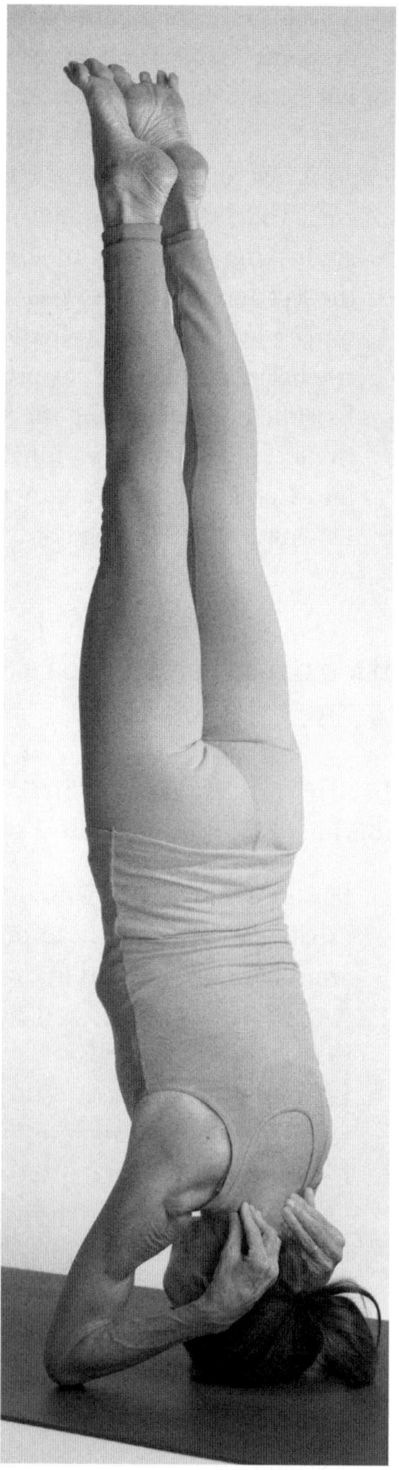

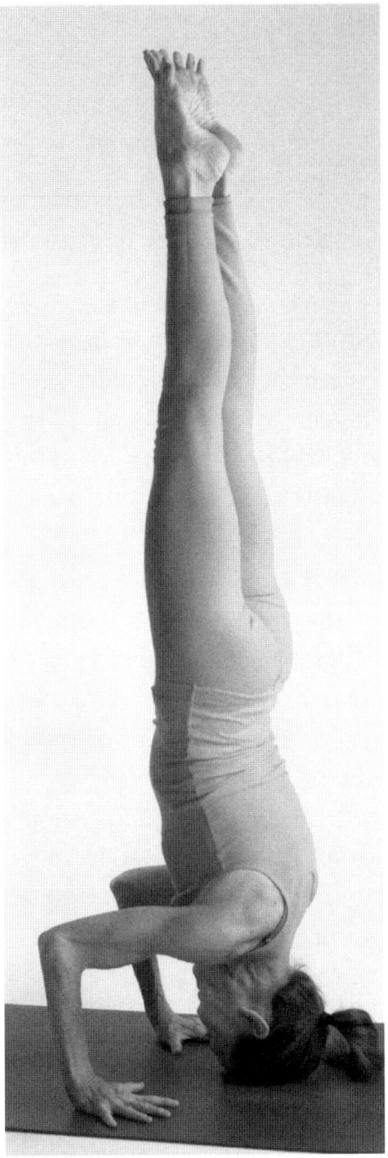

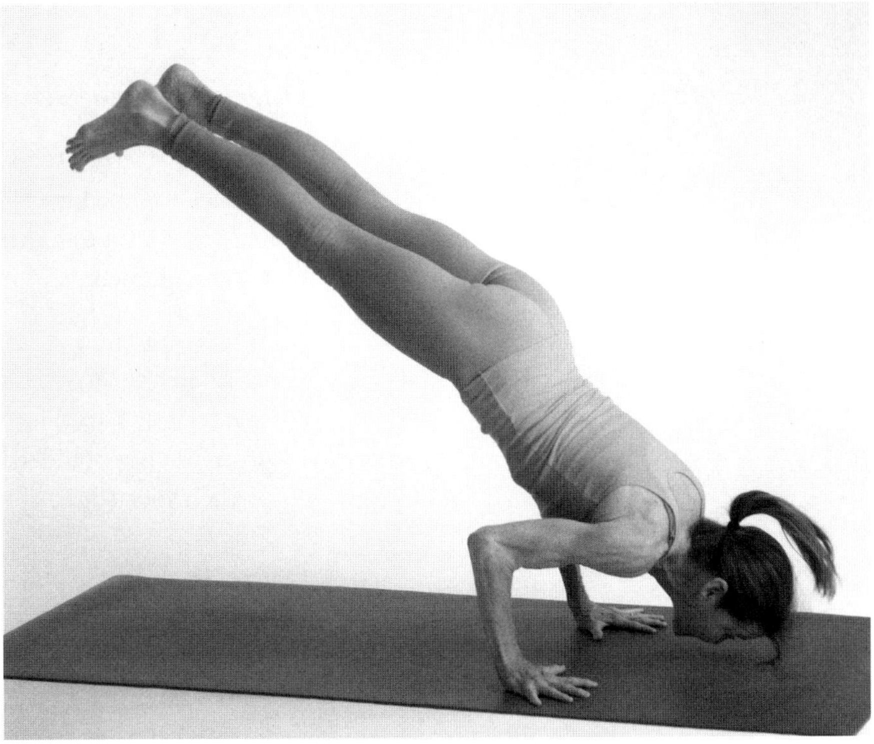

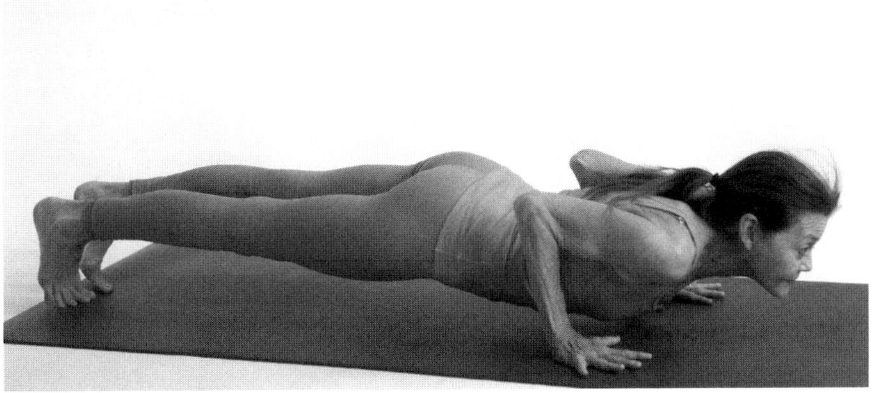

on an inhalation. Hold the form for five breaths before dropping into Catvāri.

4. For form C, place the hands as if you were preparing for Piñcha Mayūrāsana, then position the head for a headstand and lift into Śīrṣāsana on an inhalation. Hold for five breaths before moving the hands to drop down into Catvāri.
5. For form D, place the arms up by the head, with the elbows bent and the fingers gently touching the upper trapezius muscles. Again, move in and out of the pose as for other variations of this sequence of headstands. For the final exit, after moving through a Half Vinyāsa, hop through to a seated position and the next pose.

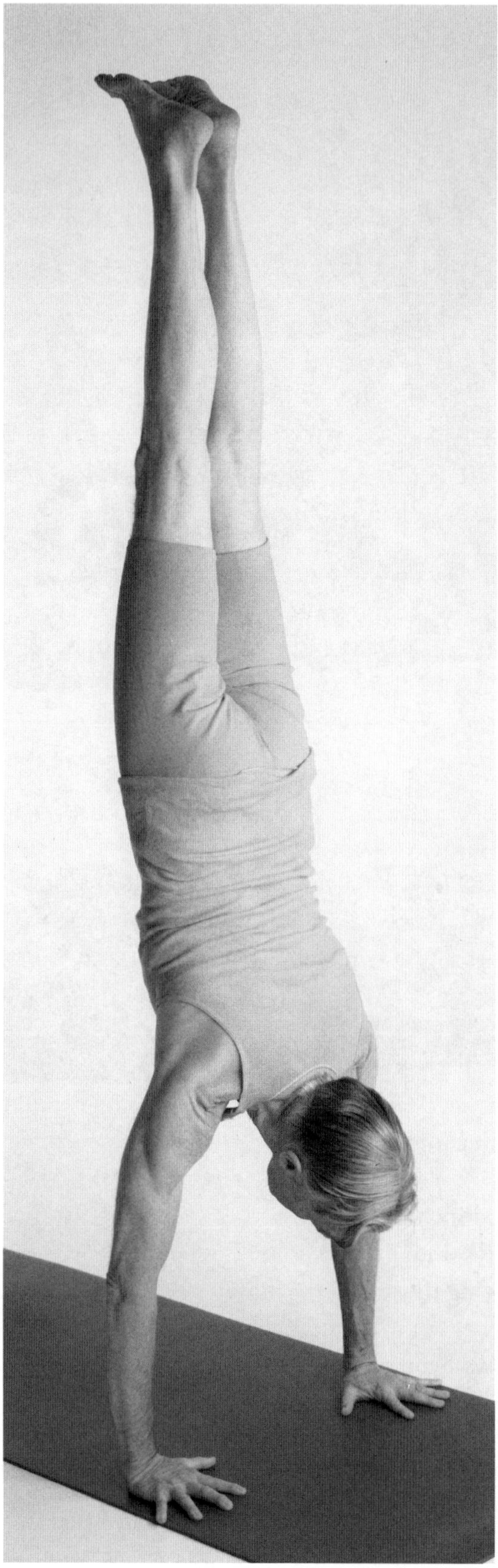

Adho Mukha Vṛkṣāsana

Downward Facing Tree Pose

Commonly referred to as Handstand, this pose can be practiced after backbends, as part of the Nāvāsana sequence, or simply on its own to build core strength and fine-tune proper shoulder alignment.

1. When you are first learning this pose, use a wall to kick up against. Lean over and place the hands shoulder-width apart about 1 to 2 feet from the base of the wall. Firmly protract the shoulder blades and confirm the grounding of the inner edges of the hands as in Downward Facing Dog Pose.
2. Exhale to set the pelvic floor. Kick up with one of legs as you inhale, leaving a slight bend in the elbows and maintaining hand and shoulder alignment as described in step 1. Your second leg will naturally follow the first, and when learning the pose you can place both heels on the wall, then begin to practice balancing without the wall.
3. At first keep the head fully behind the arms and gaze at a point on the floor just in front of the fingertips. Keep the legs stiff and awake using an inward rotation, and stretch up through the inner edges of the feet, keeping the buttocks soft.
4. The key to balancing is to be fluid with tiny back-and-forth adjustments in the belly, spine, hands, arms, legs, and (of course) pelvic floor. These constant adjustments are what makes this one of the finest yoga poses!
5. Once you have stability, you can enter the pose slowly with both legs straight and feet held together. Hold the pose for at least five breaths, then exhale to drop the feet slowly back down to the ground, placing them between the hands just in front of the face. Establishing and maintaining control entering and exiting the pose is where the juice in the pose is found. Work intelligently and slowly for lasting results. Another method of exiting the pose is to slowly bend the arms and bring the heart between the hands to exhale into Catvāri.

11

Finishing Poses

FINISHING POSES, MORE THAN ANY OTHER GROUP of poses, teach subtleties of the core of the body that lead to deep meditative states. We call them finishing poses because we generally do them at the end of an āsana practice, though under certain circumstances, they may be the entirety of the practice. Finishing poses include the whole family of poses associated with Sarvāṅgāsana (Shoulderstand) and a number of variations, which may be used therapeutically. The finishing poses also include Śirṣāsana (Headstand) and its variations as well as Matsyāsana (Fish Pose), which creates a deeply rooted set of counteractions and movements to balance the deep effects of both Shoulderstand and Headstand. There are also a number of extremely internal and meditative linking poses in the sequence, such as Balāsana (Child's Pose), Yoga Mudrā (Seal of Yoga), and Tāḍāgī Mudrā (Pond Mudra), as well as a long Śavāsana (Corpse Pose) that are included in the finishing postures.

A nice thing about this particular sequence is that it provides a good balance between the vibrant, precise state of mind that is required for any of the Aṣṭāṅga series, and the tranquil mood that allows the residue of an intense practice to be assimilated and transformative. We see that this balance makes the finishing poses important for everyone, but particularly for those with a rigorous Aṣṭāṅga Vinyāsa practice because the poses automatically induce a profound feeling of vairāgyam, or letting go. This freeing phase of the practice exposes the ritualistic and sometimes linear framework that the mind sometimes creates as a means of starting and maintaining a yoga practice. All too often, enthusiastic practitioners neglect or leave too little time for the finishing sequence as if fueled by a background fear that prevents them from entering the deeper meditative states of yoga in which there is a sense of delight in dissolving into the truth of impermanence. One of the obstacles in yoga is to circumvent the stillness and silence that proper practice of the finishing sequence necessitates. More rare in the Aṣṭāṅga Vinyāsa world is the opposite fault—that of being too attached to dissolving and being unable to create precise, radiant form in a true yoga āsana. However, some practitioners avoid the depth offered by the finishing poses, conceptualizing them as strictly therapeutic or restorative practices, which can create an imbalance toward an attachment to dissolution before there is actually anything to dissolve—in other words, before they have done the work. This can quickly become tamasic dullness in yoga. Anything within our yoga practice that creates avoidance of a vibrant, awakened, and precise state of mind should be avoided.

All of the finishing poses stretch, stimulate, and balance the myofascial sheaths of the head, chest, and neck. Thanks to this and their contemplative nature, they also make us keenly aware of multifaceted patterns of sensation in the physical structures of the body and, on a more subtle-body level, within patterns of Prāṇa that interpenetrate and connect the entire body and mind. When practicing the finishing poses, it is important to go slowly, progressing step by step, particularly because of the delicacy of the upper neck and structures of the head. The inversions require precise and correct placement of the shoulders, as well as positioning and alignment of the head in relation to the upper vertebrae of the neck so that Prāṇa moves freely throughout the core and into the periphery of the body. In this way, practicing the finishing poses creates a sense of liberation within the forms and underscores the necessity of navigating poses in an intelligent, grounded, and spontaneous manner. Even more than in all other families of poses, when working with the finishing sequence we must begin with an awareness and softening of the palate, mouth, face, and heart by using the technique of proper gazing. This way we can naturally make the correct and usually subtle adjustments to bring a pose into a pleasant, luminous balance.

The finishing poses require a highly refined sense of the entire structure and movement of the spine and the pelvic floor in order to bring them into a full form. One of the great benefits of experiencing these subtle relationships within the body is that the three bandhas will come naturally and easily when we practice finishing poses in a meditative manner. Of course, this not only has a palpable effect on our overall āsana practice and the day-to-day residue from that, but it also helps to deepen our prāṇāyāma practice.

Finishing poses are vital for all levels of practitioners. Even beginners who are physically not ready for some of the poses in the full sequence can and should practice appropriate variations. No matter the level or intensity of our practice, the finishing sequence will help us digest the residue and assimilate the physical benefits of the practice.

Paśchimottānāsana and Variation

Tuning Up the Back Pose

After finishing the full Ūrdhvā Dhanurāsana, folding the hip joints closed and elongating the spine forward provides the counterpose alignment that brings a sense of ease and balance.

1. Lying flat on the back with the knees bent, clasp the hands around the upper shins and, with the thighs apart, squeeze the knees in toward the armpits. Keep the sacrum on the floor to maintain the natural lumbar curve. Imagine that the pubic bone is heavy and dropping down toward the mat so that the PC muscle responds to hold the coccyx. Hold this for five breaths.
2. Next, draw the knees together and squeeze the legs into the chest. Resist the pull of the arms slightly through the legs so the spine is drawn into smooth, even traction. Again, hold for five breaths.

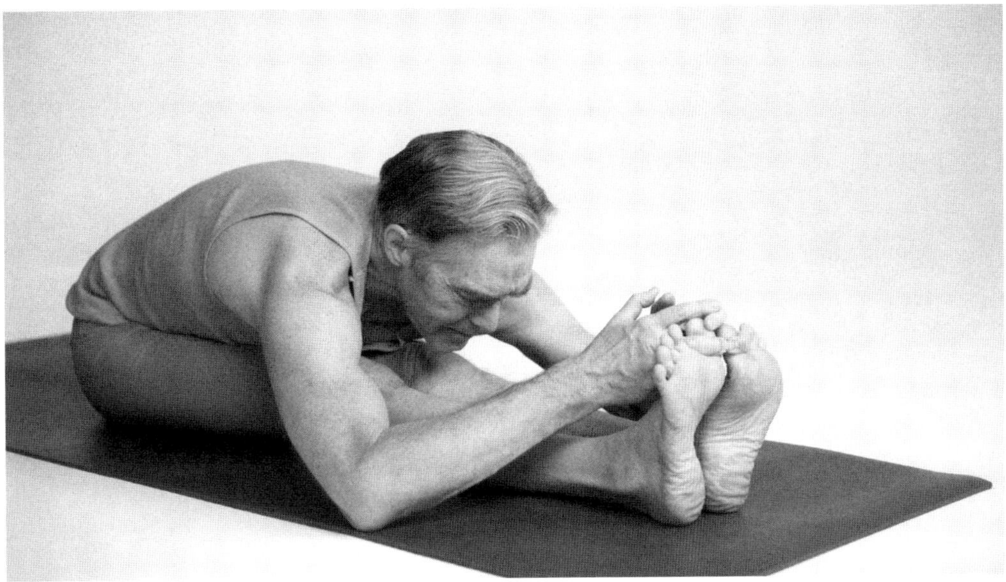

3. On an exhalation, extend the legs up toward the ceiling, then rock up to a seated position.
4. With the legs stretched straight out in front and the spine elongated, fold forward over the legs, taking your favorite hand position from the Paśchimottānāsana sequence (see pages 162–66 for full description). Hold for at least ten breaths. On an inhalation, sit up.

Sarvāṅgāsana

Shoulderstand

This pose also contains Halāsana both in preparation for the full Shoulderstand and as part of the exit from the pose.

1. Enter Sarvāṅgāsana from Tāḍāgī Mudrā (see page 27). At the end of an exhalation, start lifting the straightened legs. Once they are about 30 degrees from the floor, begin to inhale, lifting the hips and buttocks and moving the feet up toward the ceiling.
2. Follow the big toes with the eyes, but don't lift the chin, as, while exhaling, the feet disappear straight over the nose and eventually find their way to the floor above the head.

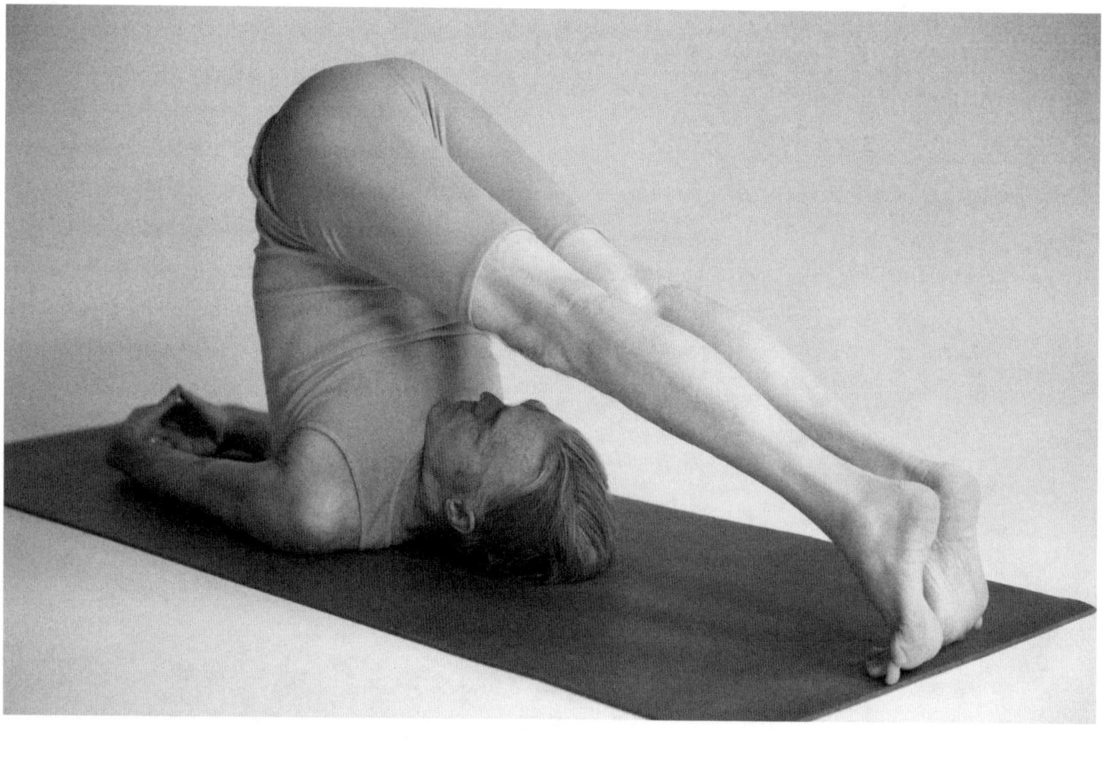

3. Walk or roll the shoulders back and under. Draw the elbows close to each other to make the upper arms parallel. Press the elbows into the floor and clasp the hands behind your back, reaching out and down through the arms and hands. Your toes may be flexed at this stage, pushing gently into the floor, which helps to keep the sitting bones lifting toward the ceiling and the spine straightening.

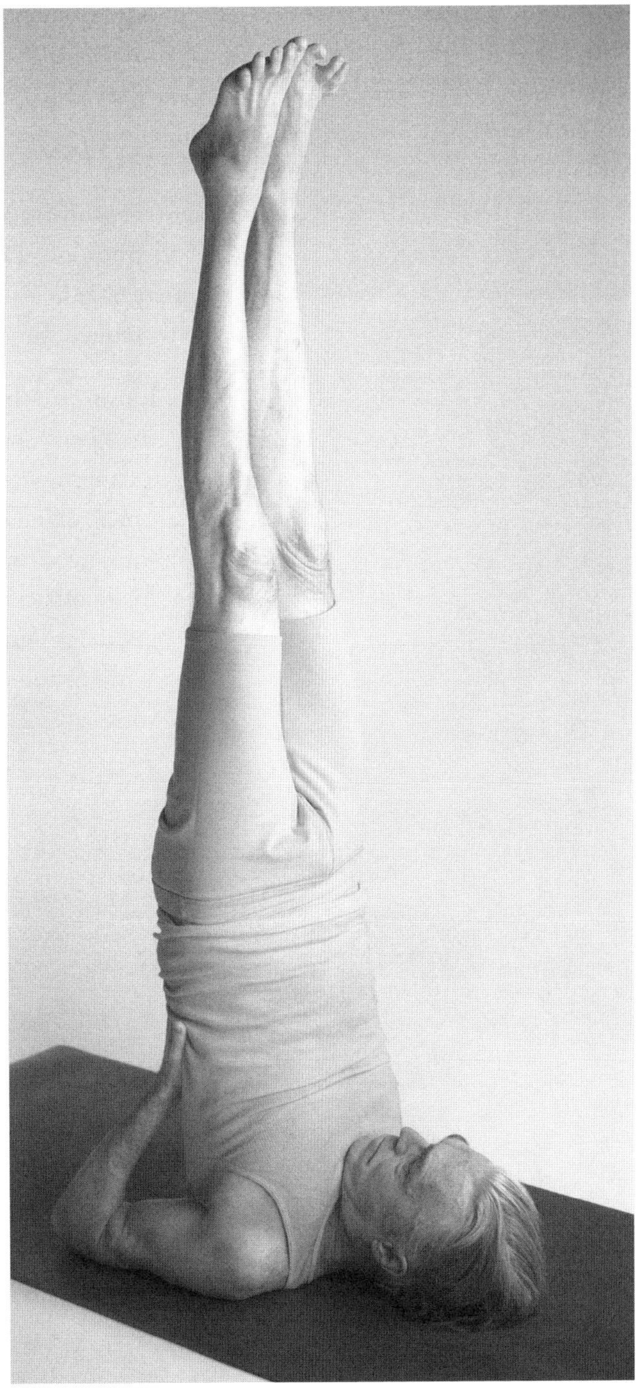

4. After a few rounds of breath, bend the elbows and work the hands up and into the back to draw the skin of the upper back toward the ceiling. Roll the shoulders even farther back into the floor; this should position the neck and chin correctly. Maintain the cervical curve in the neck, but keep the neck, chin, jaw, and tongue soft.
5. Draw the whole spine into the body. Make the legs firm and with an inhalation lift them, together or one at a time, flexing the feet slightly so the inner edges of the feet are reaching up to the ceiling. Keep both legs engaged and alive as you work more deeply into the pose, working the hands high up the back, as close to the upper shoulder blades and neck as possible. Stretch out through the heels before pointing the toes.
6. Gaze at the big toes. Keep the feet above the hips rather than allowing them to drift forward over the face.
7. Do not press the back of the neck into the floor or draw the chin in toward your throat! The large vertebra at the base of the neck (C7) is drawn up into the body. Your upper chest should expand, bringing the top edge of the sternum toward—and eventually to gently touch—the chin. Do *not* actively draw the chin toward the sternum.
8. Remain in Sarvāṅgāsana for at least fifteen breaths, if comfortable.
9. If you experience discomfort during or after the pose and/or cannot keep the back of the neck off the floor, place a folded blanket(s) under the shoulders and arms. The shoulders and elbows will then be elevated on the firm, flat surface, while the head remains down at floor level. If

using a blanket, be sure to have it folded neatly with the folded edge (not the raw or fringe edge) beneath the neck. The shoulders should be positioned so that when in the pose, C7 just grazes the edge of the folded blanket. A qualified teacher can demonstrate the details of this technique. There should be no discomfort or pain in any of the Finishing Poses.

Setu Bandha Sarvāṅgāsana

Bridge Shoulderstand

For beginning students or those with neck injuries, this variation of full Shoulderstand is a good alternative as part of the finishing sequence. It is also an excellent restorative pose for anyone, in or out of this sequence.

1. Lie on your back in Tāḍāgī Mudrā (see page 27) for five breaths. Draw the knees up and place the feet on the floor at the outer edges of the buttocks.
2. On an exhalation, lift the sacrum about 3 inches off the floor, working the knees forward toward the toes. On the next inhalation, engage the quadriceps and lift the pelvis off the floor, with the sacrum moving in and up.
3. Walk or roll the shoulders back and down, clasping the hands behind your back. The sternum will move toward the chin, but keep the chin

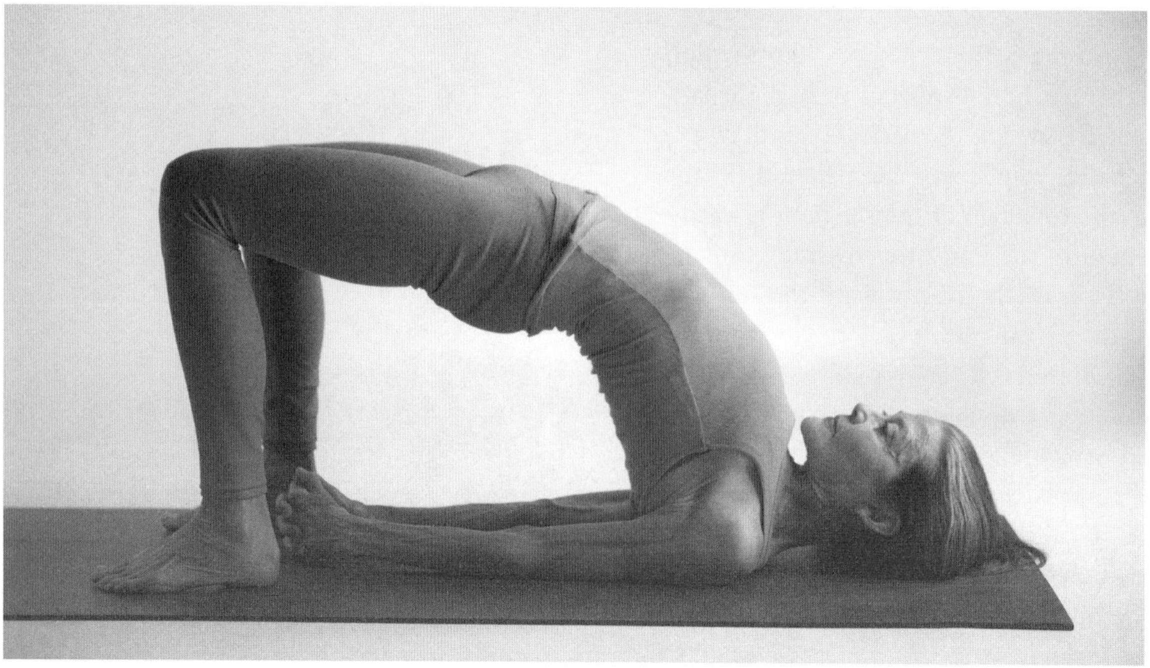

and face neutral. Keep the legs engaged, as if squeezing a block between the thighs, and keep the feet parallel.

4. Gaze along the line of the nose, and hold the pose for at least ten breaths. Exit on an exhalation, releasing the hands to unroll the spine so that the sacrum is the last part to come down to the floor.

Halāsana

Plough Pose

Halāsana is often practiced as a stage while working through Sarvāṅgāsana, but it can also be practiced on its own as a meditative and restorative form.

1. Lying on the back in Tāḍāgī Mudrā, gazing down the nose, exhale fully as you begin to lift the straightened legs away from the floor. When they are about 30 degrees from the floor, begin to inhale as the hip joints fold more deeply. Keep the head neutral, but gaze at the feet as they move over the head to the floor.
2. Clasping the hands behind your back, roll the shoulders completely back into the floor and make the spine straight, moving the sitting bones up toward the ceiling. You may bend the elbows at first, but

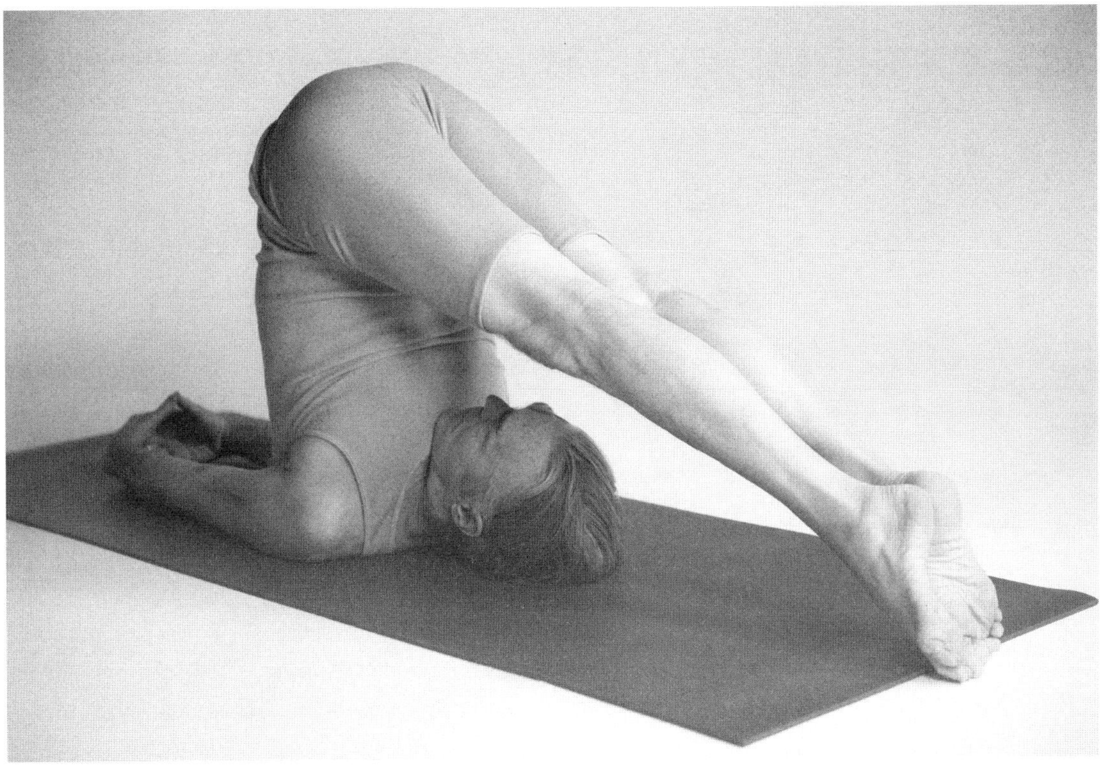

work toward straightening the arms to further guarantee that the shoulders roll under.

3. Shift the softened gaze to the tip of the nose. The back of the neck remains off the floor, and the throat stays soft.
4. Straighten the spine, keeping the legs firm. This is an excellent opportunity for cultivating Uḍḍīyāna and Mūlabandhas. Point the toes only if you can keep the legs absolutely straight.
5. Remain here for ten breaths. To exit, continue into Karṇa Pīḍāsana or release the hands and, exhaling, roll down onto the back. Move into Catvāri via Cakorāsana.

Karṇa Pīḍāsana

Squeezing the Ears Pose

This deeply meditative pose incorporates flexion of the spine into the shoulder structure that is used in Sarvāṅgāsana, an alignment that creates a feeling of safety within a strong form. Cupping the knees next to the ears focuses attention on *listening* to the breath so that breathing becomes smooth, even, and deep.

1. Begin in Halāsana. Exhaling, bend the knees and lower them toward the floor next to the ears. Releasing the palate as you exhale

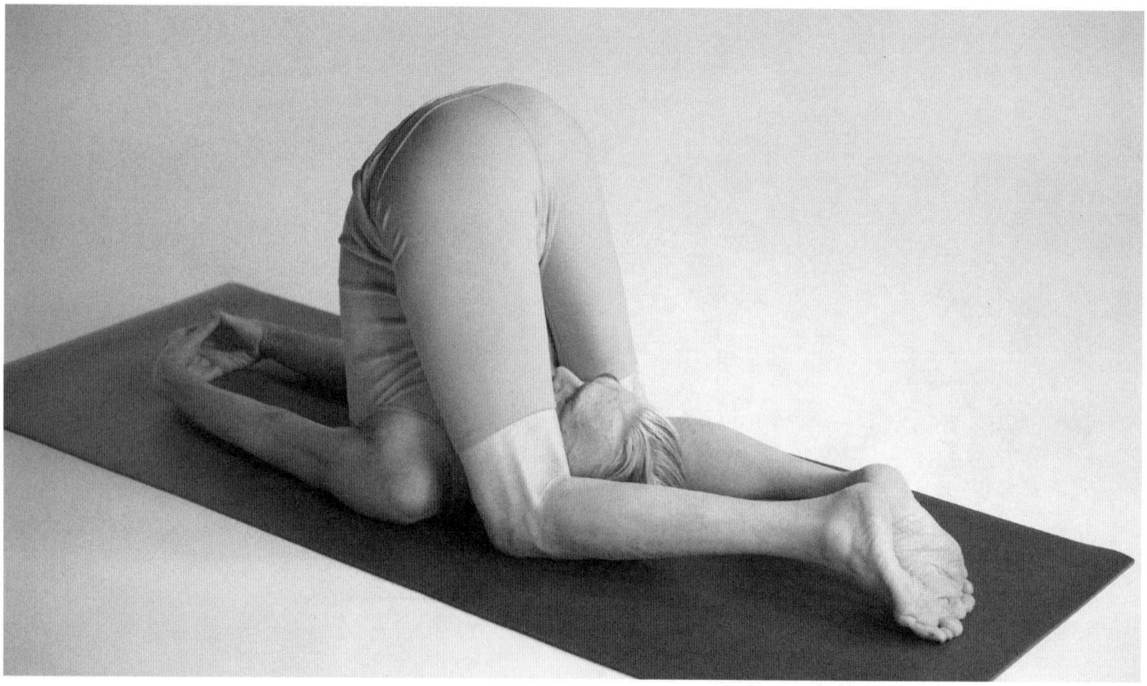

will lengthen the entire spine in both directions. If the knees reach the floor, gently cup the ears with the inner knees. If they do not reach the floor, do not strain, but allow gravity and consistent practice to slowly deepen the pose until they can touch the ears. This may take a long time (years), but you should not strive too much for it.

2. Keep the hands clasped behind the back, and press the straight arms down into the floor. Gaze at the tip of the nose. Relax the ears. Soften and steady the eyes. Empty the palate as if softly smiling. Circulate the breath evenly through the entire field of perception as you hold the pose for ten breaths.
3. To exit, either roll down onto the back on an exhalation, or step back up into Sarvāṅgāsana to complete the full finishing sequence.

Ūrdhvā Padmāsana

Upturned Lotus Pose

This pose is an excellent opportunity to begin to feel movement in the pelvic floor at the ends of the breath. It is great training for Uḍḍīyāna and Mūlabandhas and also for keeping the PC muscle toned at will.

1. From Karṇa Pīḍāsana or Halāsana, place the arms back in Sarvāṅgāsana position behind the back with the elbows bent and the hands on the upper back. Inhaling, step back up into Sarvāṅgāsana.
2. Still in Sarvāṅgāsana, cross the legs into Padmāsana. Use one of the hands for assistance if needed to position the feet and legs. If you cannot yet do Padmāsana, simply cross the legs or place the soles of the feet together as in Baddha Koṇāsana.
3. Place the hands on the ends of the femur bones at the medial edges of the knees. Straighten the arms. Press the knees into the hands, while pushing back with the hands against your knees. Gaze softly along the line of the nose, holding the pose for five breaths. To exit move immediately into Piṇḍāsana on an exhalation.

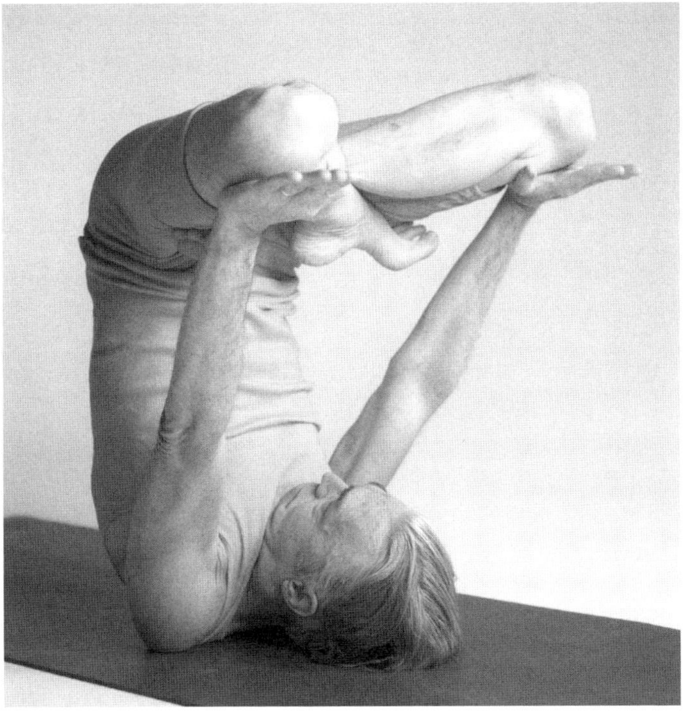

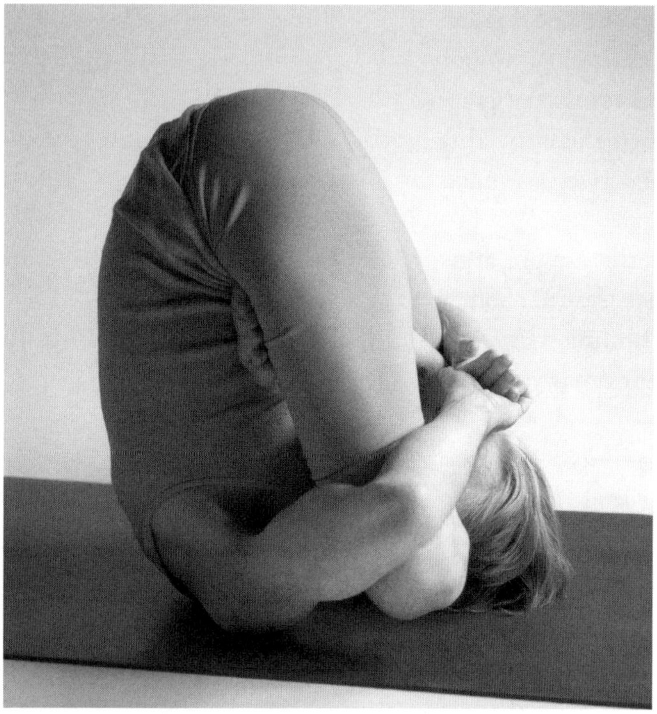

Piṇḍāsana

Embryo Pose

This is an excellent counterpose for the spine after Sarvāṅgāsana and Halāsana, and it also serves as a threshold to awaken the spine for counteractions required for the subsequent cervical backbends in the Finishing Sequence.

1. From Ūrdhvā Padmāsana, on an exhalation fold at the hip joints to draw the knees down toward the fronts of the shoulders and, if possible, gently reach them to the floor, then inhale to set the pose.
2. Exhaling again, take the arms around the backs of the legs and clasp the hands, if possible. Make the body into an even ball, curling the spine and releasing the shoulders and neck completely. Leave the shoulder blades rolled back into the floor. Notice that this movement lessens the angle of flexion in your neck, preparing the body for its descent.
3. Gaze internally along the line of the nose with the eyes half closed. Stay in this position for ten breaths.
4. To exit, exhale while rolling down onto the back and placing the arms down along the sides of your body. Move immediately into Matsyāsana.

Matsyāsana

Fish Pose

Due to the sense of a heavy coccyx, which is necessarily maintained by the legs being in Padmāsana (or crossed), this strong backbend opens the heart area and thoracic spine with less chance of excessive folding in the lumbar spine than with other deep backbends. Gazing down the nose keeps the neck properly extended and the pose integrated.

1. Lying on your back, keep the legs in Padmāsana or easily crossed. Take the outsides of the upper thighs with your hands. Ground the elbows, lift the head, and glance toward the navel as you complete an exhalation. Hold the seed of the exhalation in the center of the pelvic floor as you begin to inhale to unroll the spine into a backbend. Initially push

the sacrum up and in, unroll up to the heart, and then up to extend the lower neck. Finally the head is allowed to rotate back at the very top of the inhalation. Exhale as you place your head down to the floor. Inhaling, activate the pose, release the palate, and gaze down the nose.

2. Use the elbows to adjust the shoulders, positioning the center of the crown of the head onto the floor. Take the elbows away from the floor and clasp the feet. Either pull back slightly through the hands or push with the hands and arms to pull or stretch the skin at the crown of the head in different ways. Notice the effects of these actions. Push down toward the floor through your knees. Give yourself time in this pose to position yourself comfortably and on the wave of the breath, inhaling as you push through the elbows and lift the heart area into a backbend and exhaling as the head is repositioned on the floor until it is in exactly the right, most comfortable place for your particular circumstances. If Padmāsana is not possible, leave the legs stretched out straight, and still work through the elbows to open the heart area into a backbend.

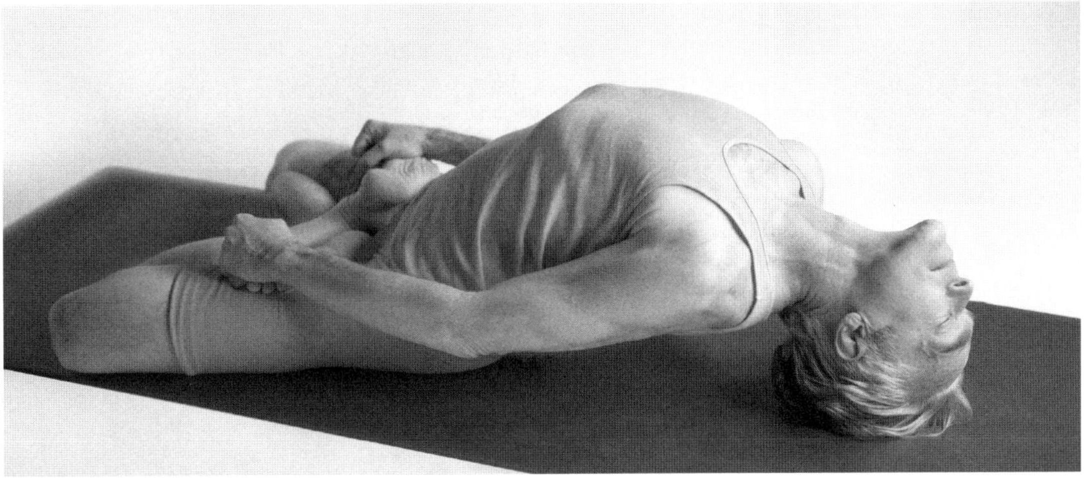

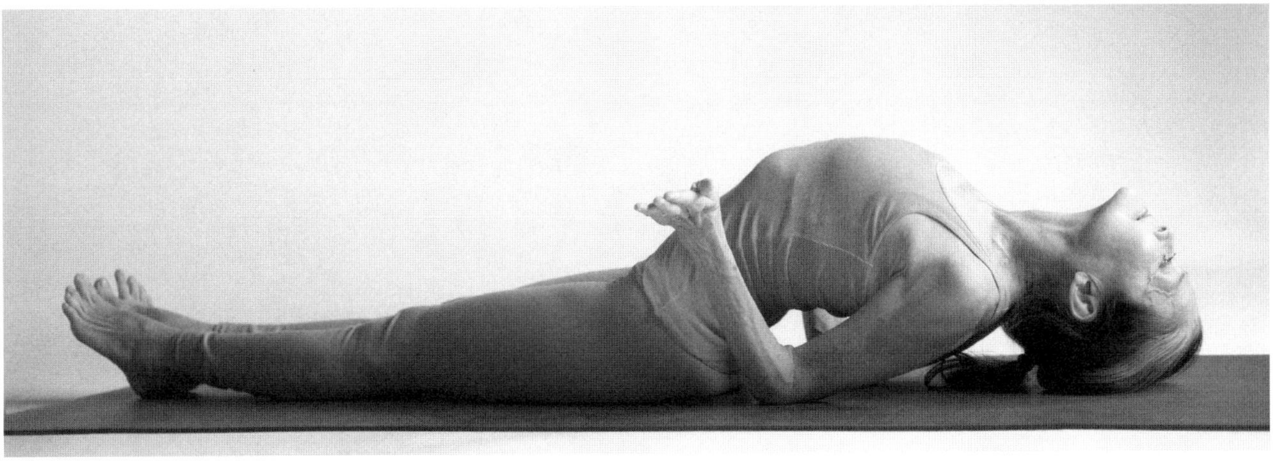

3. Continue to gaze down the nose as you drink nectar from the root of your palate. Silence the tongue, release the ears, and sink the sitting bones as the heart opens. Stay here for at least ten breaths rather than moving immediately into Uttāna Pādāsana. If you prefer to exit Matsyāsana, release the feet with the hands and place the elbows on the floor near the waist. Push through the elbows to lift the heart and then exhale, lift the head to look at the navel. Inhaling, lower the back onto the floor from bottom to top, placing the back of the head down last. Unravel the legs and then exit through Cakrāsana.

Uttāna Pādāsana

Upwardly Stretched Legs Pose

This pose is reminiscent of an enthusiastic fish. Maintaining the form of Matsyāsana in the upper body, the legs are straightened and angled from the floor so that it you were a fish doing Uttāna Pādāsana, you'd be flying!

1. Move directly into Uttāna Pādāsana from Matsyāsana, leaving the top portion of the body in Matsyāsana.
2. With the legs still in Padmāsana (or crossed), flex the hip joints to lift the knees off the floor so the thighs are at about a 60-degree angle

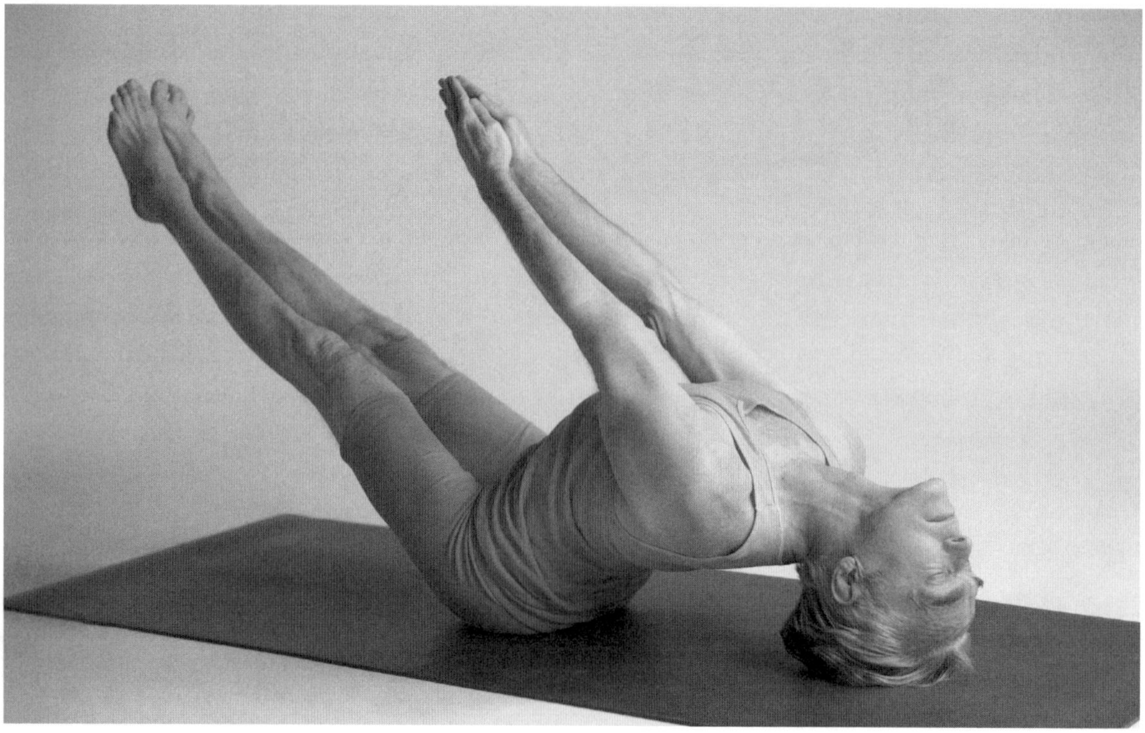

from the floor. Unravel the legs and straighten them into the air, reaching out through the feet. The legs act to ground the sitting bones even more.

3. Choose a comfortable angle for the legs. If you are a beginner, you might keep them at 45 degrees or higher, while more advanced practitioners could lower them closer to the floor.
4. Straighten the arms out in front of the chest, placing the palms together and keeping the arms at about the same angle as the legs.
5. Gaze down the line of the nose and stay in the pose for eight breaths.
6. To exit, on an exhalation, place the arms along the sides and bend the elbows, hands pointing toward the ceiling. Exhale deeply and push through the elbows to lift the chest and the head off the floor, curling the neck to look at the navel, then inhaling, lower the spine to the floor as you lift the legs to vertical. Place the hands up by the ears, fingers pointing toward the tops of the shoulders and roll back through Cakrāsana into Catvāri and on through a Half Vinyāsa.

Śīrṣāsana

Headstand

One of the most important poses in any yoga practice is Śīrṣāsana. It takes time to learn the pose well, but even for beginners, it can offer the immediate benefit of changing their perspective. Over time, it becomes clear that this pose relies on proper shoulder alignment and arm strength, in addition to a trust in gravity. The pose is meditative, bringing form and focus into the plumb line, as well as connecting forces of movement and form out through both the feet and the crown of the head to invite awareness into subtleties that arise moment by moment. It is truly Samasthitiḥ upside down. Once stable in it, visualization of deities and internal forms reveals the central channel beautifully.

1. Create the foundation of the pose carefully. Place the outer edges of the lower arms on the floor and draw the elbows in so they are exactly shoulder-width apart with the forearms parallel. Interlace the fingers. Press the roots of the index fingers together and pull the roots of the little fingers slightly apart. Touch the tips of the thumbs; pull the wrists away from each other isometrically but keep them parallel and upright as they ground down through the ulnae. The palms should remain vertical (not cupped under). A few practitioners with proportionally short arms find that pressing the heels of the hands together allows the elbows to bear weight correctly in the pose.

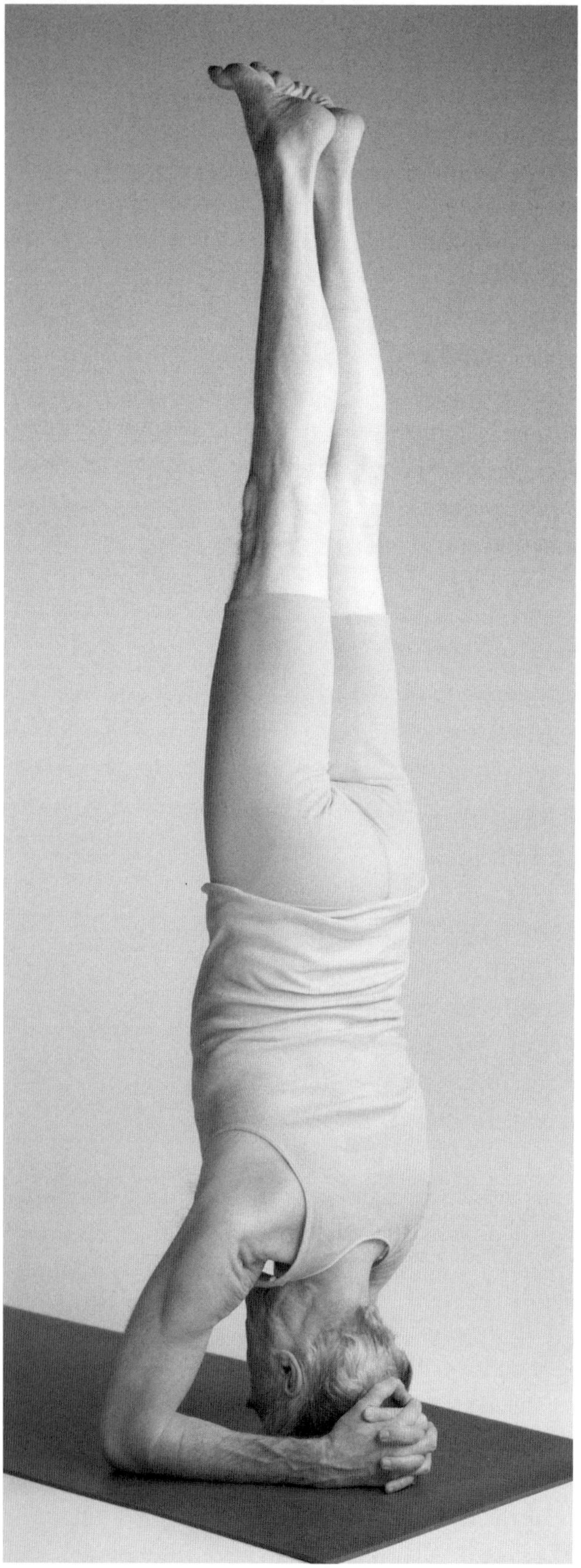

2. Lift the hips and walk the feet in toward the shoulders to place the center of the crown of the head lightly down on the floor. The exact point that should be touching is an individual matter, and you should experiment with it intelligently so there is no strain created in the neck or head. It is important that the majority of the weight for the pose be held through the base of the arms—especially if you are first learning the pose. So you must work out the placement of the head (the angle and exactly where it should be within the nest of the hands) for your individual circumstances.
3. The heels of the thumbs should evenly touch the back of the head. Spread the shoulders as wide as possible, and lift them as far from the floor as possible. When the center of the crown of the head is down, you will be able to see the ceiling, just as you are able to see the floor in Samasthitiḥ when the head is level. Again, the Headstand is similar in form to Samasthitiḥ.
4. Distributing the weight within the broad frame of the arms and shoulders, walk the feet toward the face. Exhale and then, with the elbows grounding, inhale to draw the straightened legs up. Stretch the inner edges of the legs through the inner edges of the heels during the ascent. This will give you control and will give the elbows a greater share of the weight. If a straight-legged ascent is not possible, bend your knees and curl partway or completely up into the pose. Alternatively, you may lift the legs one at a time. If you are a beginner, you can do this pose against a wall until the balance becomes natural.
5. Hollow (draw back) the groins as in Samasthitiḥ; do not push out through them across the room. Stretch the inner heels as high as possible before pointing the toes. The legs are held together with an inward rotation in each leg. Throughout the pose, keep the inner edges of the feet together, constantly lengthening the inner seams of the legs toward the ceiling. Imagine holding a hollow straw between the legs as if holding the plumb line at the center of the pelvic floor, the mūla.

6. Widen the front edges of the armpits as if drawing the skin back and together around the backs of the shoulders. Pull the shoulder blades firmly down the back (when you're upside down, this means they are going up toward the ceiling), keeping the kidney area broad. The back of the neck should be long and strong but without tension. There should be no discomfort in the head or neck.
7. Press the sides of the hands and the edges of the forearms into the floor. Spread the weight wide through your whole body. It will feel light at the crown of your head as you push the plumb line into the floor using only your sense of dignity. The heart and throat feel spacious and there will be a sense of openness in the ears, and brightness at the root of the palate.
8. When you are stable and happy in the pose, gaze at a point straight out from the eyes or eventually gaze at the tip of the nose. It should be easy to keep the gaze strong, soft, and steady, and the breathing should be smooth and even. This is a great Mūlabandha pose. Hold for at least twenty-five breaths.
9. If you are an advanced student, you can finish by lowering the straight legs to a horizontal position with legs parallel to the floor. Reach out through the heels and inseams of the legs while gazing

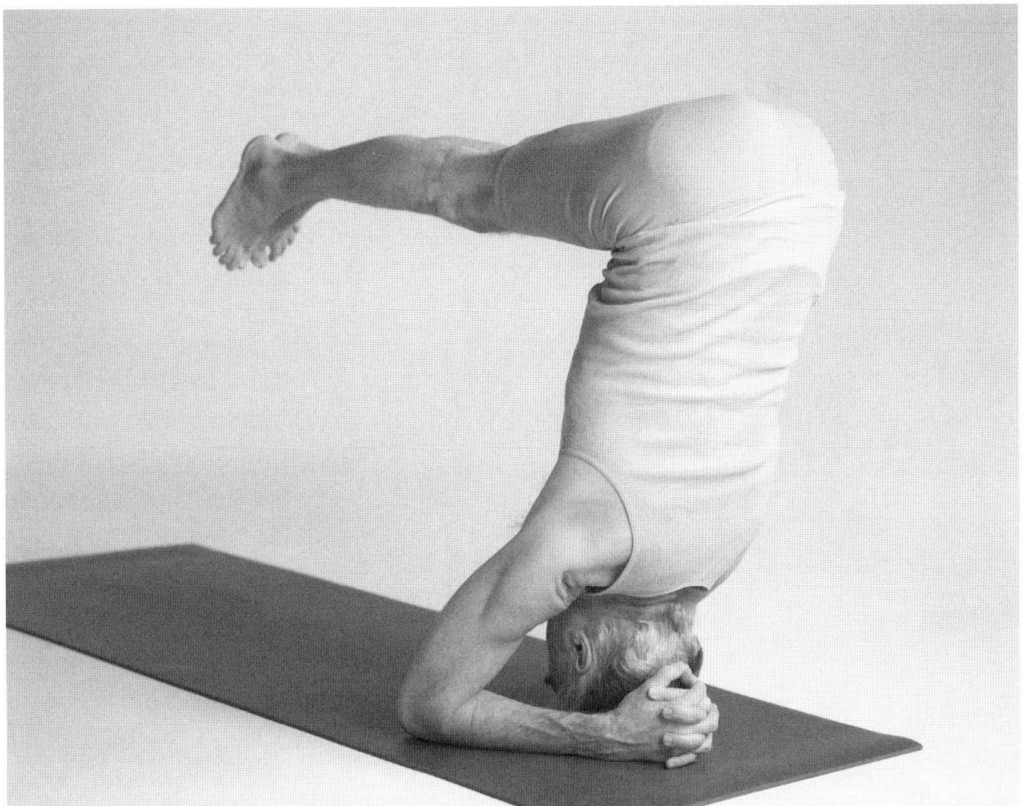

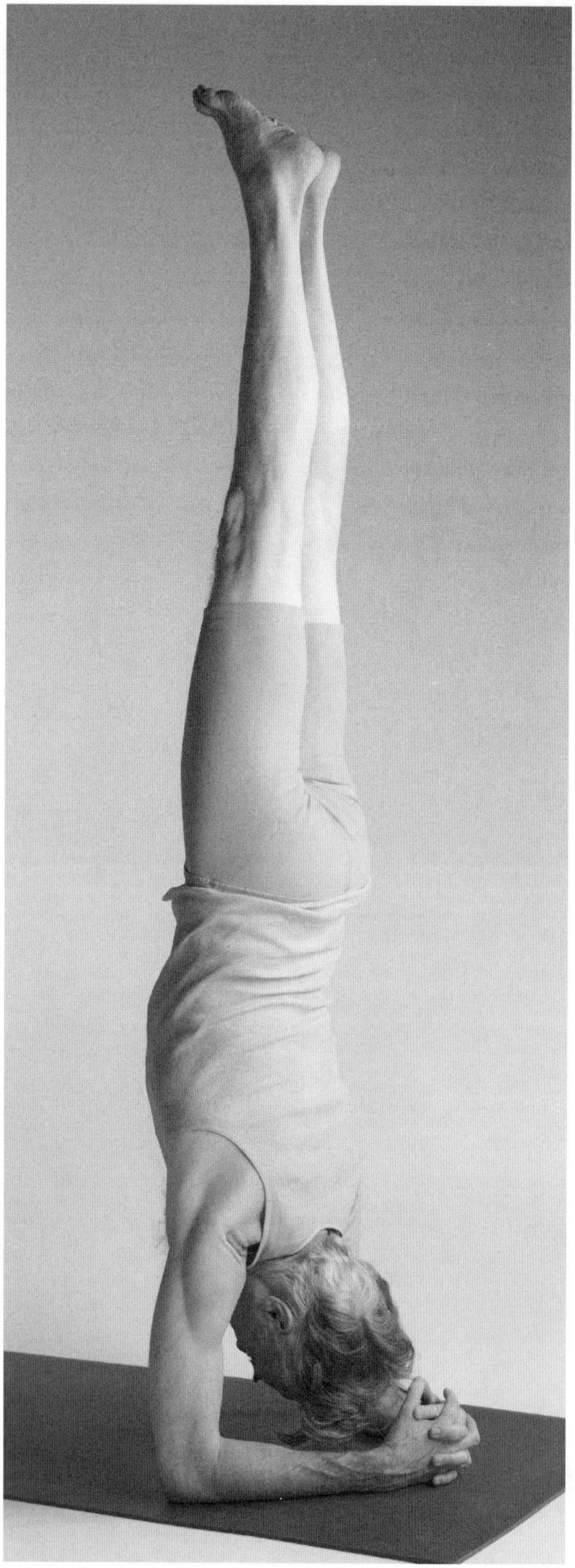

at the big toes for five breaths. Keep the lower belly hollowed back at the edges of the pubic bone and the shoulders stretched high and wide. Do not wrinkle the skin on the back of the neck as you lower into or hold this form.

10. Inhale and lift the legs back up into full Śīrṣāsana. Exhaling, activate the legs and push down through the frame of the arms, while shifting the weight toward your elbows without allowing the wrists to ascend. On an inhale push evenly down through elbows and wrists to effortlessly lift the head entirely off the floor. Do not do a backbend here. Rather, keep the legs vertical. Hold for ten breaths, then lower carefully back down into Śīrṣāsana for one breath before lowering the legs to the floor to rest in Balāsana.
11. If you are a beginner, you can finish by coming slowly down from Śīrṣāsana on an exhalation without lifting the head off the floor and resting in Balāsana.

Balāsana

Child's Pose

It is very important to practice this deeply restorative pose after Śīrṣāsana to reestablish smooth circulation and absorb the residue from the pose. It is also an excellent pose to take when stressed, tired, or on one's moon cycle.

1. Sit on the mat with the legs folded back and the feet under the buttocks. The knees may be almost touching or as far as hip-width apart, depending on what feels best. Do not open the hips extremely wide for this pose. If you experience pain in the knees, place a folded blanket behind them for support.
2. Fold forward at the hip joints to place the forehead on the floor. If your head does not reach the floor, place a soft block or blanket to support the forehead in a position so as not to interfere with breathing.

3. Relax the arms. You can take various arm positions, each creating a slightly different effect. One or all may be practiced on any given day. The most common arm position is to reach up along the floor over the head with the elbows bent and the forearms resting on the floor. Or you may drape the arms along the sides of the body, with the palms facing up.
4. A third variation that is particularly good to practice after Śīrṣāsana is to rest the head in the hands and place the neck in a gentle traction. To do this form, with the arms reaching out in front, lift the head and bend the elbows so the hands easily reach the head. Walk the elbows forward on the mat, and place the hands along the sides of the head with the roots of the fingers along the temples, between the tops of the ears and the corners of the eyelids.

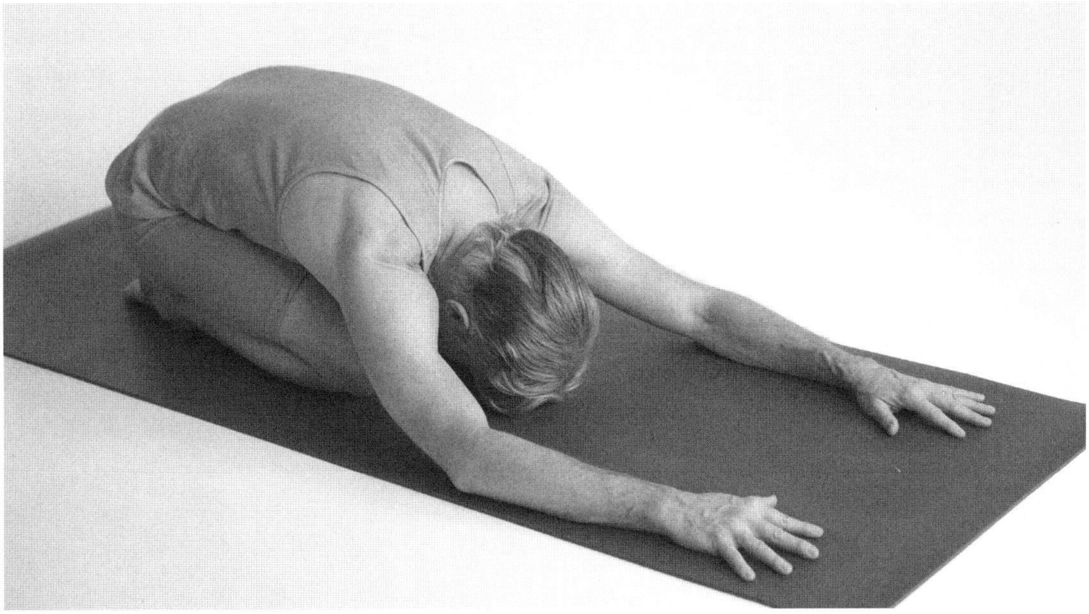

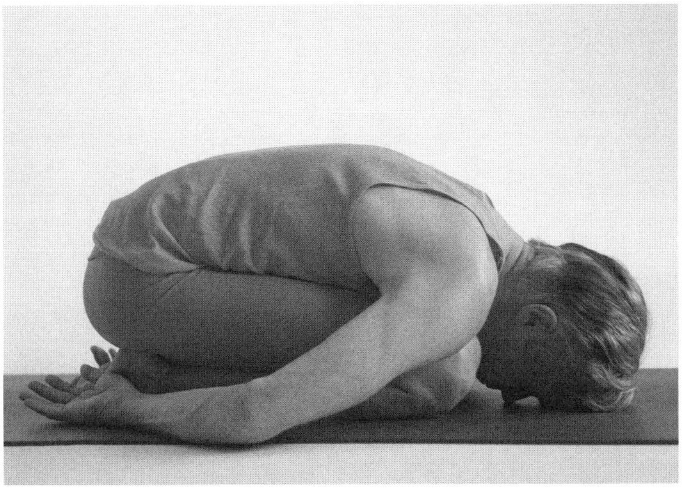

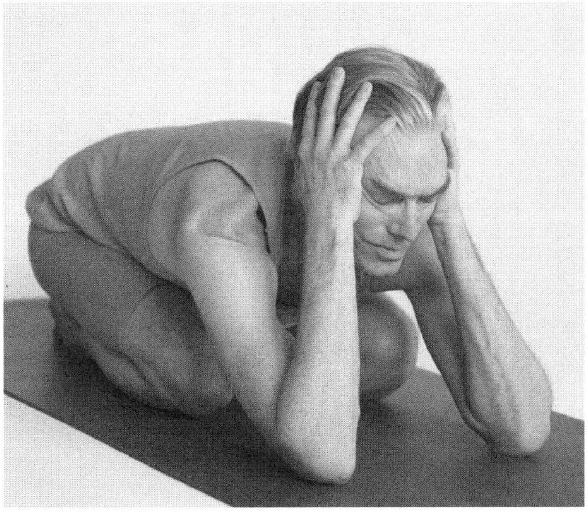

5. In this form, bring awareness to the spot on the head where you were in contact with the floor when in Śirṣāsana. Concentrate on the quality of the breath cycle, with a soft gaze toward the tip of the nose. Imagine that prāṇa and apāna have linked together deep in the navel and practice umbilical breathing to release all residue.

Padmāsana

Lotus Pose

If you cannot grab the toes, hold the forearms behind your back and whether holding toes or not lower the shoulders. If you cannot cross the legs into Padmāsana, sit in a comfortable cross-legged position.

1. Sit and tilt the pelvis slightly back as you bend the right knee and use the hands to draw the right foot back, bringing the heel toward the lower left side of the belly in the psoas button area. Be careful with the knee and do not force the placement of the foot if there is knee discomfort. Press the right knee toward the floor using the hip muscles.

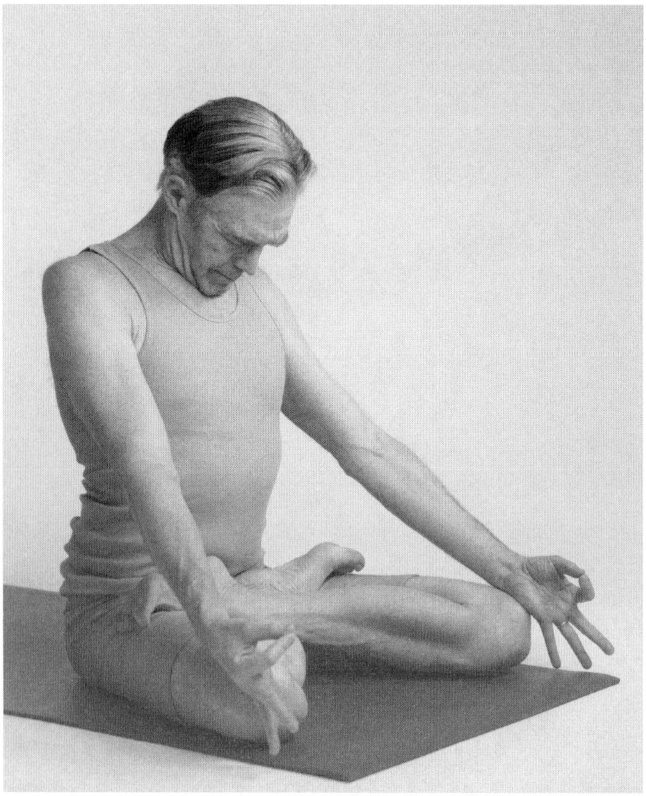

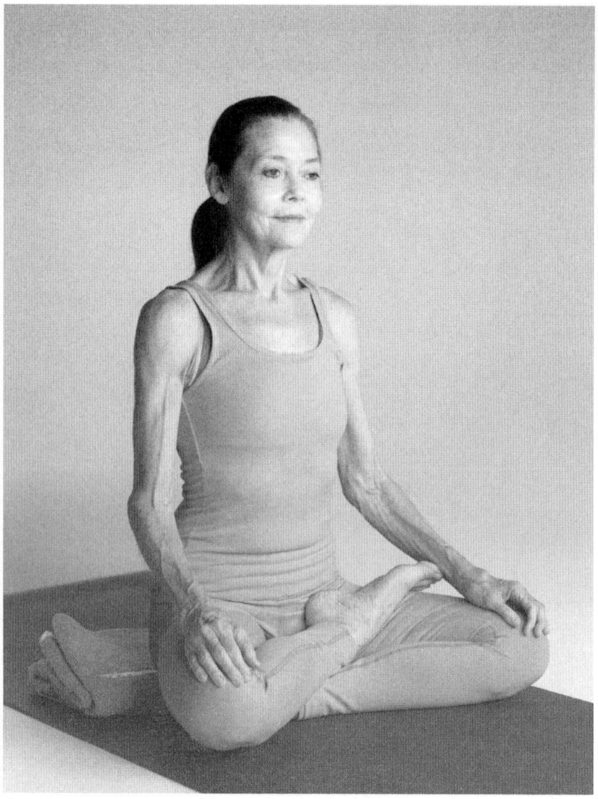

2. Bring the left foot in over the right toward the lower right side of the belly and the psoas button on that side. Once the feet are in place and the heels are touching or close to the lower abdomen, flex or turn the feet out so the ankles do not collapse and the bottoms of the feet begin to look out to the sides.
3. Fine-tune the pose so you have no discomfort in the knees or ankles. Do this first by softly turning the skin on the top of the ankle outward so the front of the tibia can rotate slightly toward the floor. Once in the pose, draw the knees closer together or keep some active outward rotation and flexion, pulling the knees slightly apart, to set the pose properly. Keeping the heels in contact with or close to the lower abdomen keeps the knees closed properly and comfortably. A good Padmāsana should naturally stimulate Uḍḍīyāna and Mūlabandhas. When beginning to learn the pose, do not grit your teeth in order to sit through any pain in the knees or ankles as if to train the body. This will only result in distracted mind and potential injury. Instead, you may try the posture for a few breaths only and then move into Half Padmāsana (below) for the remainder of your time in the pose.
4. Padmāsana should be used for meditation and prāṇāyāma only after it is very comfortable for a long period of sitting. Otherwise the knees or ankles could be damaged. You should be able to move the ankles and feet easily in a full, comfortable Padmāsana. If full Padmāsana is too difficult, you may sit in Half Padmāsana—with one foot up and the other leg folded under and supporting the Padmāsana leg and knee.

Baddha Padmāsana

Bound Lotus Pose

This is a meditative form of Padmāsana that encourages the kidney area to open and allows a deep meditative state to spontaneously arise upon the releasing of the binding of the arms.

1. Sit comfortably in Padmāsana, Half Padmāsana, or a simple cross-legged pose. Squeeze the knees closer together slightly more than you would if you were merely sitting. Both knees will eventually come to the floor when your flexibility has developed. However, do not sacrifice the symmetrical grounding of both sitting bones to bring the knees down.

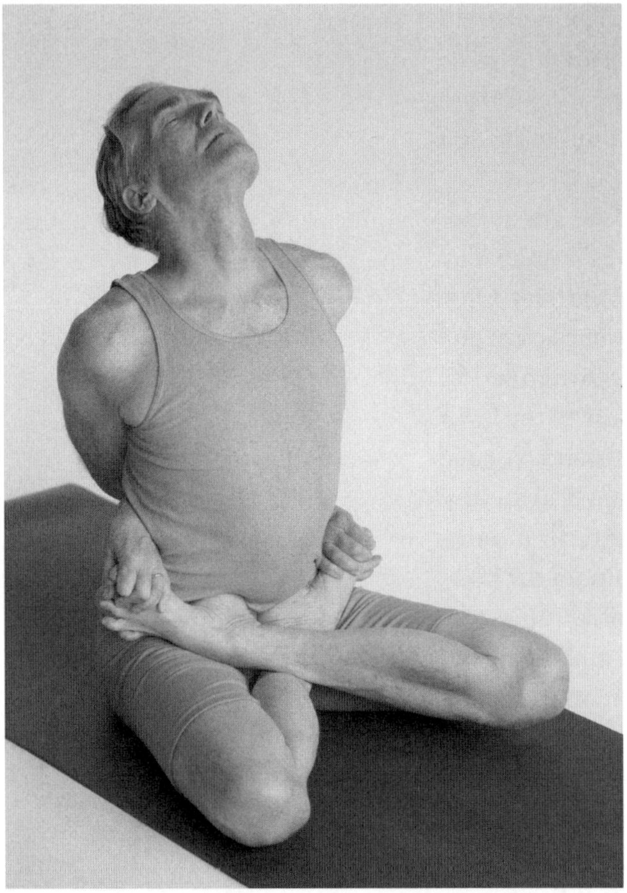

2. Exhaling, wrap the left arm behind the back and take hold of the left big toe. After an inhalation, exhale strongly again to wrap the right arm around the back to grab the right big toe. Balance the shoulders as best you can, considering the asymmetry.
3. At the top of an inhalation, lift up the front of the spine and place the chin down on the heart in Jālandhara Bandha position for a few breaths to establish the Uḍḍīyāna and Mūlabandhas activity under your belly.
4. Lift the head and gradually roll it back so the face is parallel to the ceiling, but do not collapse the cervical spine. Look down the nose, empty the palate, and carefully stretch the front of the neck holding this form for at least three breaths. Move immediately into Yoga Mudrā.

Yoga Mudrā

Seal of Yoga Pose

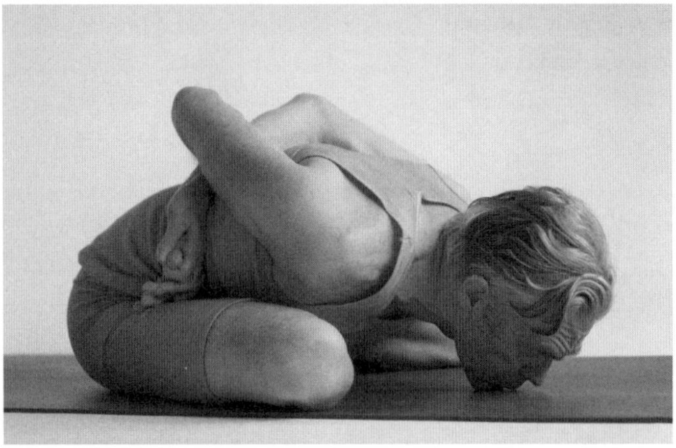

1. From the previous pose, keep the head up and back while looking down the nose. For a few breaths, release the palate as if to spread the front of the throat on the ceiling. Drop the front edges of the sitting bones deep into the earth using Mūlabandha. Imagine you are drinking the nectar of compassion from the root of the palate as each wave of inhalation crests.
2. Fold forward on an exhalation. Touch the chin to the floor, if possible. Otherwise, take the forehead down to the floor. You may place a block under the forehead if the head does not reach the floor.
3. Draw down the back surface of the body to bring the sitting bones toward the floor and to maintain the apānic base. Complete each exhalation while internally stretching the middle line from the heart through the crown of the head. You should feel the palate-perineum reflex in the full cycle of inhaling and exhaling.
4. If the chin is on the floor, gaze between the eyebrows and keep the front surface of the spine flowing upward in contrast to the strong

downward sealing action of the sitting bones dropping and the PC muscle toning. If your forehead is on the floor or a block, softly gaze down the nose. Stay here for ten breaths and after a full exhalation then inhale to sit up straight. Release the hands to move into Padmāsana with Ujjāyī Prāṇāyāma for at least ten breaths.

Padmāsana with Ujjāyī Prāṇāyāma

Lotus Pose Variation

This straight-arm form is held in response to the powerful residue left in the arms and shoulders from the previous pose. If you sit longer, the straightness of the arms and the exaggeration of the Jñāna Mudrā can be relaxed.

1. Sit in Padmāsana (or with your legs crossed). Place the hands in *Jñāna Mudrā* (Seal of Wisdom) with index fingers and thumbs touching and the middle, ring, and little fingers extended and awake. Straighten the arms and place the hands on the knees turning the palms up and spreading the three outer fingers on each hand.
2. Lift and widen the fronts of the armpits as you pull down and widen the backs of the armpits. The arms should be lightly stiffened at this point. This helps to set the shoulders down into the correct position. The whole front of the spine seems to rise.
3. Draw the lower belly, 2 inches below the navel, back and tone the perineum as its center lifts.
4. Drop the chin to rest it on the upper edge of the sternum, as the collarbones lift and widen. This is Jālandhara Bandha position. It is similar in form to a swan resting its head on its chest. If your chin does not easily rest on the sternum, use a folded washcloth for support, placing it on the sternum and resting the chin on the cloth.
5. Practice ten rounds of full Ujjāyī Prāṇāyāma in this position. Gaze softly down toward the tip of the nose, and use only natural, pleasant retentions of a few seconds at the ends of the breaths. Listen carefully to the quality

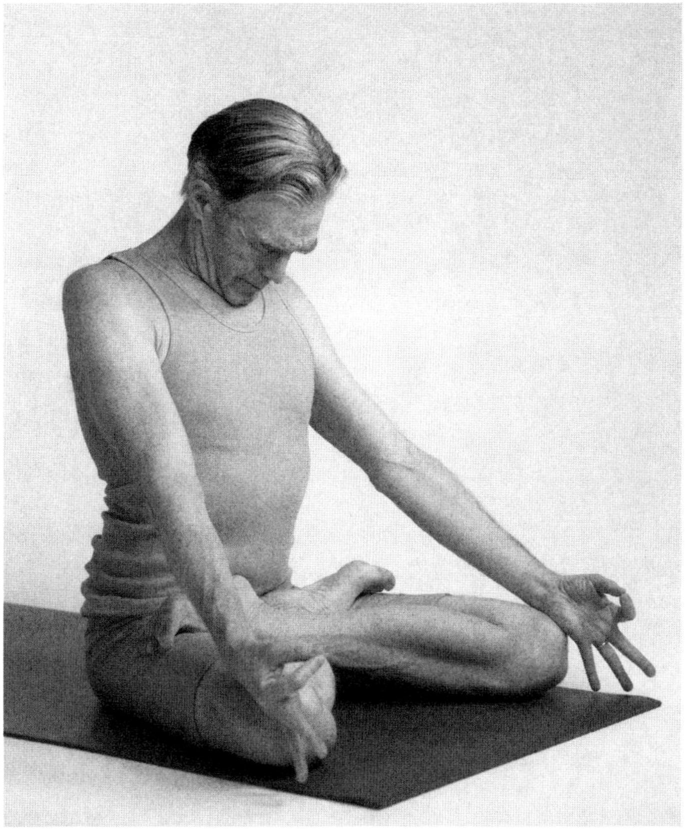

of the breath. Such breathing is extraordinarily pleasant. Do not strain! This pose may be practiced on its own when practicing a gentle or moon day practice, or as part of the finishing sequence in a more active practice, in which case move directly into Utplutiḥ after completing the final exhale of this pose.

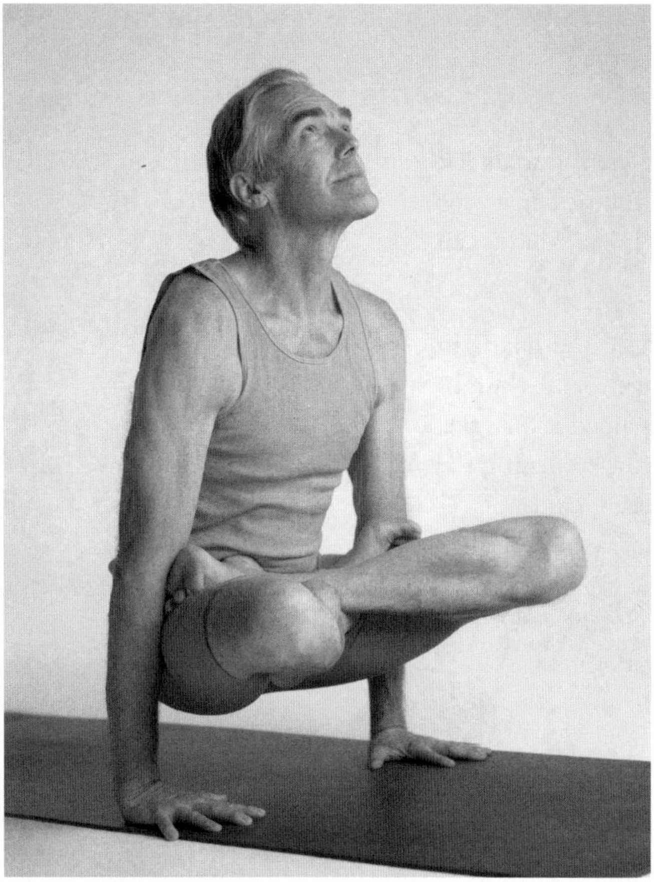

Utplutiḥ

Uprooting Pose

1. Still in Padmāsana, place the hands on the ground next to the hips and lift the knees off the floor. On an inhalation, lift the buttocks off the floor for ten breaths. Turn the face up toward the sky, but gaze down along the line of the nose to release the back of the neck. It might take some practice to stay for ten breaths or even to lift at all. That is not a problem. The attempt to lift will contract the necessary muscles and produce the desired result, eventually leading to the ability to lift.
2. While lifting, keep the hands evenly rooted into the floor, the jaw released, and the tongue soft. Maintain a sense of the shoulder blades flowing down the back as you lift.
3. After completing the pose, exhale as you swing the legs, still in Padmāsana, back through the arms and unwrap them quickly to land in full Catvāri position. Or lower down to the floor on an exhalation and unwrap the legs into a simple cross-legged position. Inhale to lift up, and exhale as you swing back through into Catvāri and a Half Vinyāsa.

Śavāsana

Corpse Pose

Sri K. Pattabhi Jois used to say that Śavāsana is the most difficult pose. Many students thought he was kidding, but once you've been practicing for a while, this sentiment rings true. The essence of the pose is to embody complete balance in all directions but also to find equanimity between the state of being completely alert and that of being absolutely relaxed. In more advanced Śavāsana, one does not fall asleep, but a calm and removed, yet alert, open feeling pervades the body and mind. In Śavāsana, all of the residue within the body, mind, and nervous system has time to be assimilated. Depending on the intensity of the particular practice and nonpractice circumstances, it may be necessary to hold Śavāsana for anywhere from ten to twenty minutes until everything has settled and has been integrated properly

1. Lie on the back as if in Samasthitiḥ. Lightly stiffen the arms and legs. Roll the shoulders back and down to the floor. Draw the lower tips of the shoulder blades up into the body as the kidney area falls back and widens. Lightly press the back of the head into the floor with the chin a hair's breadth lower than the eyebrows.
2. Gaze, with the eyes closed, down the line of the nose. Feel the seed of a smile to "empty" the palate, as the breathing pulls the Mūlabandha like a steady flame.
3. This is the formal Tāḍāgī Mudrā pose and should be practiced before dissolving into full Śavāsana. Carefully arrange the body so it is symmetrical. Remain for one to five minutes in this position, breathing smoothly. Allow the breath to fine-tune the subtle alignment of the body.
4. Now relax. Let the breath go. Leave everything alone and as it is in the present moment. The mouth releases. The hands and feet release. The eyes soften. The heart floats up, bright and empty. The palms of the hands and the soles of the feet soften. Let the ears relax into listening. The tongue is silent, letting everything be, just as it is.

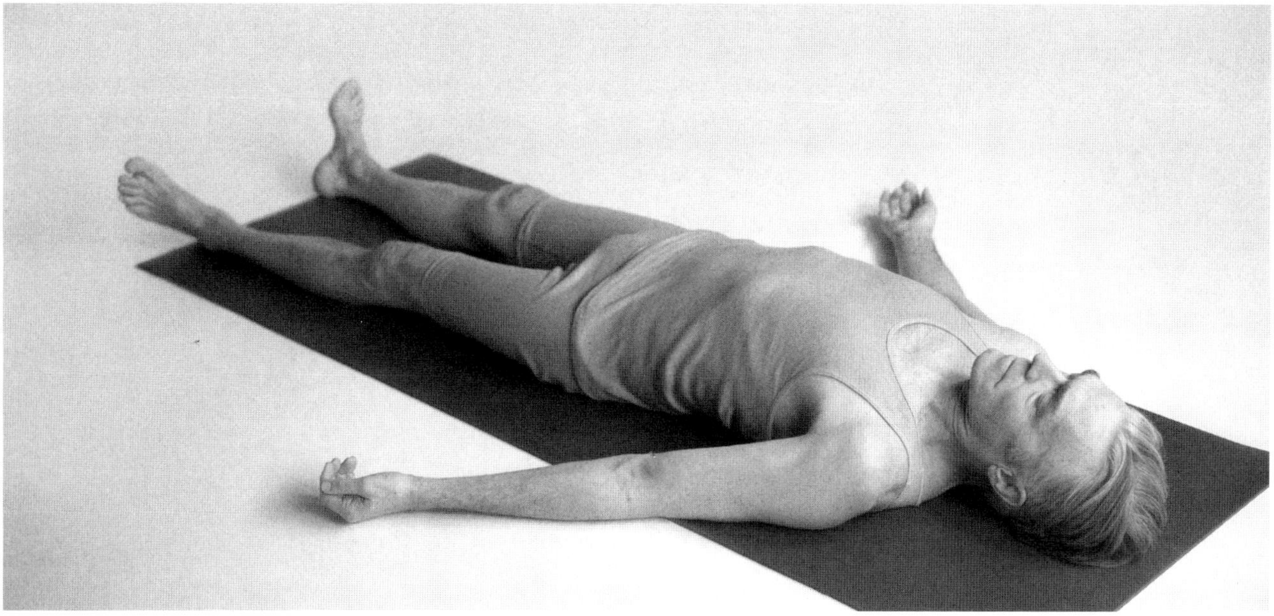

Acknowledgments

We would like to thank all those wonderful people who have inspired us and who have contributed to the production of this book. First, we thank our son Gabe who drew the concise anatomical drawings and then the beautiful illustrations that capture the feeling of the subtle internal practices described in the text.

We appreciate the hard work, enthusiasm, and remarkable patience of Sara Bercholz of Shambhala Publications in getting this project to finally take shape. Other members of the closely knit Shambhala team have also played instrumental roles in bringing the book to life. Beth Frankl, our editor, has given support, insight, and encouragement at just the right moments along the way. Julia Gaviria has worked tirelessly with the details of editing when the two of us have gone cross-eyed looking for correct spelling, diacritical markings, and general form. We have benefited from the fine aesthetic of Shambhala's art department and those who worked carefully with us, Lora Zorian, Hazel Bercholz, Jim Zaccaria, and the book's designer, Steve Dyer. The project literally took form because of our photographer Robert Muratore, whose work with light and composition was so quick, brilliant, and spontaneous that even a couple of aging yoga teachers found the three-day photo shoot easy.

We also thank the worldwide Aṣṭāṅga Vinyāsa yoga community—our friends who are remarkably kind and humorous, being so grounded in themselves and their tradition that the synthesizing of the many traditions and views presented here is a natural process. We salute the broader background of our lineage in the brilliant work of Sri T. Krishnamacarya, B. K. S. Iyengar, T. K. V. Deshikachar, and so many others. And we are continually thankful to our teachers and friends in many manifestations of the Buddhist tradition who keep us sharp by holding up a brilliant mirror to the many practices and philosophies of the yoga tradition.

APPENDIX I

Ancient Wisdom, Contemporary Circumstances

We find ourselves in this day, this time, this very moment. If we're lucky, we awaken to the circumstance—the beauty of what is before us, an astonishing, open kaleidoscope of interconnected patterns of perception. Waking up may happen by chance, or we may decide it's worth the time and effort to lay the groundwork for it to occur. Through yoga, meditation, and prāṇāyāma, we practice with open hearts and inquisitive minds, and occasionally there's a moment of clarity or insight as we touch the foundation (primordial immediacy) of breath, dṛṣṭi, bandha, and mudrā. Sometimes it all falls into place easily, like a puzzle just waiting to be solved; at other times, the pieces of form, movement, mind, and attention seem to be parts of disparate stories jumbled together. Yet we still return to whatever arises and the practice with a strand of faith that there's more to it all than we will ever know. We understand that all we really *must* do is show up.

When things are going your way, it's simple to show up, and that's good. But the test is when things aren't going so well. When life throws the unexpected, complex, or difficult circumstance in your path, what then? Can you practice if you have only limited time, if everything is in flux, if habitual patterns of mind and body seem to have taken over your entire existence, or if you're ill or injured? Of course! In fact it's in those times of complexity, transition, difficulty, and doubt when practice is paramount.

Remember that the mind is always looking for an excuse not to practice, because the more we practice, the more the mind itself (our ego structure) starts to dissolve. You tell yourself, "I'm too stiff / too sore / too tired." You think the practice just isn't for you, it's too difficult, you can't practice because you're an emotional wreck, you're too old or too sick. And when you've proven each of these to be untrue, you come up with more excuses because somehow the easiest solution for the wandering mind is not to practice. That makes sense. The mind's full-time job is to take in information, organize the data, make decisions, construct theories of "you" and guide you smoothly through time. For a responsible, intelligent mind, the most disastrous prospect is to give up its identity—to dissolve. The same rational mind that gets dragged into a practice eventually begins to notice that *after* practicing, there's a feeling of safety, happiness, clarity, and a lack of tension. During practice, the mind forms a relationship with its complementary partner, the breath, and in this context, it gradually softens to trust process rather than conceptualization. Eventually, you see that the mind's razor-sharp intellect and ability to discriminate are necessary, but when you grasp ideas too tightly, these very same ideas are a hindrance.

These appendices offer support material for a daily practice. The traditional sequences for Primary and Intermediate Series, the names of dṛṣṭi points, Sanskrit counting, and alternative practices for when you run into complex situations that might provide the out your mind is looking for to abandon the practice.

APPENDIX 2

Invocation

vande gurūṇāṁ caraṇāravinde
sandarśita svātma sukhāva bodhe
niḥśreyase jāṅgalikāyamāne
saṁsāra hālāhala moha śāntyai

I bow to the two lotus feet of the [plurality of] gurus, which awaken insight into the happiness of pure being, which are the complete absorption into joy, the jungle physician, eliminating the delusion caused by the poison of samsāra [conditioned existence].

ābāhu puruṣākāraṁ
śankha cakrāsi dhāriṇam
sahasra śirasaṁ śvetaṁ
praṇamāmi patañjalim

I prostrate before the sage Patañjali who has thousands of radiant white heads [as the divine serpent, Ananta] and who has, as far as his arms, assumed a human form, holding a conch shell [divine sound], a wheel [a discus of light or time], and a sword [discrimination].

Oṁ

APPENDIX 3

Sequencing

Primary and Intermediate Series

When practicing within the Aṣṭāṅga Vinyāsa tradition, we begin the practice with five Sūrya Namaskāra As and Bs, followed by the standing sequence. Sometimes the standing sequence is shortened to allow time for the more difficult poses in some of the advanced series. After the standing sequence, poses in a particular series (Primary, Intermediate, and so on) are practiced. Then the finishing poses are performed to absorb the practice fully.

When learning the Primary Series, poses are added one at a time, tacked on to the end of one's usual practice. When moving into a new series, poses are added to the end of the practice until the next series is complete. Then the two series can be practiced independently of one another. Once the Intermediate Series is learned, one should still maintain the skills of the Primary Series. If one knows all six of the basic series, then all of them should still be practiced on a rotational basis. Pattabhi Jois would even divide the series into segments and combine different segments to create special skills within the student.

One should stay with the series as a method of discovering the inner principles (forms) upon which the series have been constructed. These inner principles carry the value, interest, and purpose of the practice.

INTRODUCTORY SEQUENCE

Samasthitiḥ
Sūrya Namaskāra A and B (see Appendix 5)

STANDING SEQUENCE

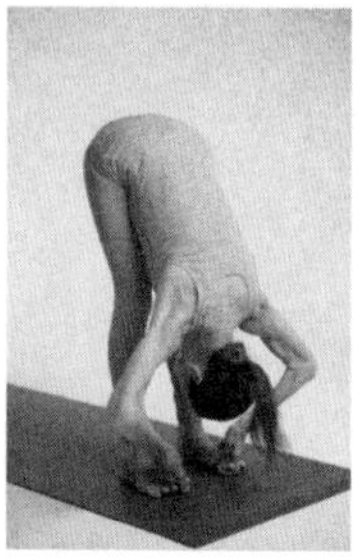
Pādāṅguṣṭh-āsana

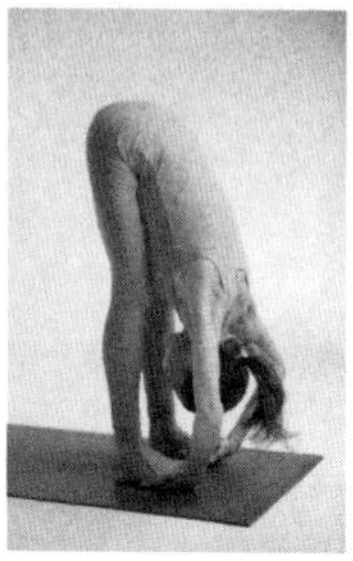
Pādahast-āsana

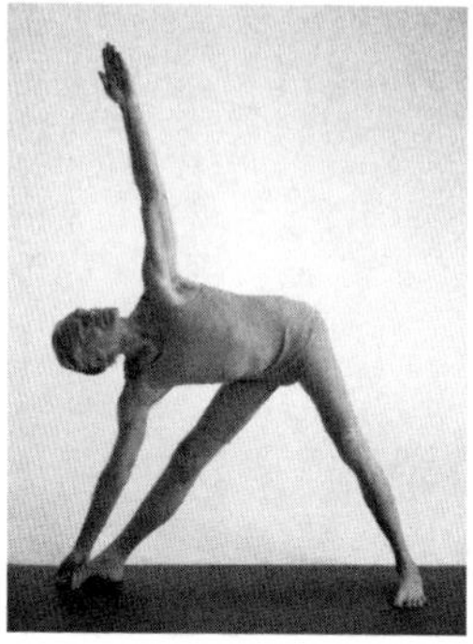
Trikoṇāsana

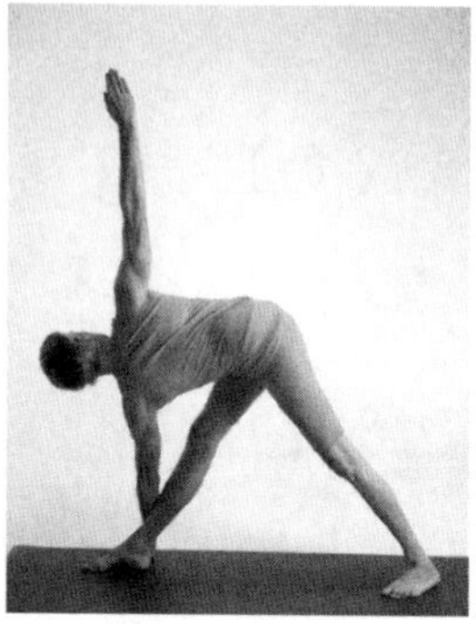
Parivṛtta Trikoṇāsana

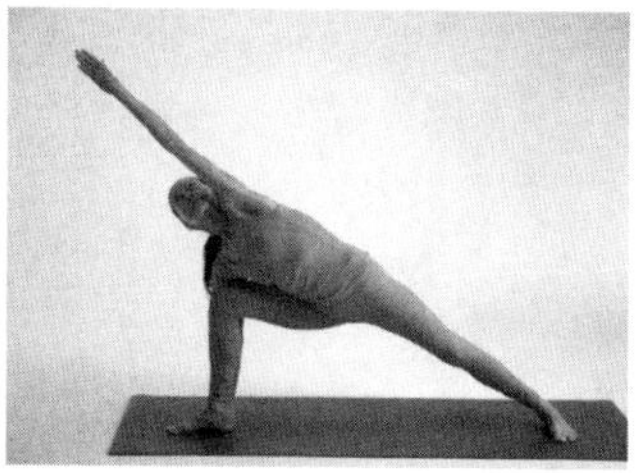
Pārśvakoṇāsana

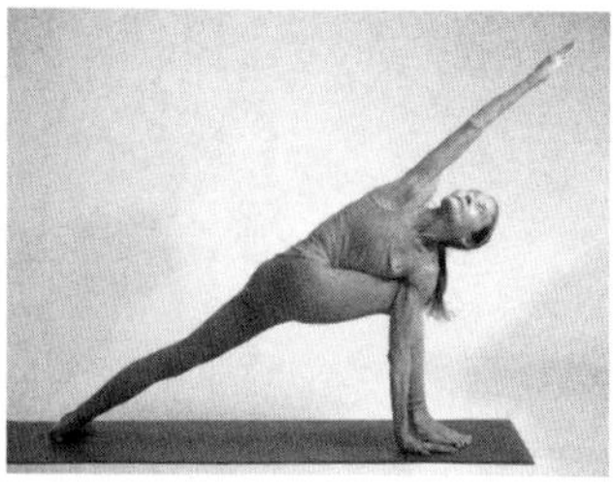
Parivṛtta Pārśvakoṇāsana

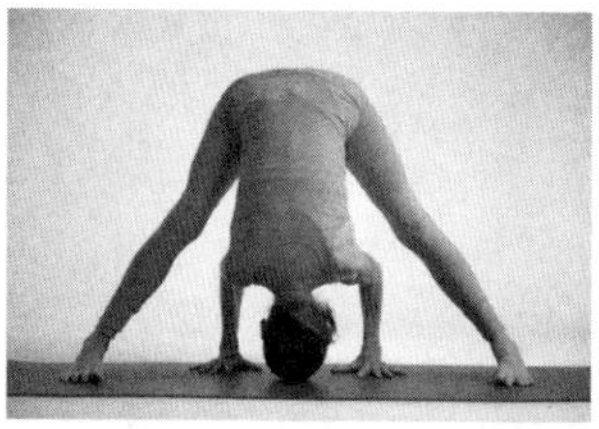
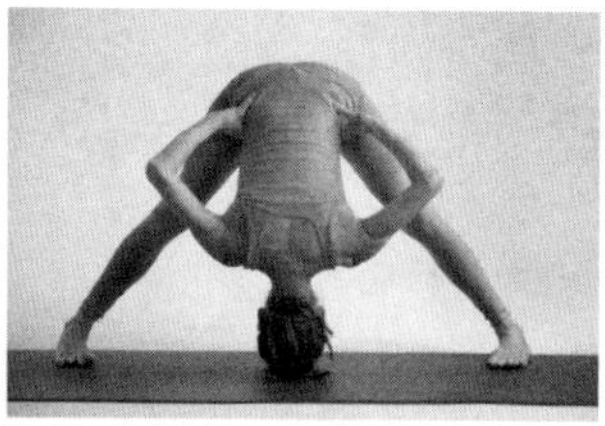
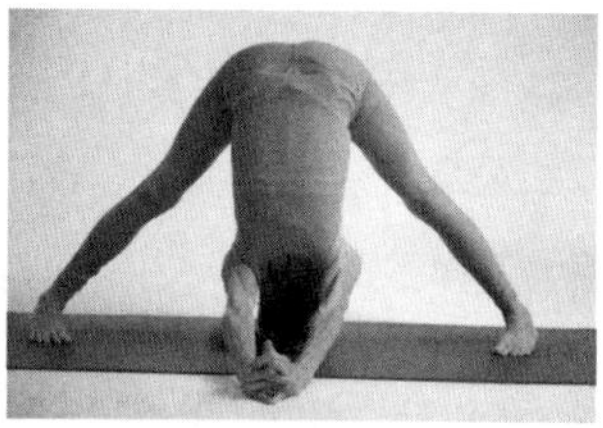
Prasārita Pādottānāsana A, B, and C

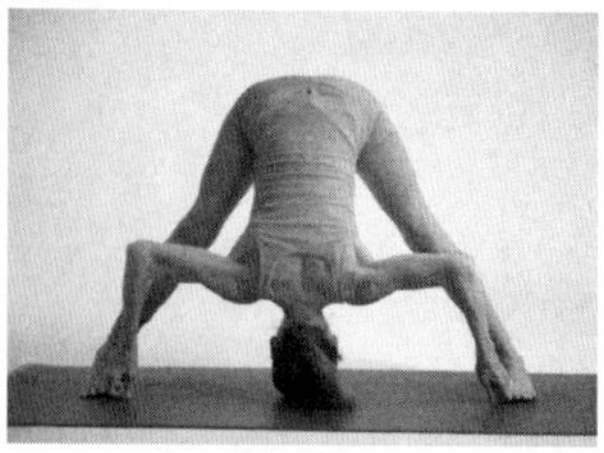
Prasārita Pādottānāsana D

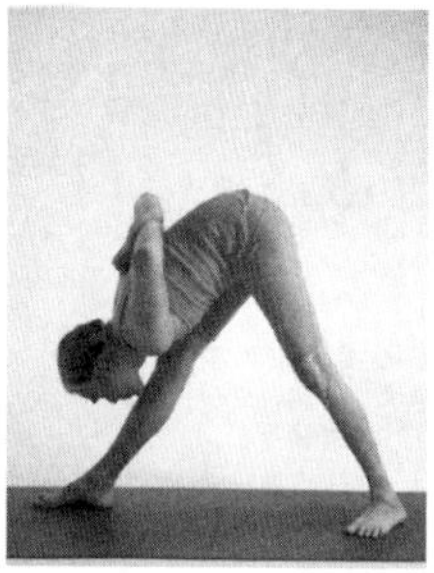
Pārśvottānāsana

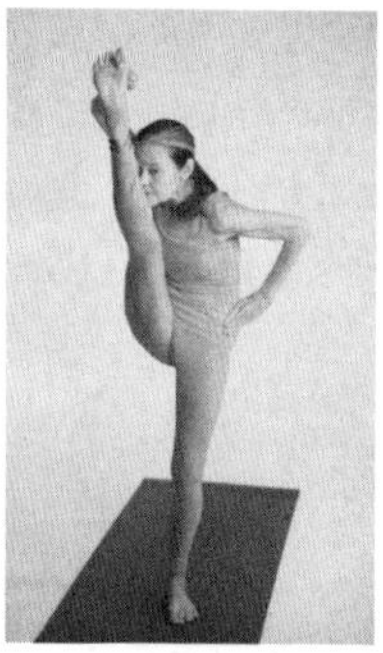
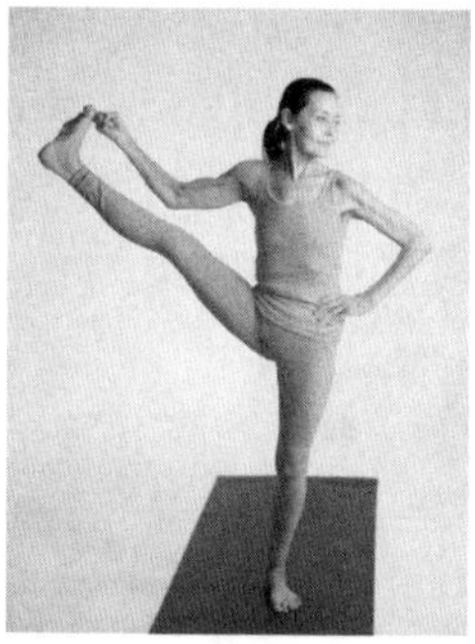
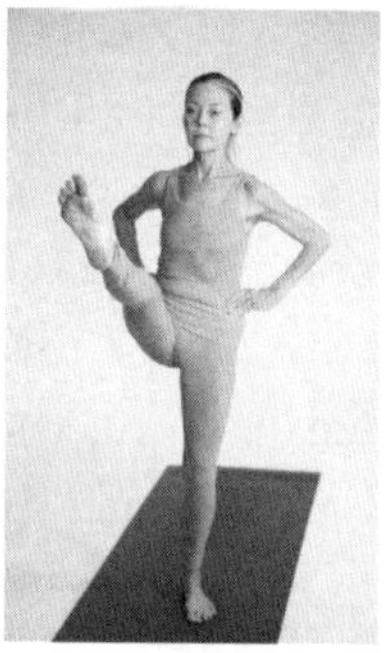
Utthita Hasta Pādāṅguṣṭhāsana

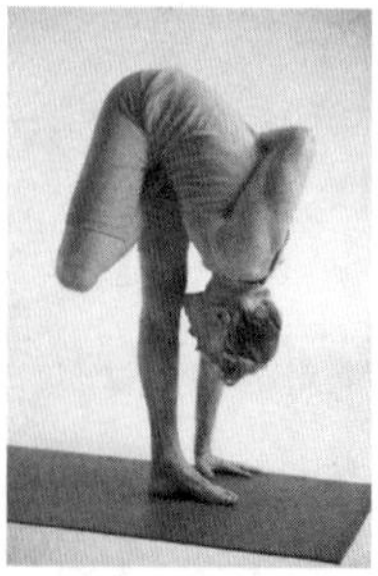
Ardha Baddha Padmottānāsana

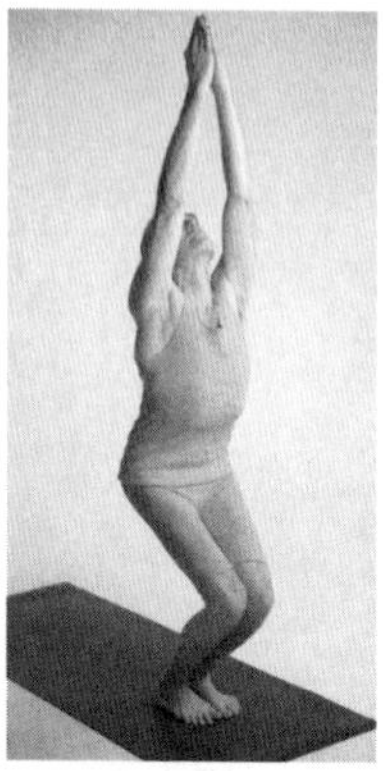
Utkaṭāsana

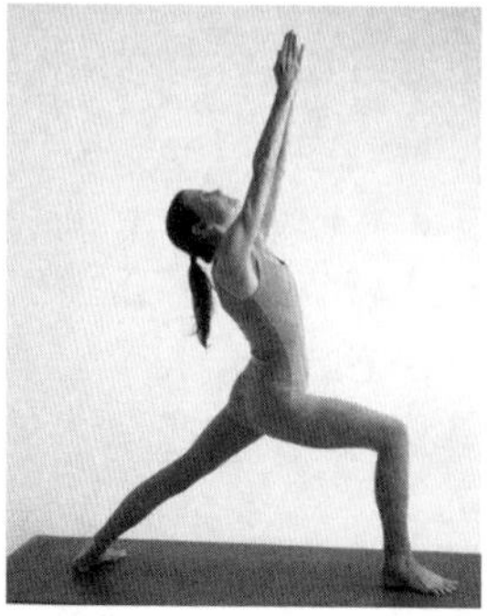
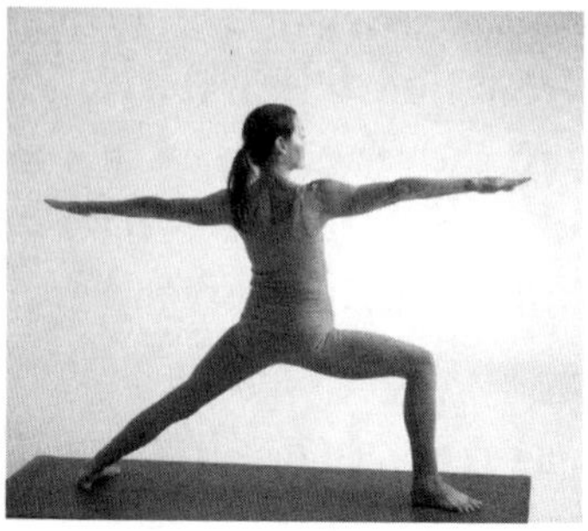
Vīrabhadrāsana A and B

BACKBENDS AND FINISHING POSES

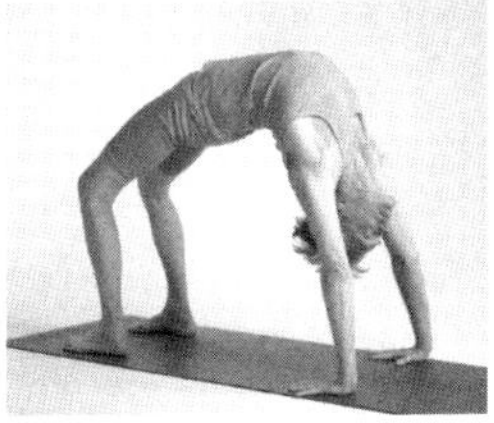

Ūrdhvā Dhanurāsana

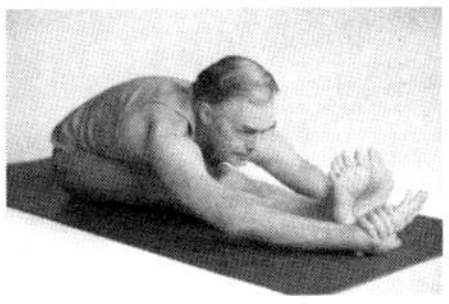

Paśchimottānāsana

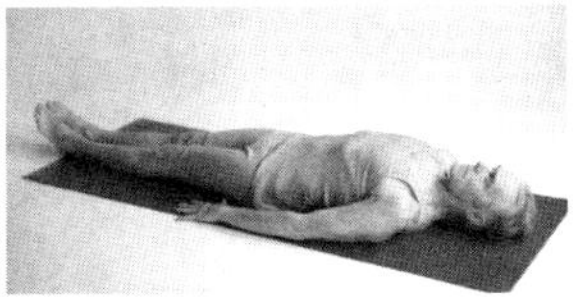

Tāḍāgī Mudrā

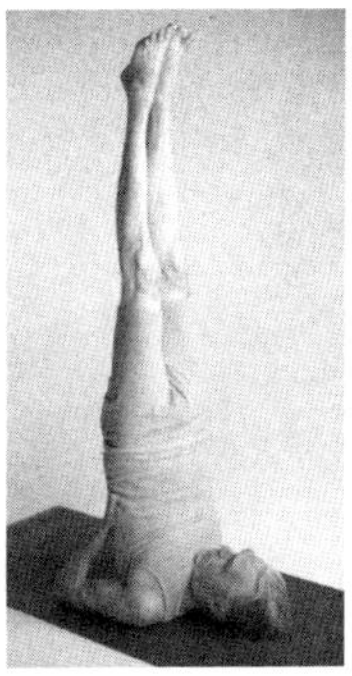

Sarvāṅgāsana

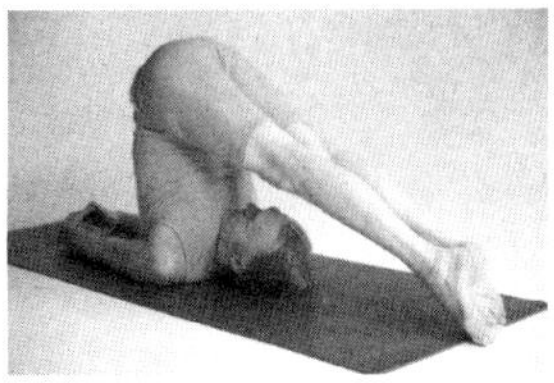

Halāsana

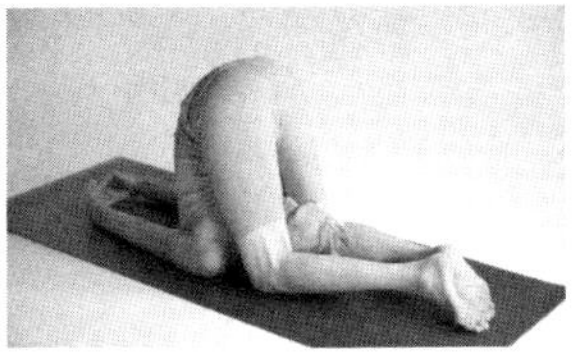

Karṇa Pīḍāsana

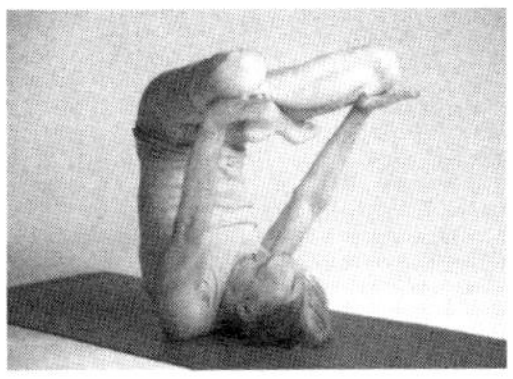

Ūrdhvā Padmāsana

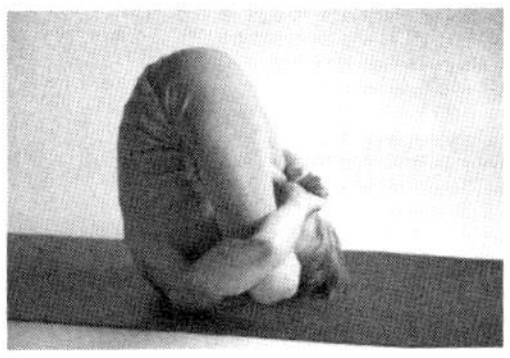

Piṇḍāsana

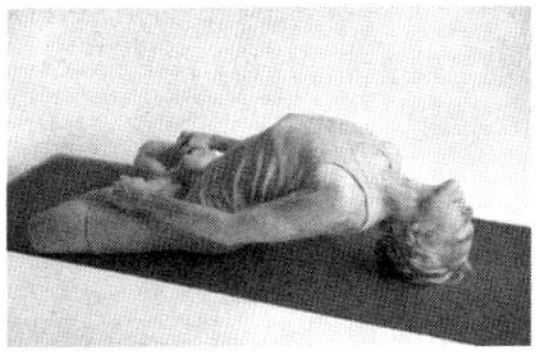

Matsyāsana

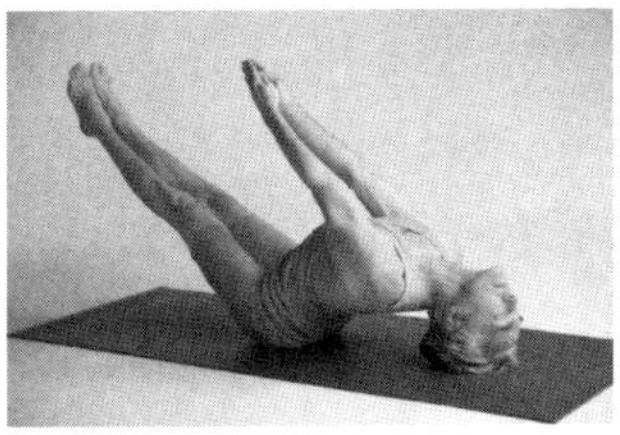

Uttāna Pādāsana

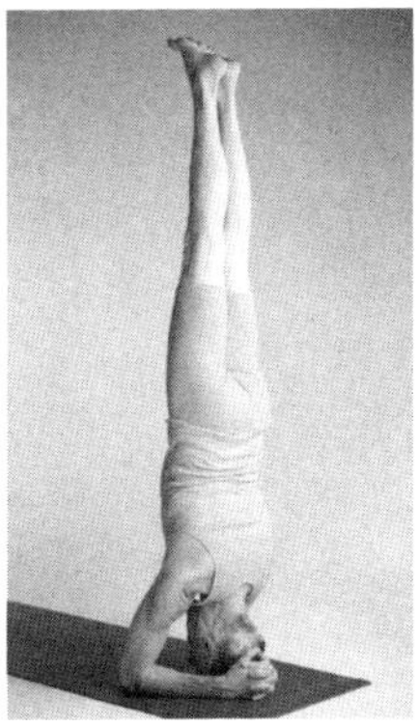

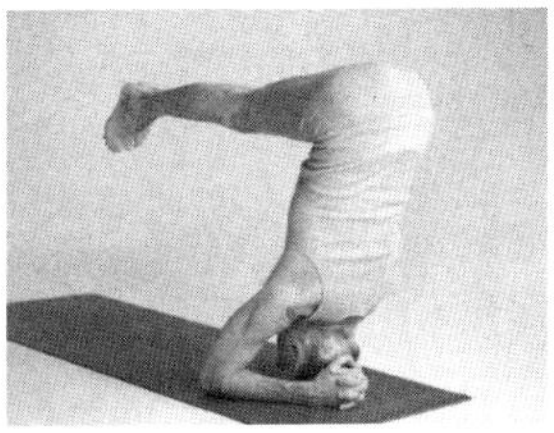

Śīrṣāsana

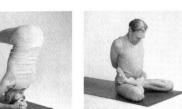

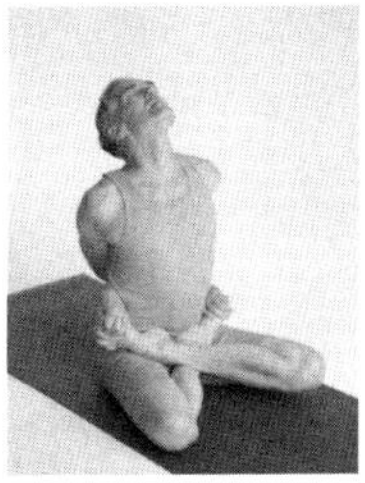

Baddha Padmāsana

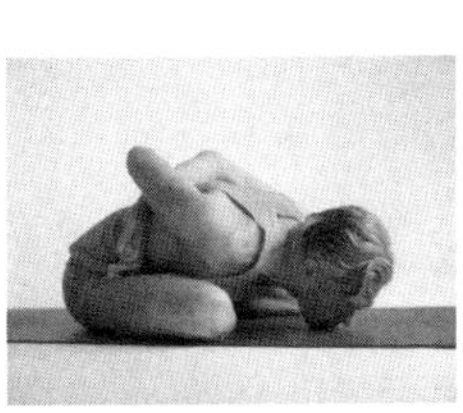

Yoga Mudrā

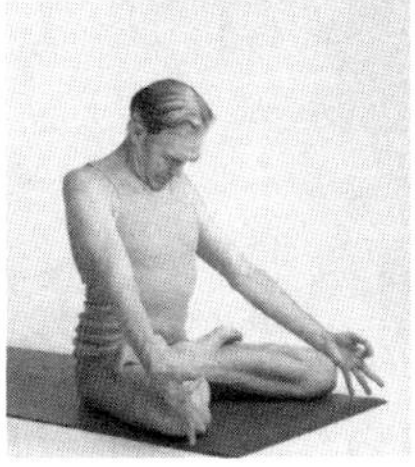

Padmāsana

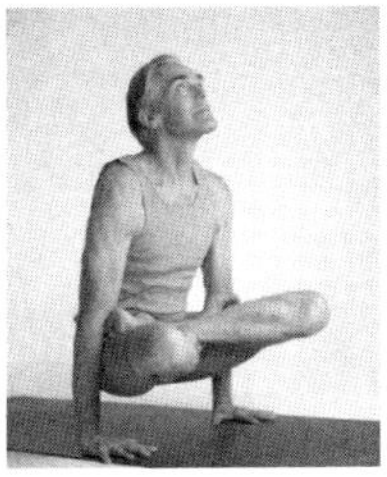

Utplutiḥ

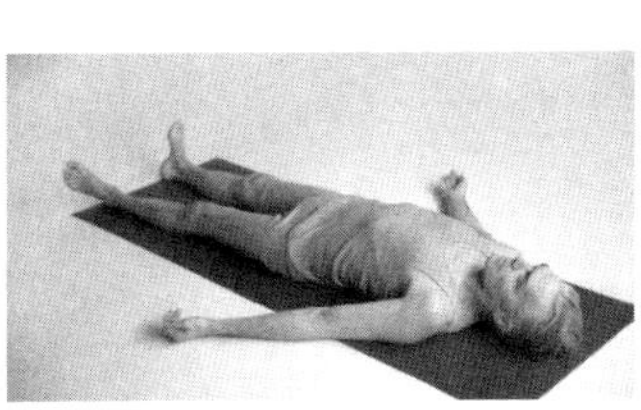

Śavāsana

PRIMARY SERIES

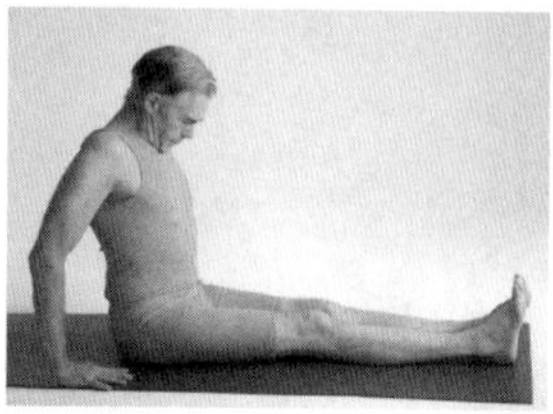
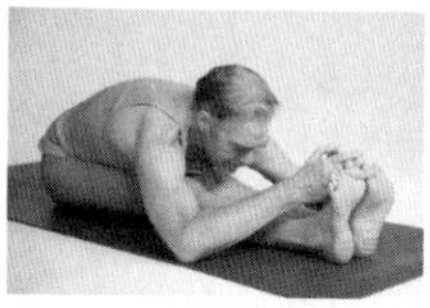
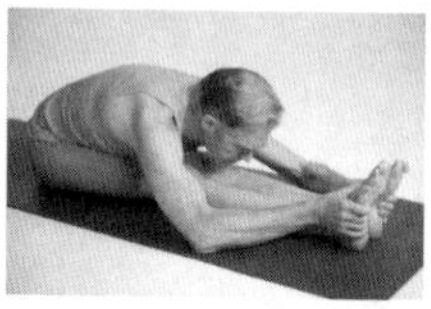
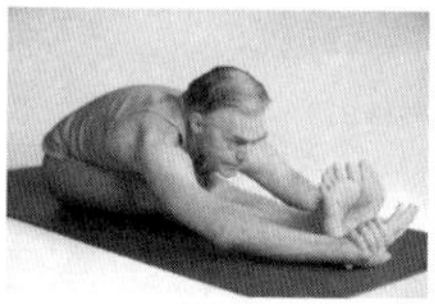
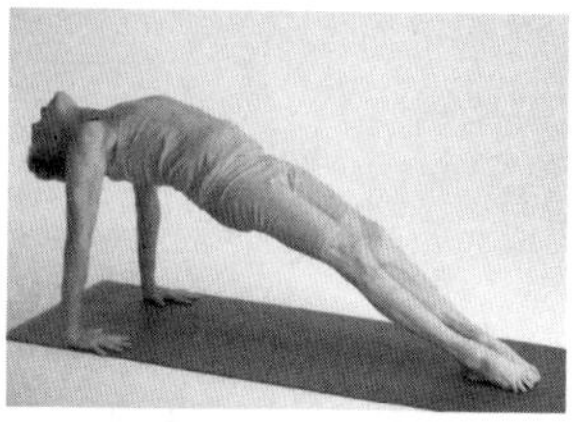

Daṇḍāsana

Paśchimottānāsana A, B, and C

Pūrvottanāsana

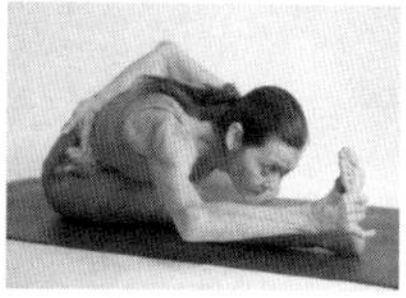
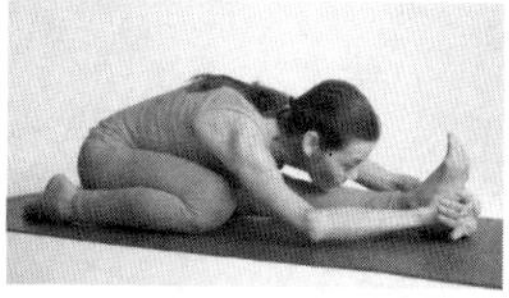
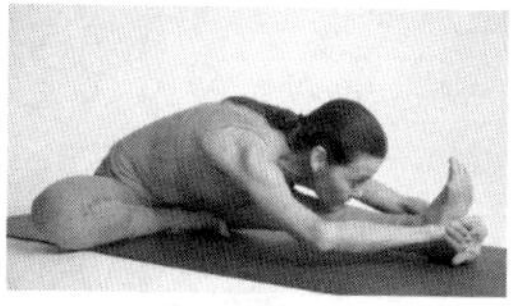
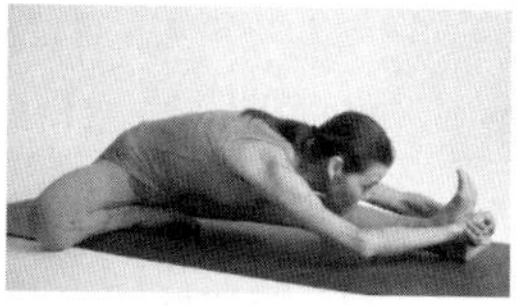
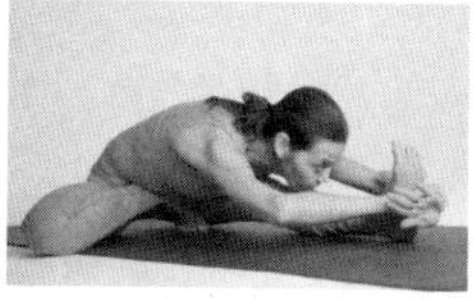

Ardha Baddha Padma Paśchi-mottānāsana

Tiryang Mukha Eka Pāda Paśchimottān-āsana

Jānuśīrṣāsana A, B, and C

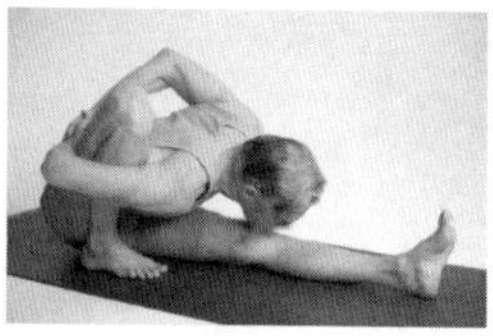
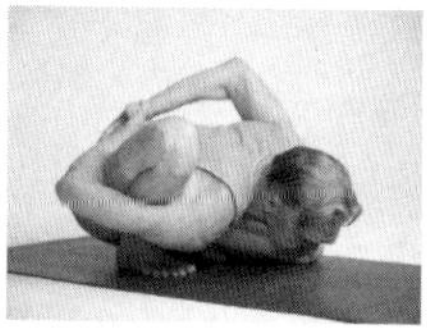
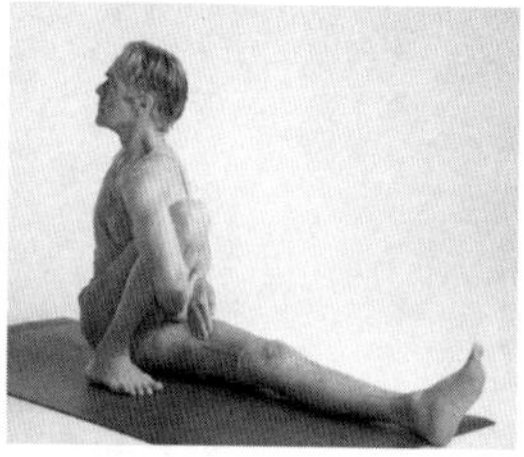
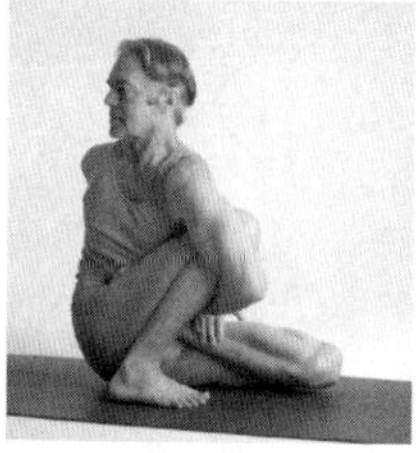
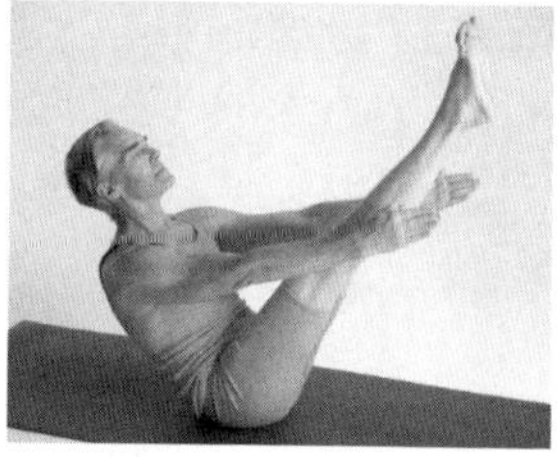

Marīchyāsana A, B, C, and D

Nāvāsana

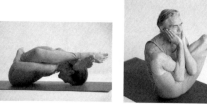

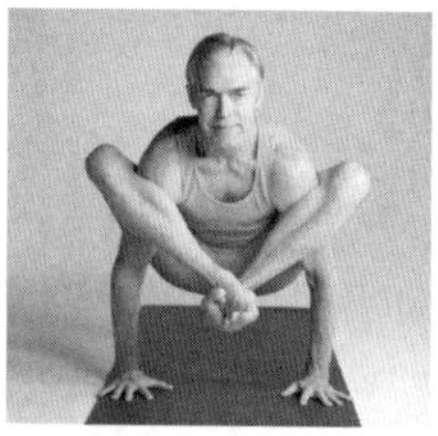
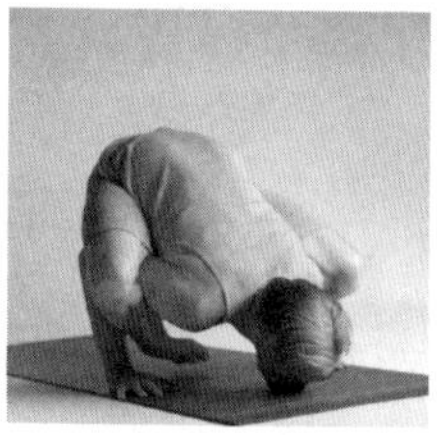
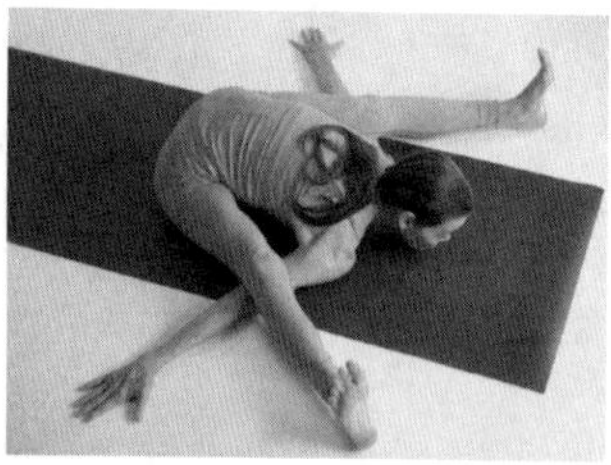
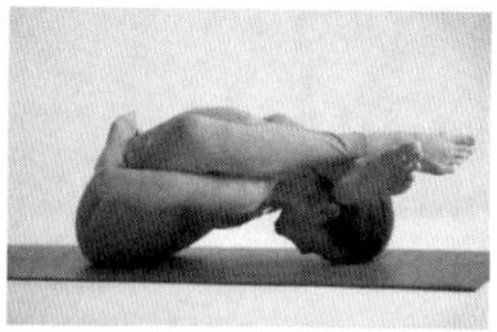

Bhujapīḍāsana

Kūrmāsana

Supta Kūrmāsana

Garbha Piṇḍāsana A

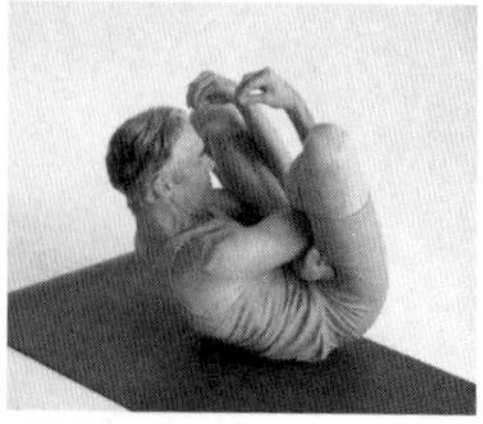
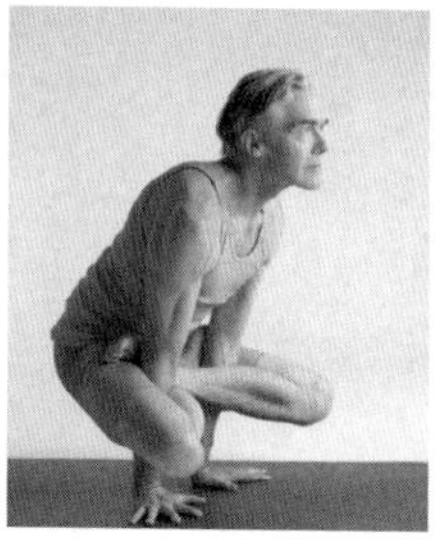
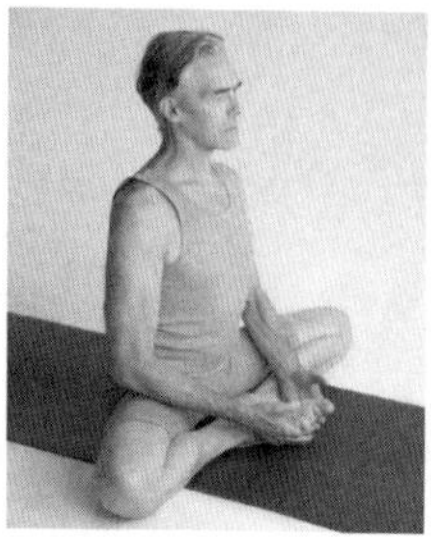
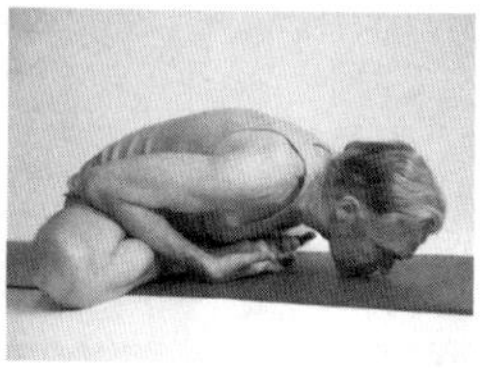
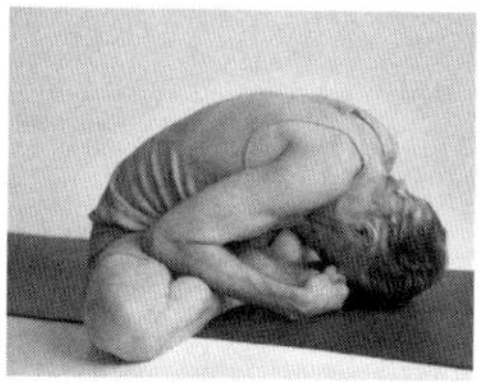

Garbha Piṇḍāsana B

Kukkuṭāsana

Baddha Koṇāsana A, B, and C

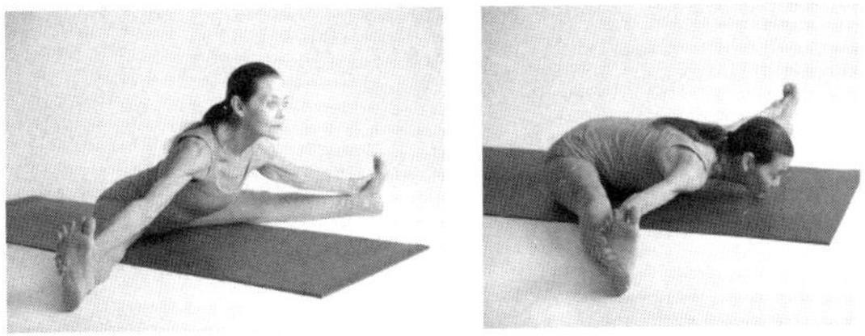

Upaviṣṭha Koṇāsana

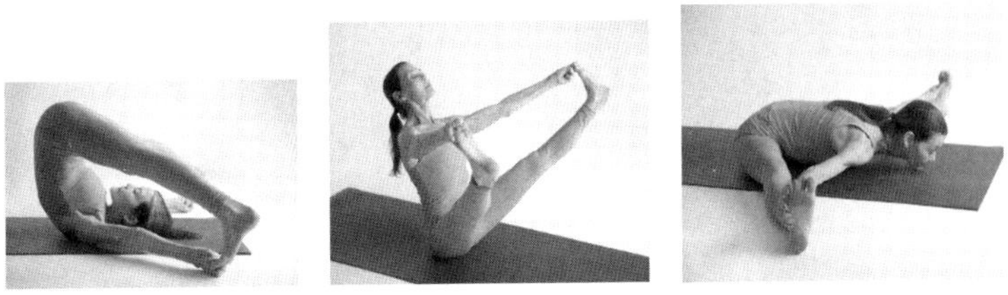

Supta Koṇāsana

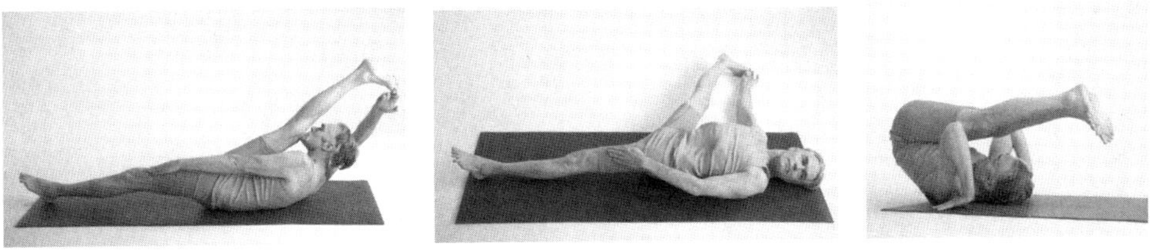

Supta Hasta Pādāṅguṣṭhāsana

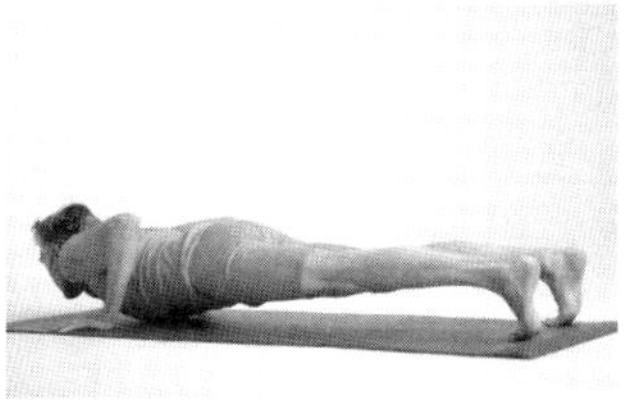

Cakrāsana

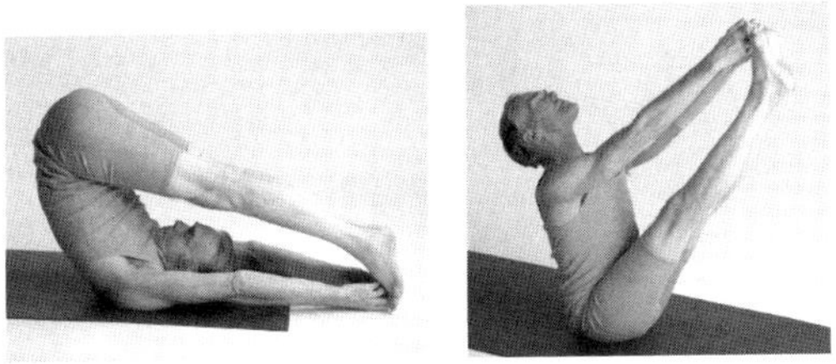

Ubhaya Pādāṅguṣṭhāsana

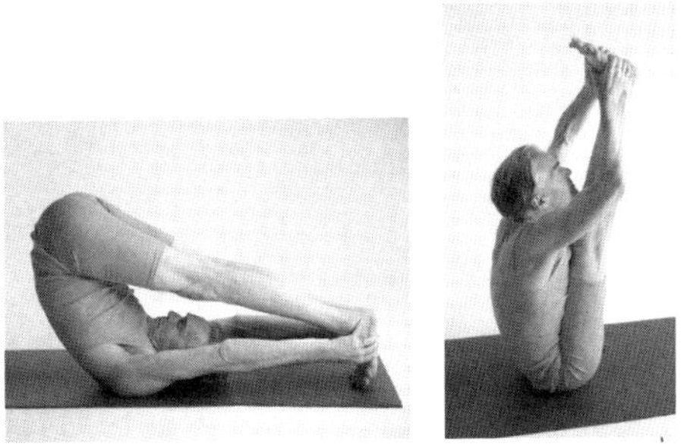

Ūrdhvā Mukha Paśchimottānāsana

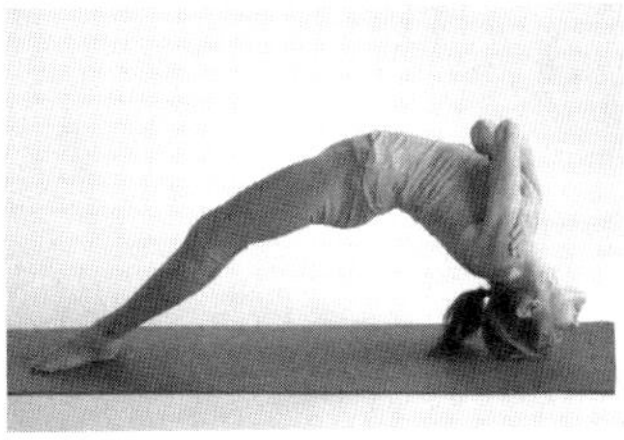

Setu Bandhāsana

INTERMEDIATE SERIES

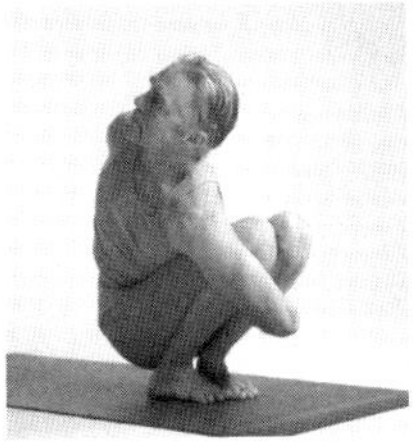

Paśāsana

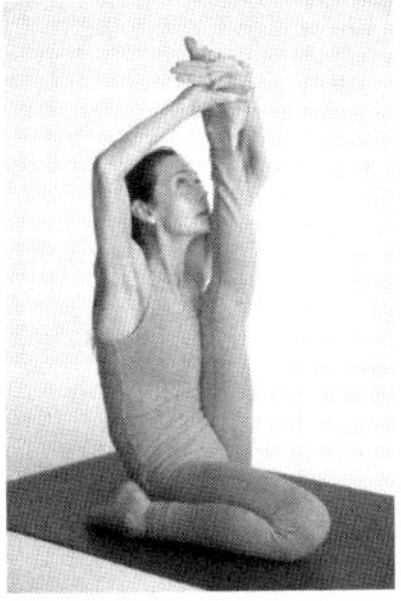

Krauñchāsana

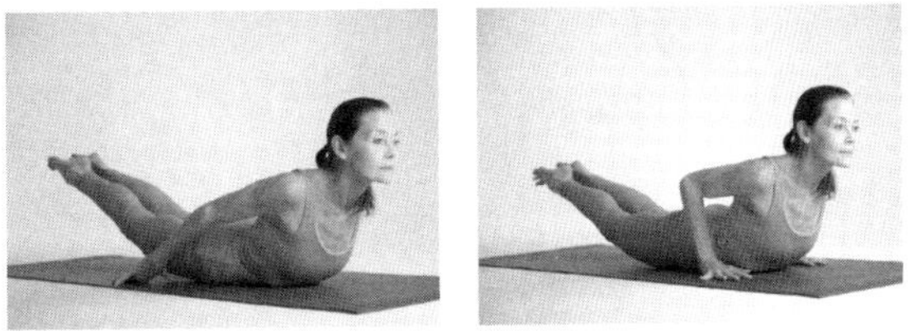

Śalabhāsana

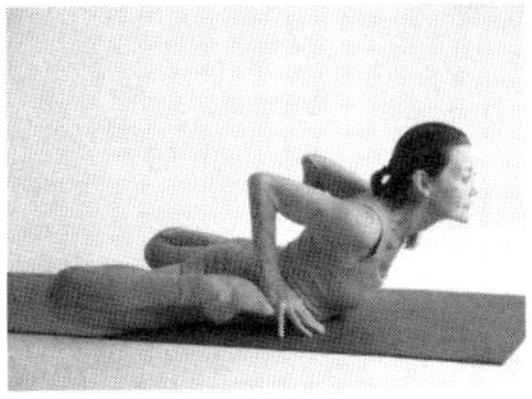

Bhekāsana

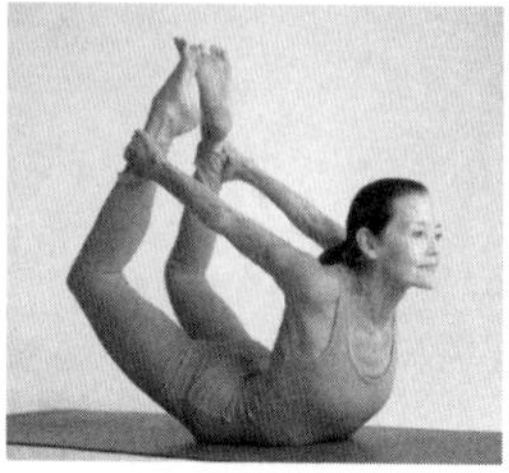

Dhanurāsana

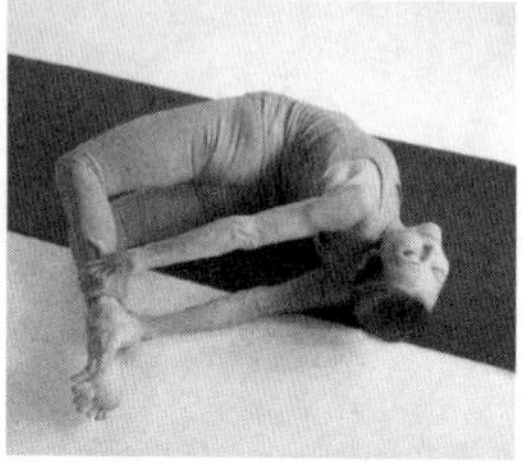

Pārśva Dhanurāsana

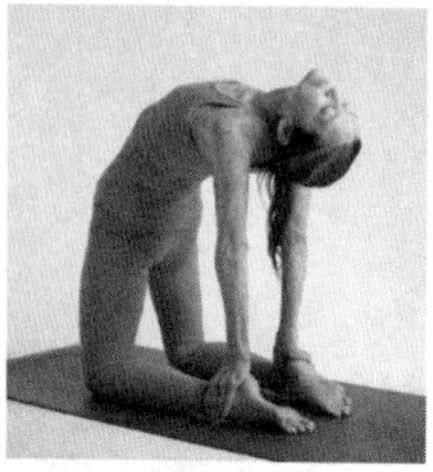

Ūṣṭrāsana

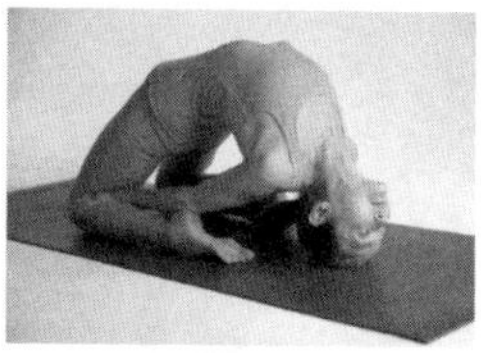

Laghu Vajrāsana

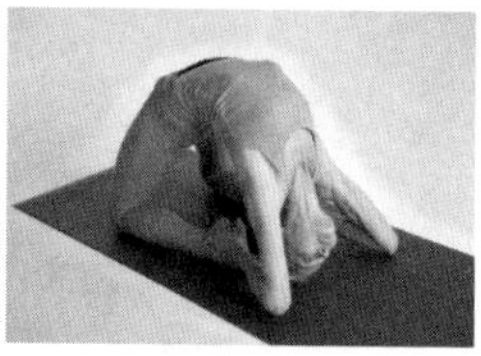

Kapotāsana A

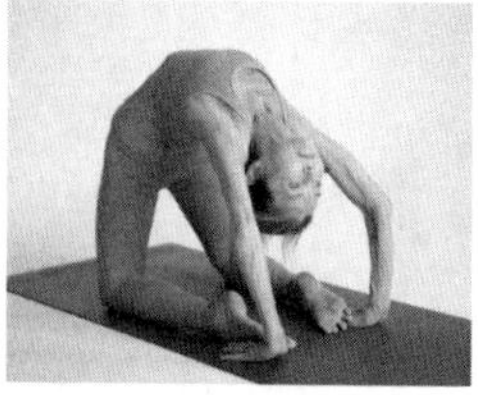

Kapotāsana B

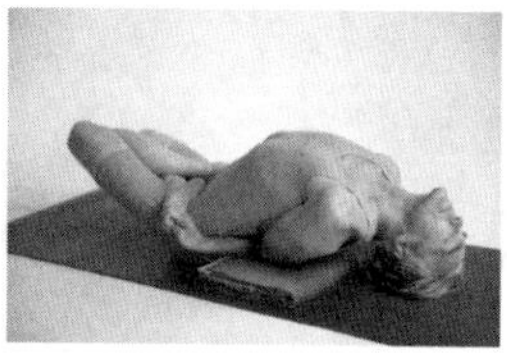

Supta Vajrāsana

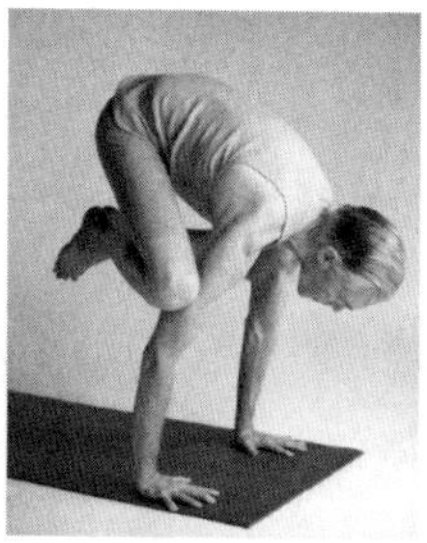

Bakāsana

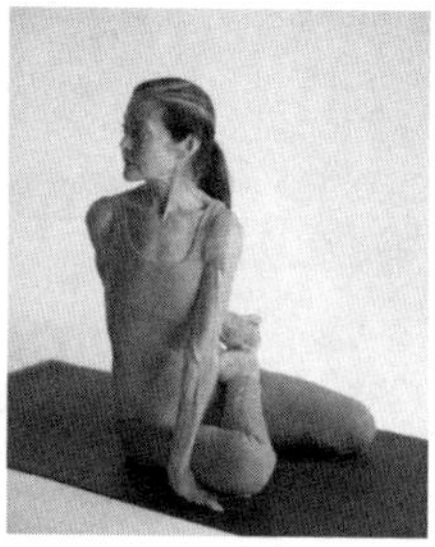

Bharadvājāsana

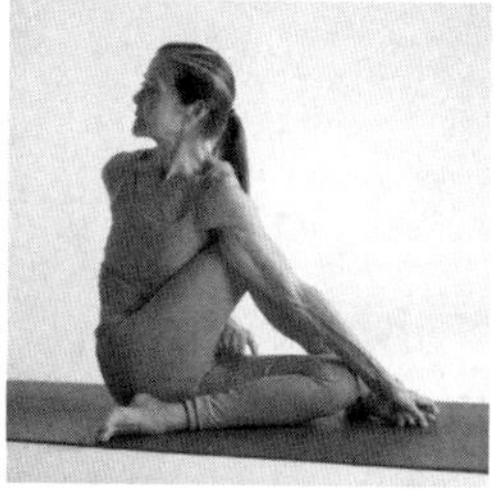

Ardha Matsyendrāsana

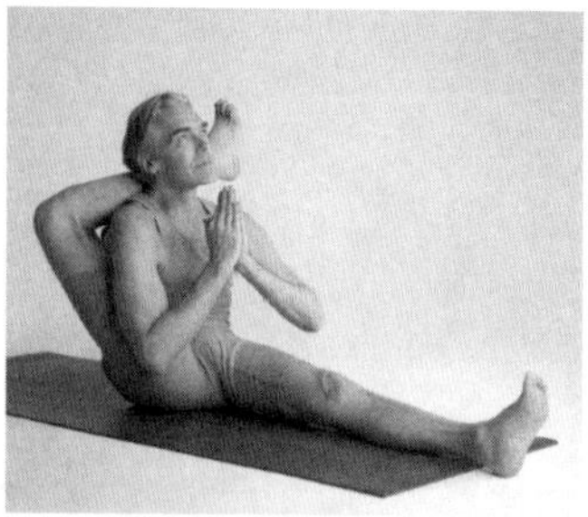

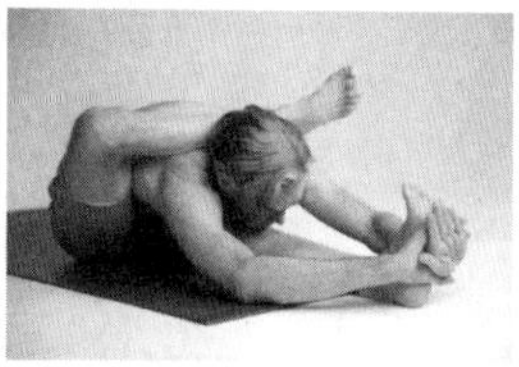

Eka Pāda Śīrṣāsana

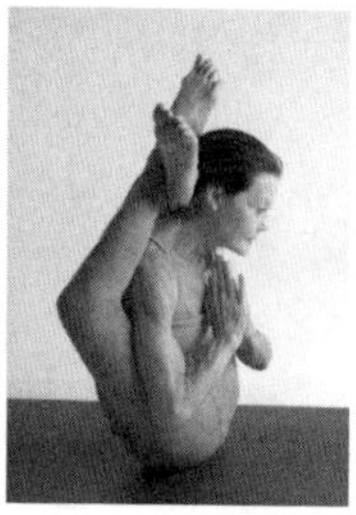

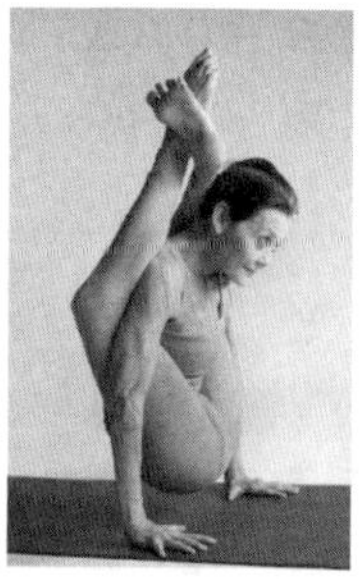

Dvi Pāda Śīrṣāsana

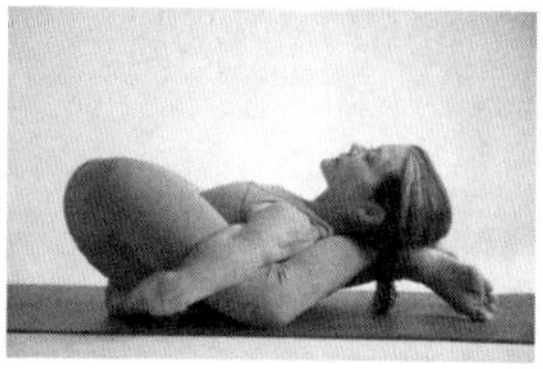

Yoga Nidrāsana

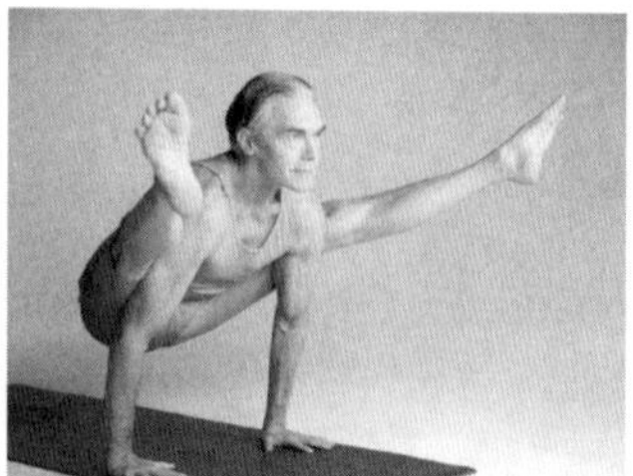

Ṭiṭṭibhāsana

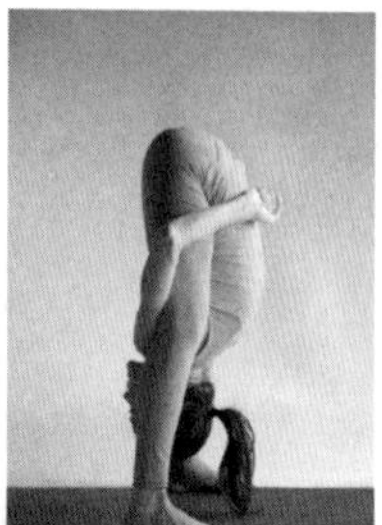

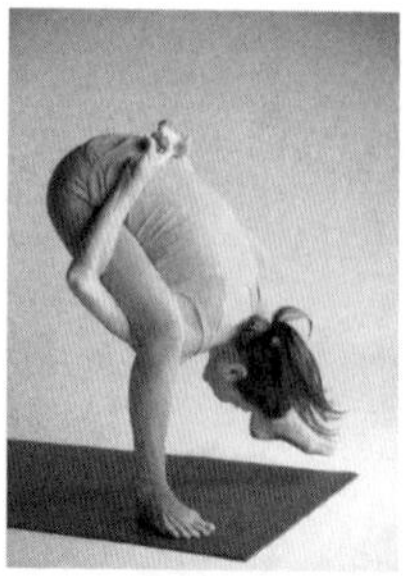

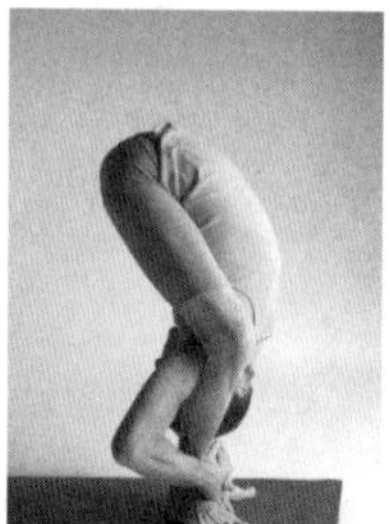

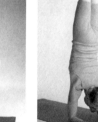

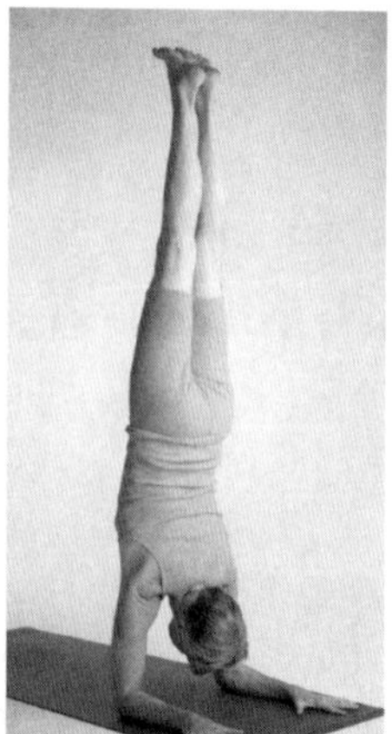

Piñcha Mayūrāsana

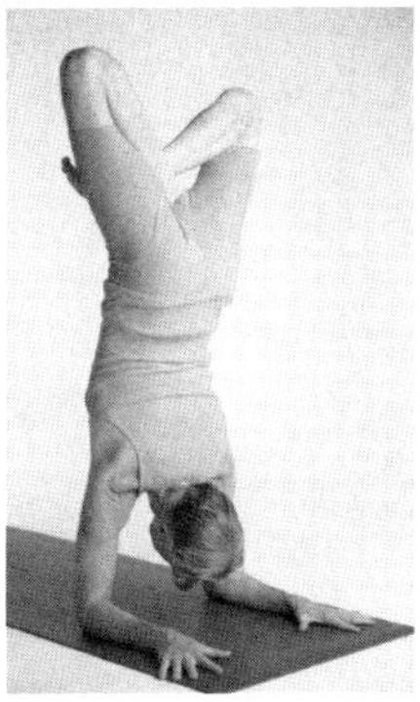
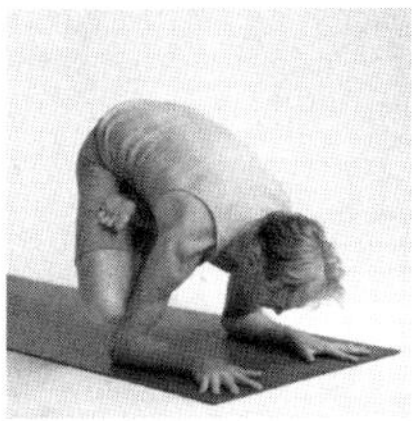

Karandavāsana

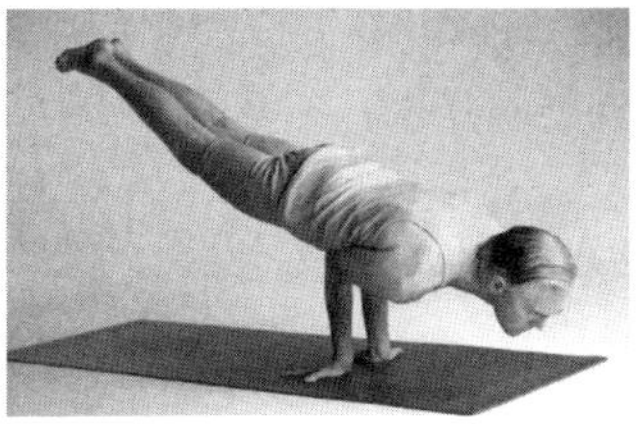

Mayūrāsana

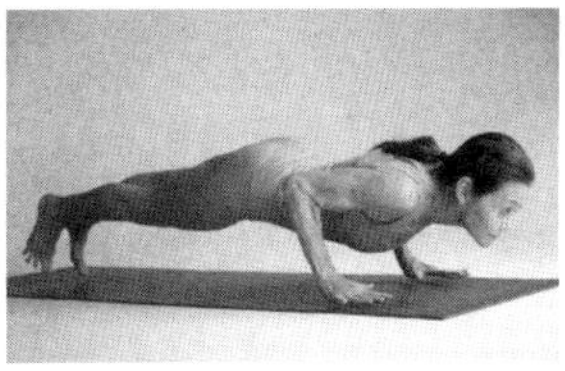

Nakrāsana

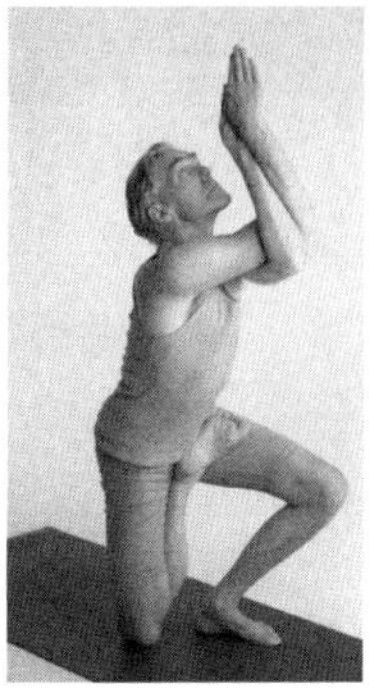

Vatayanāsana

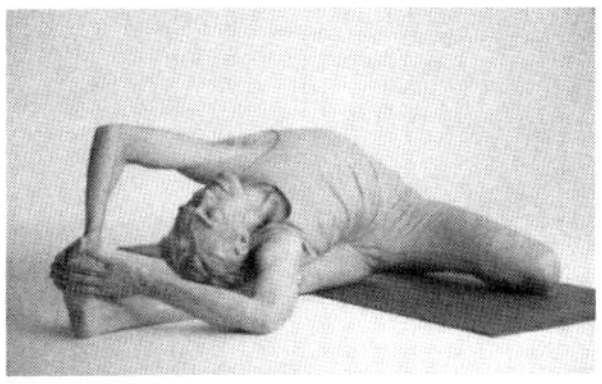

Parighāsana

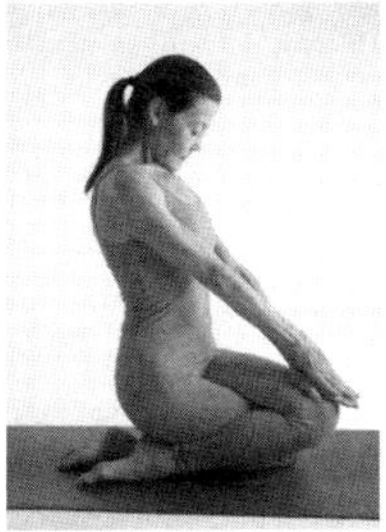
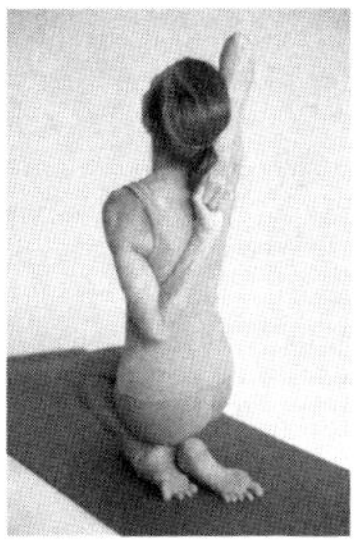

Gomukhāsana

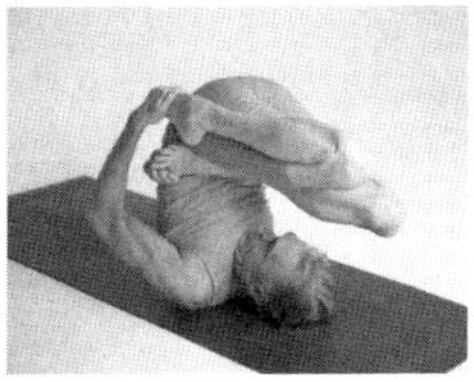
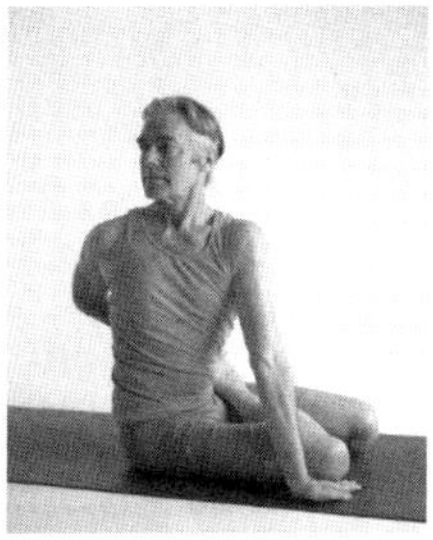

Supta Ūrdhvā Pāda Vajrāsana

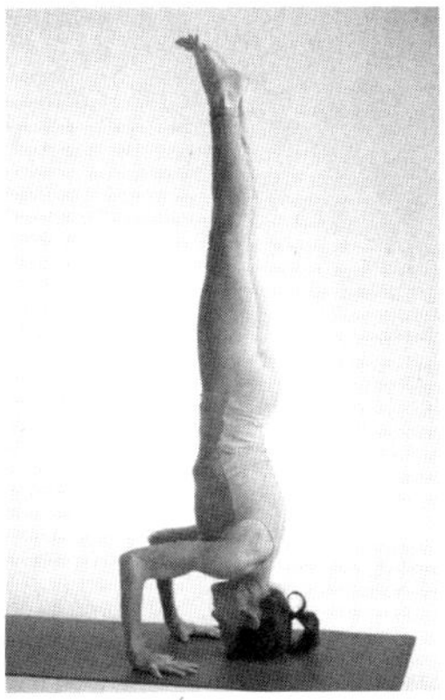
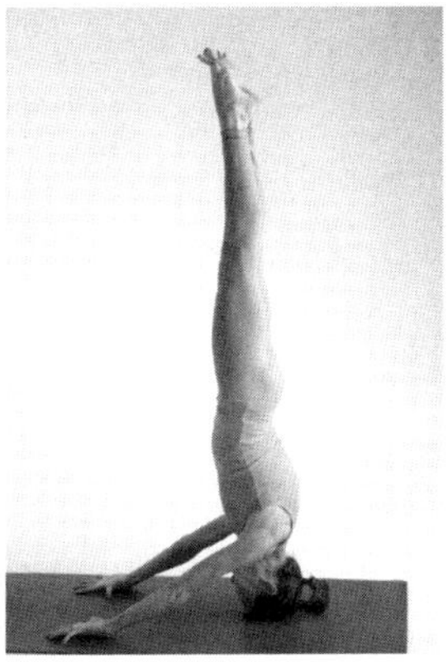
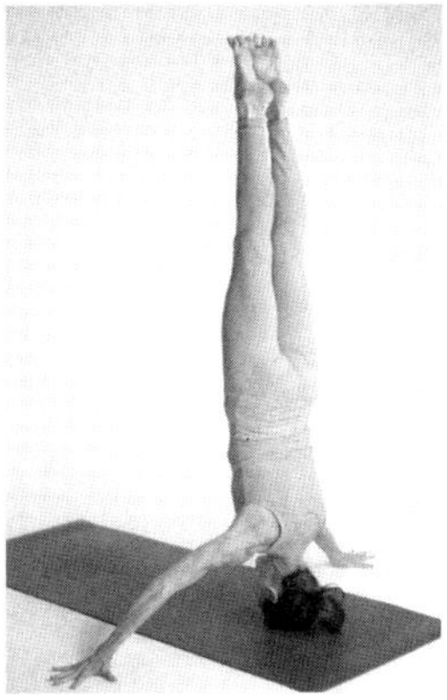

Mukta Hasta Śīrṣāsana A, B, and C

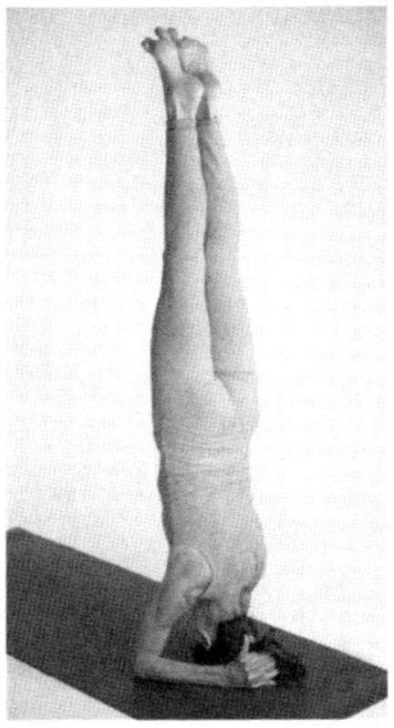
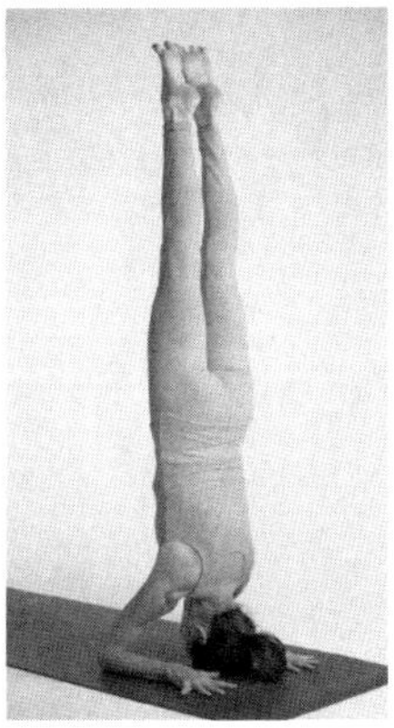
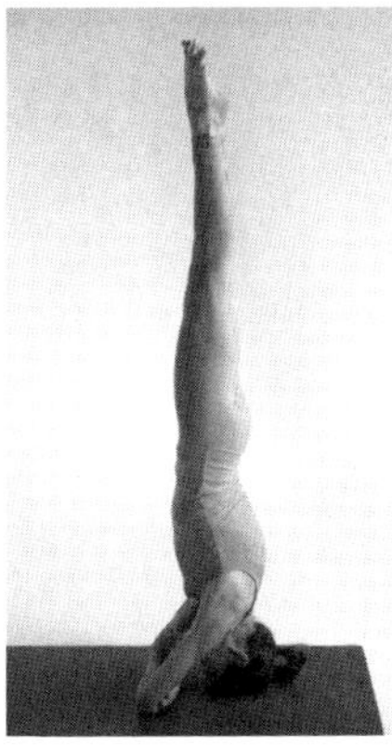
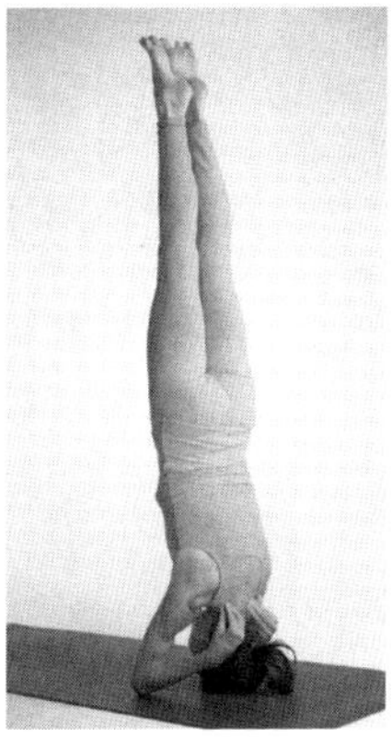

Baddha Hasta Śīrṣāsana A, B, C, and D

Sanskṛit Counting

One: ekam
Two: dve
Three: trīṇi
Four: catvāri
Five: pañca
Six: ṣaṭ
Seven: sapta
Eight: aṣṭa
Nine: nava
Ten: daśa
Eleven: ekādaśa
Twelve: dvādaśa
Thirteen: trayodaśa
Fourteen: caturdaśa
Fifteen: pañcadaśa
Sixteen: ṣodaśa
Seventeen: saptadaśa
Eighteen: aṣṭādaśa
Nineteen: ekoṇaviṁśati
Twenty: viṁśati

Eight Traditional Dṛṣṭi or Gazing Points

aṅguṣṭha (the middle of the thumb)
bhrūmadhya (between the eyebrows)
nāsāgra (the end of the nose)
hastāgra (the tip of the hand)
pārśva (the side—right or left)
ūrdhvā (upward)
nābhi cakra (the navel)
pādayoragra (the tip of the foot)

TWO ADDITIONAL GAZING POINTS

antara dṛṣṭi (internal)
ātmā dṛṣṭi (pure awareness, free of construction of subject and object)

APPENDIX 4

Illustrations of Mūlabandha, Kidney Wings, and Cobra Hood

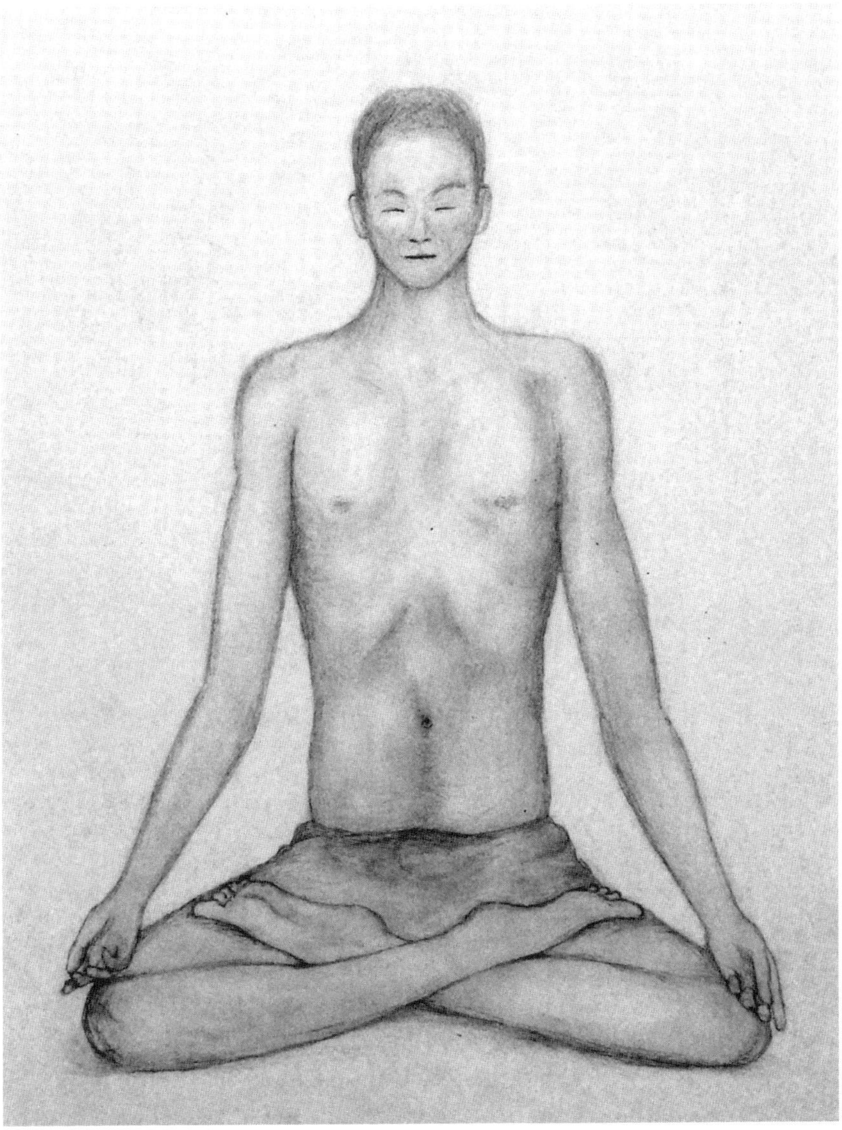

Mūlabandha is associated with an astonishingly deep concentration of the mind, initially causing a strong drawing up of the center of the pelvic floor along the central axis under the plane of the navel. Its effect is felt profoundly throughout the body and eventually causes a wonderful release starting in the soft palate and going up and back into the crown of the head, balancing and grounding all tensions and sensations of the body around the central axis. All this gives the subjective experience that the body and its surroundings are vibrant and joyous.

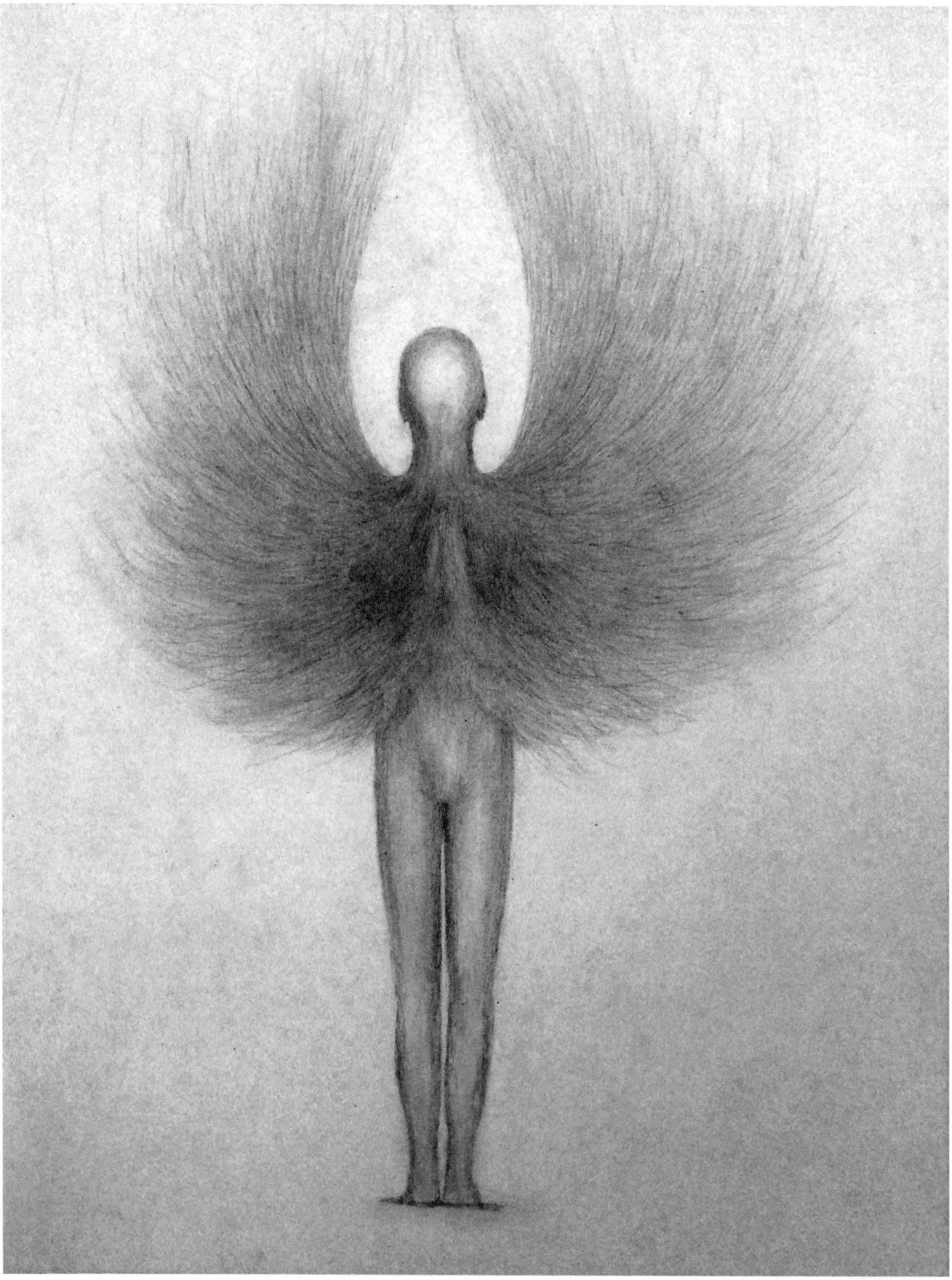

When *kidney wings* finally open to spread back, out, and up, they balance the natural buoyancy and spreading of the open heart. This makes the flame of pure attention just above the center of the pelvic floor replicate itself at stations up along the central axis until finally it unfolds in full form just above the crown of the head.

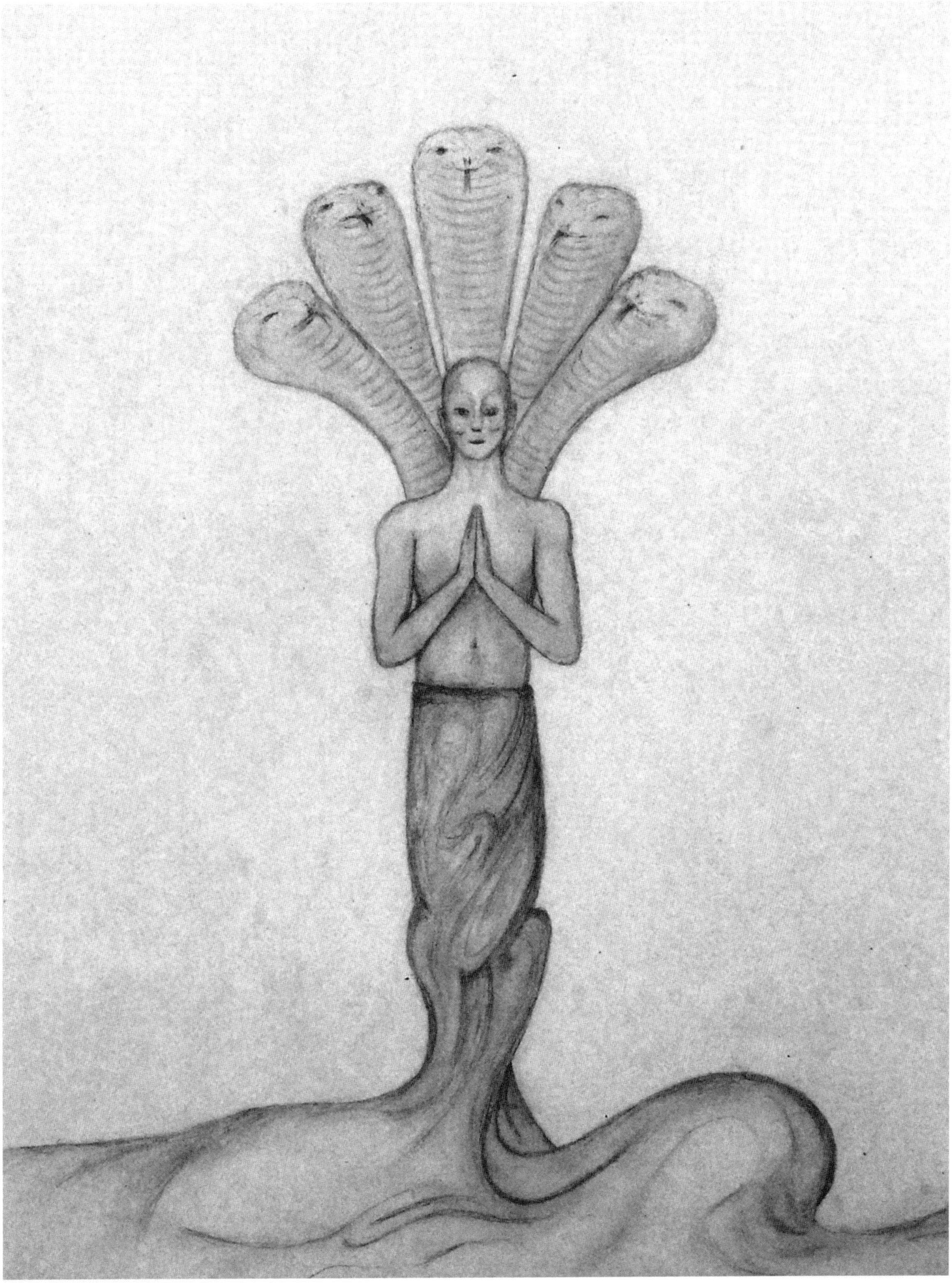

The *cobra hoods* are represented in the half-human and half-serpent (Nāga) deity form of the sage Patañjali. Here the apāna pattern manifests as the grounding tail of infinity, which in turn makes endless numbers of effulgent cobra heads open their hoods to shelter the beloved prāṇa pattern of the heart.

APPENDIX 5

Sūrya Namaskāra A and B

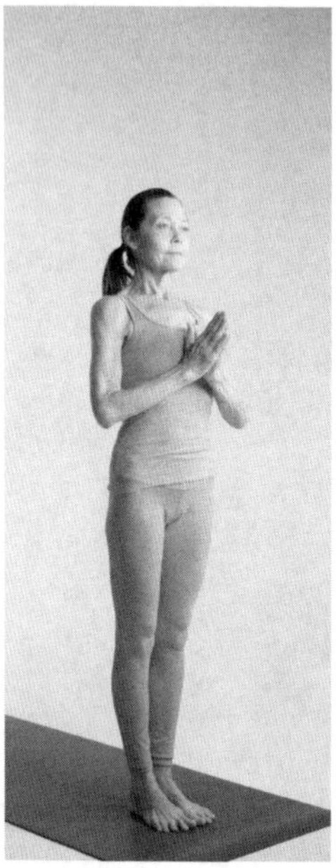
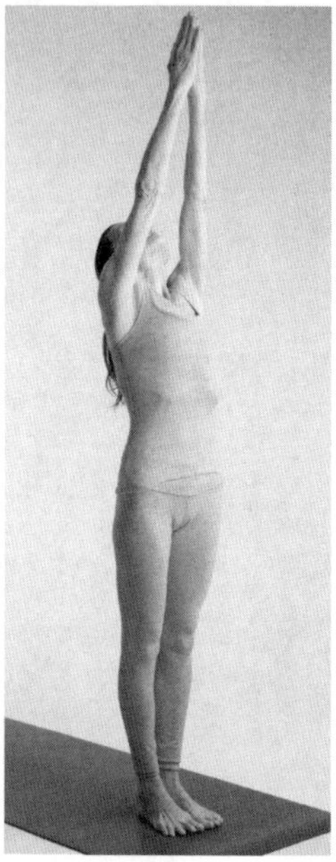
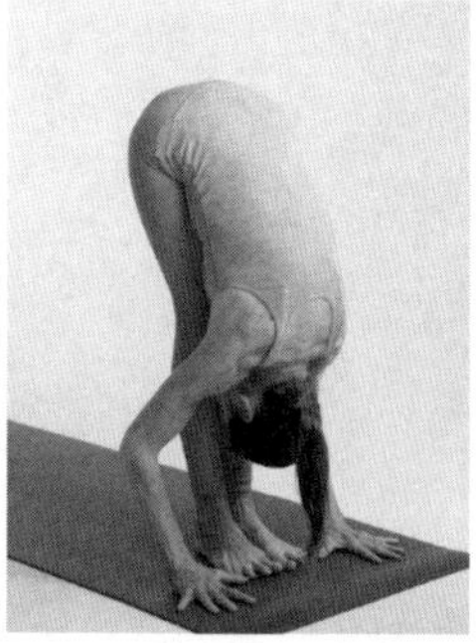

SŪRYA NAMASKĀRA A

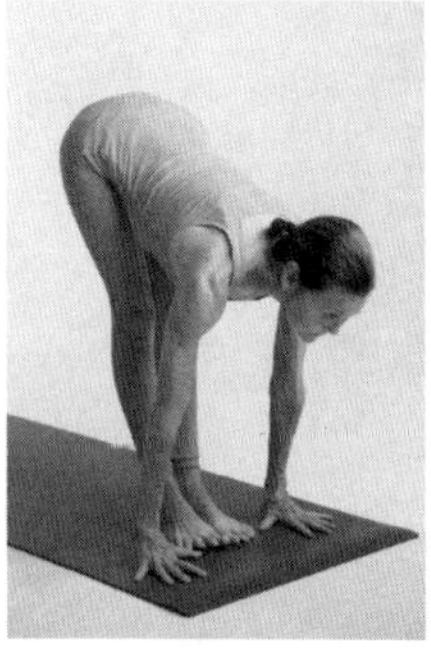
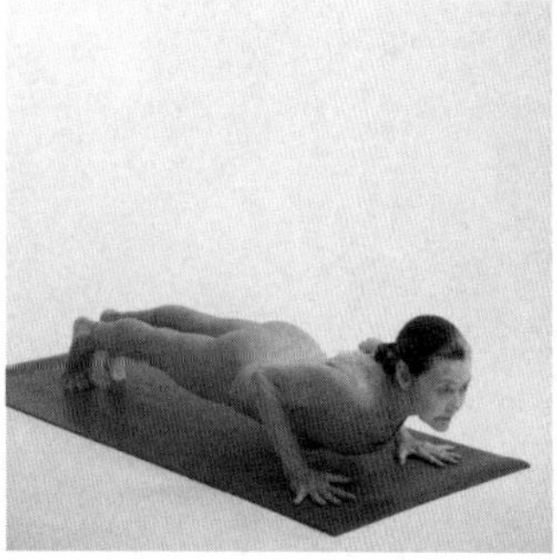
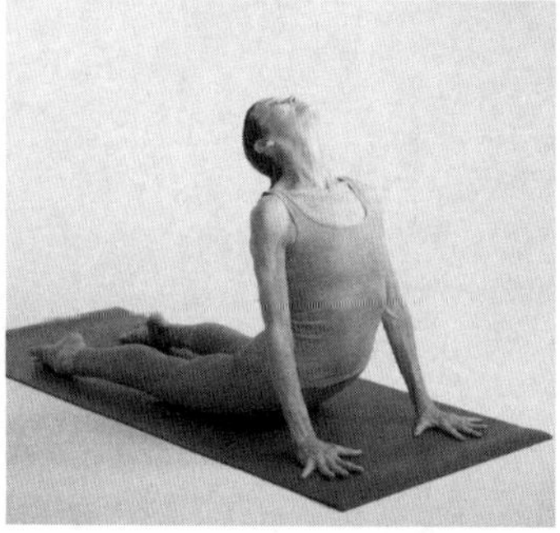
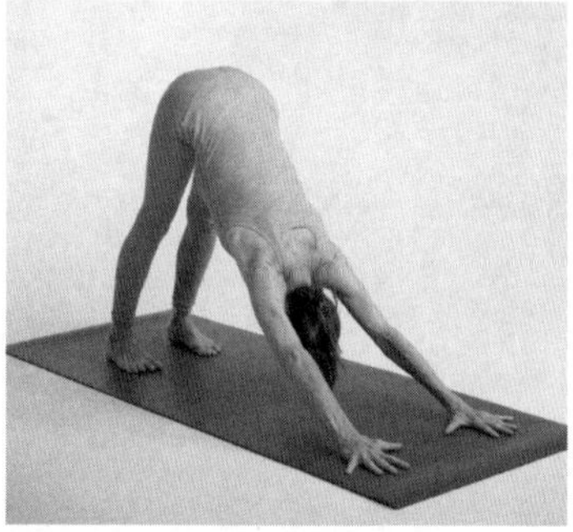
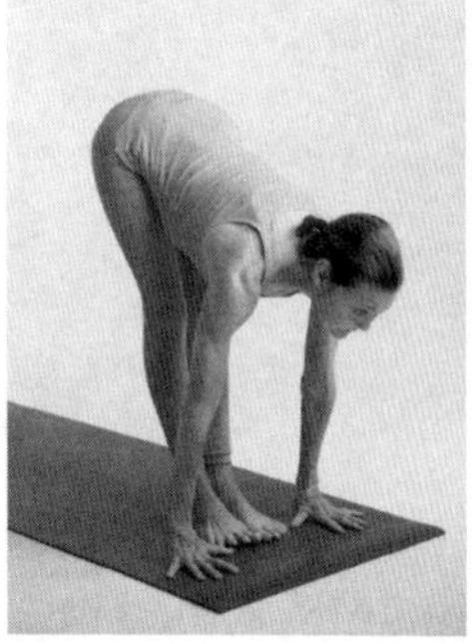
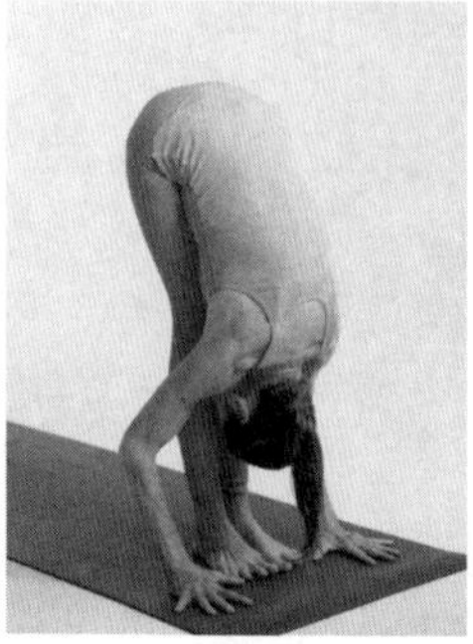
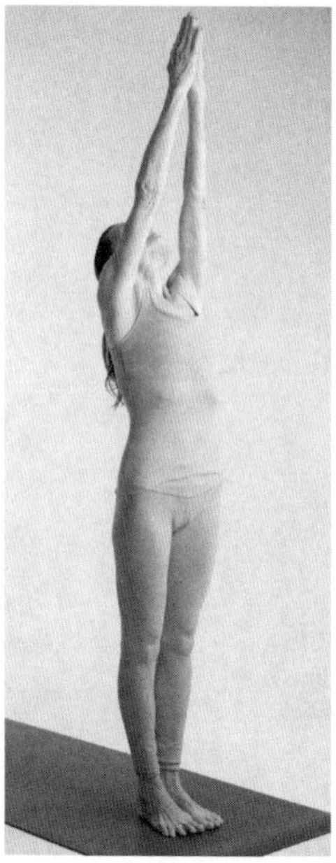
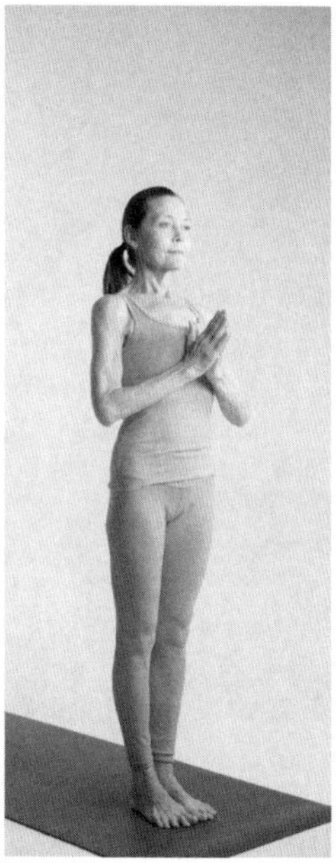

SŪRYA NAMASKĀRA B

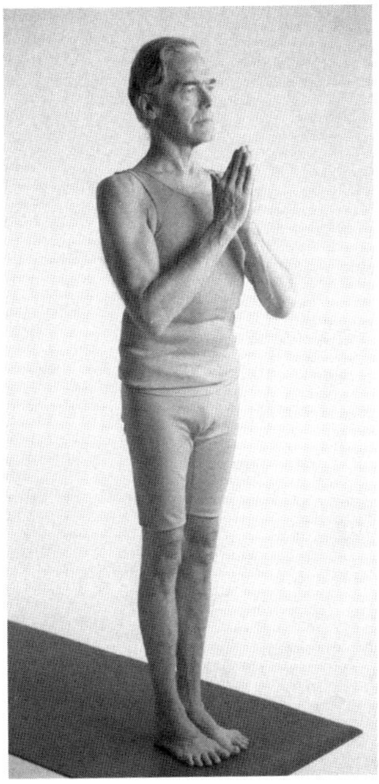

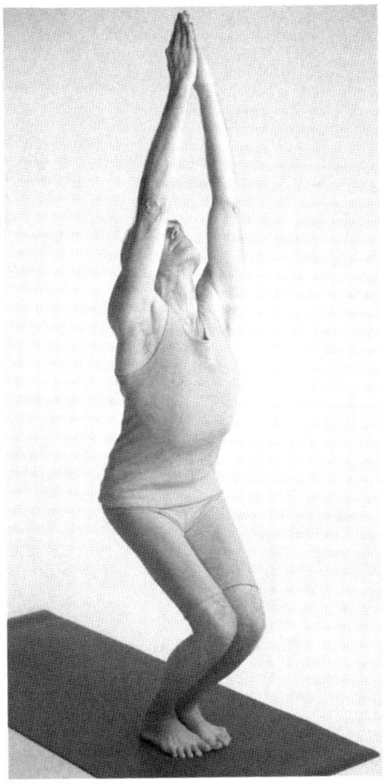

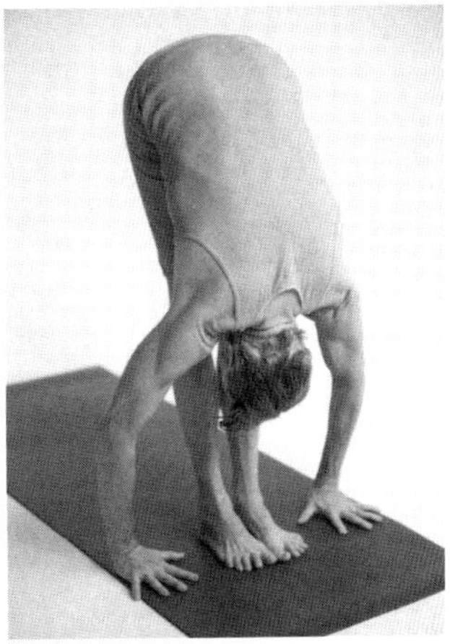

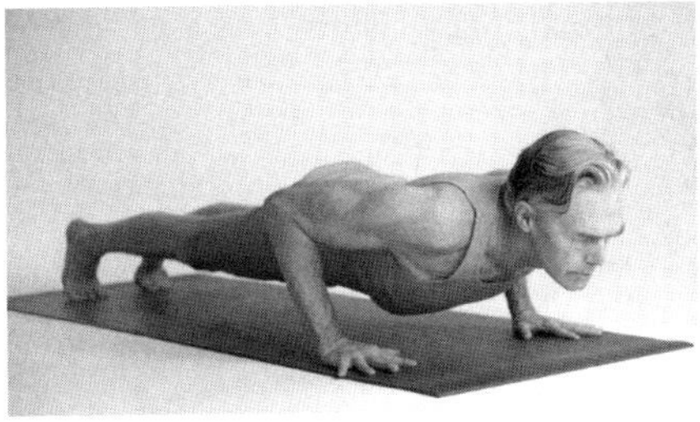

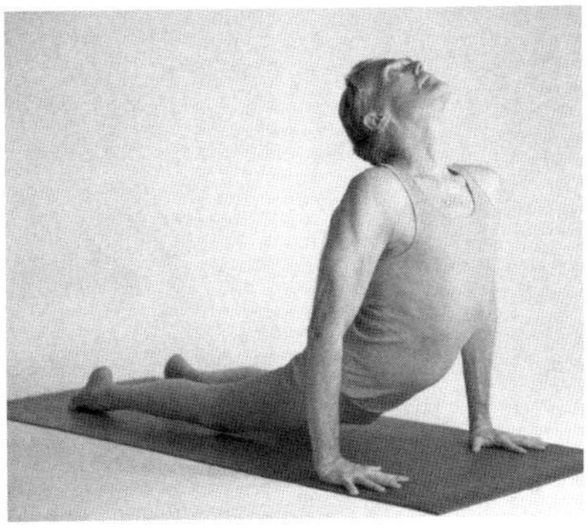

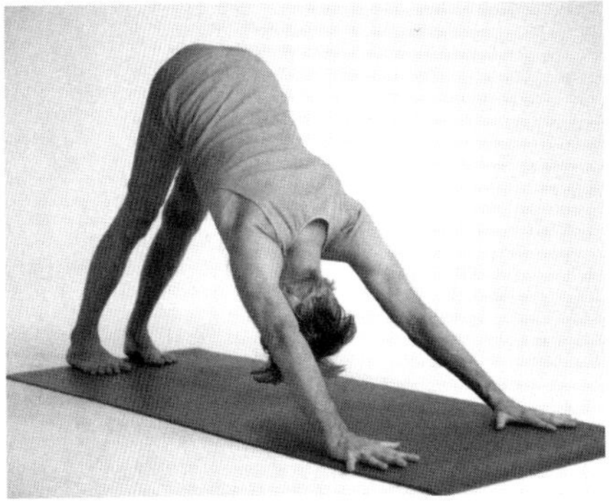

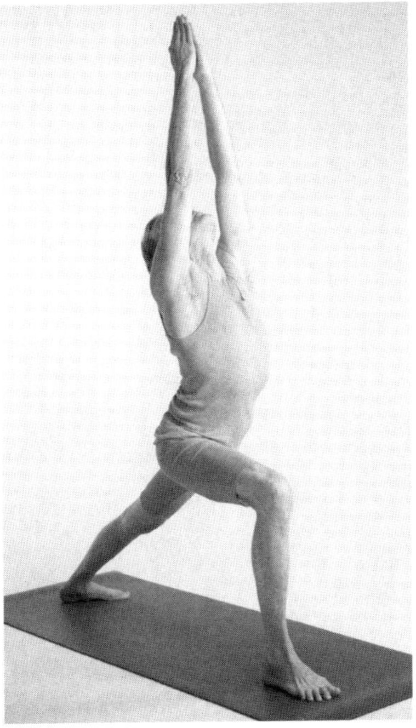

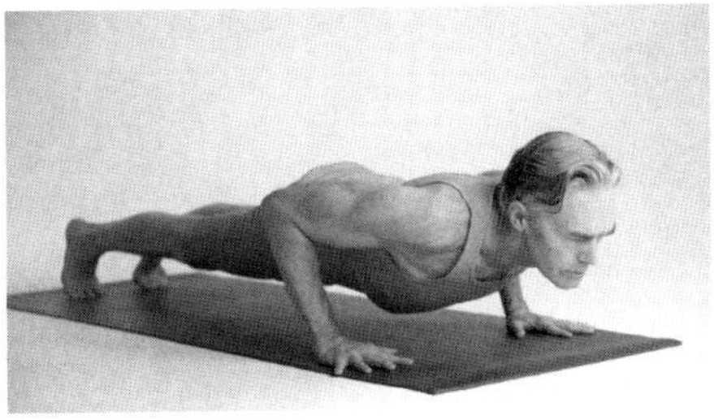

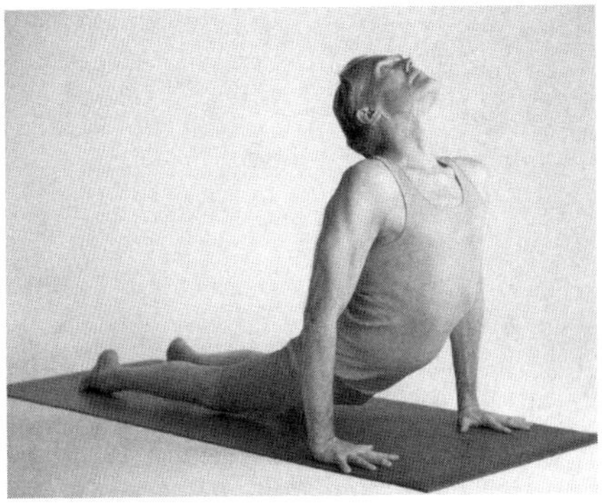

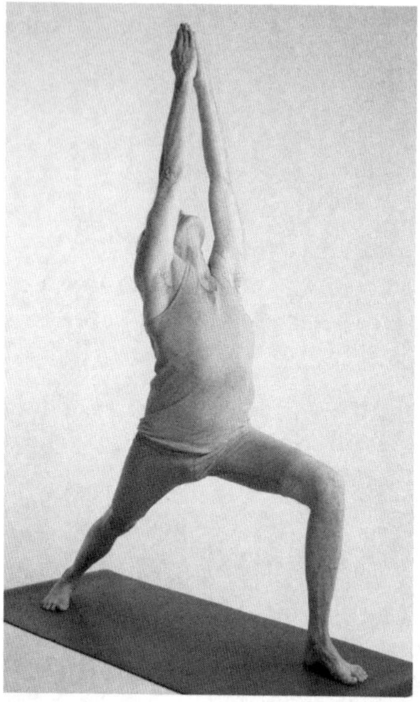

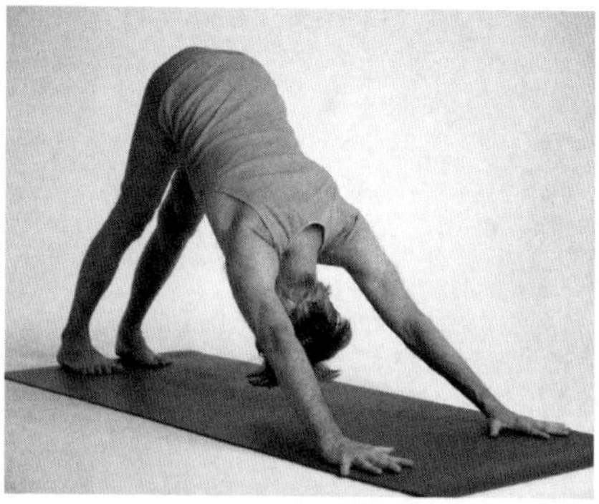

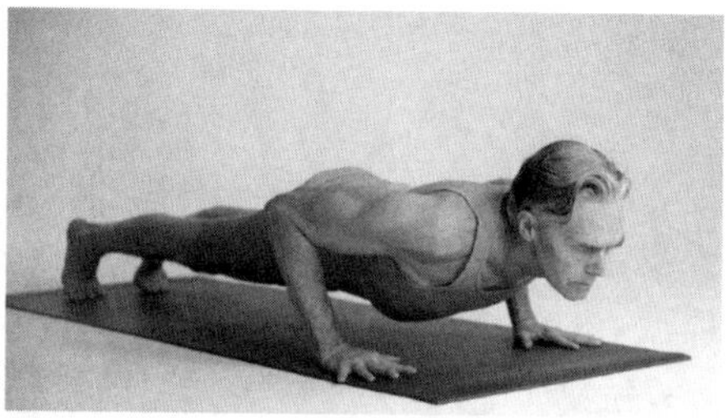

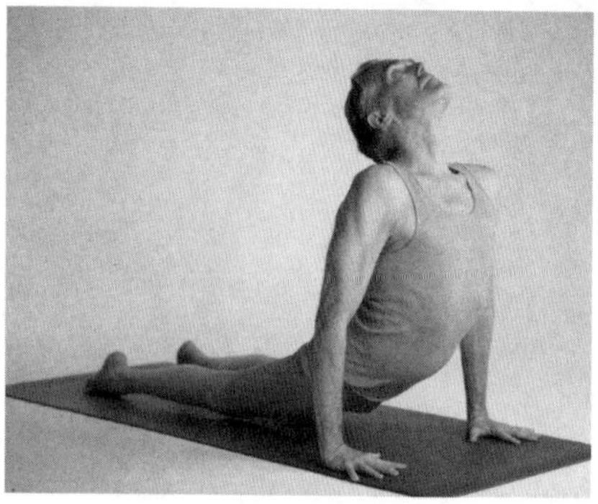

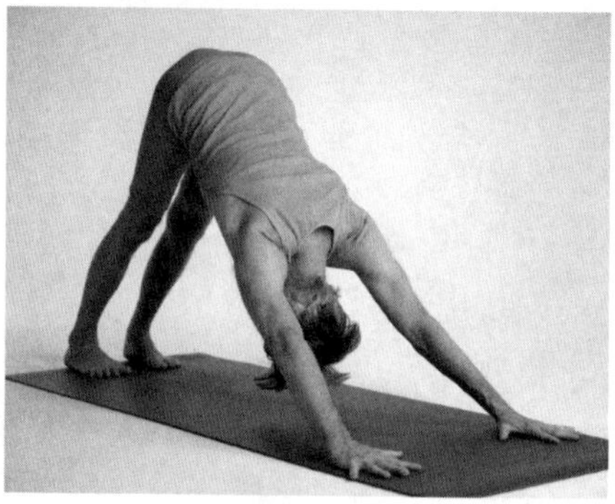

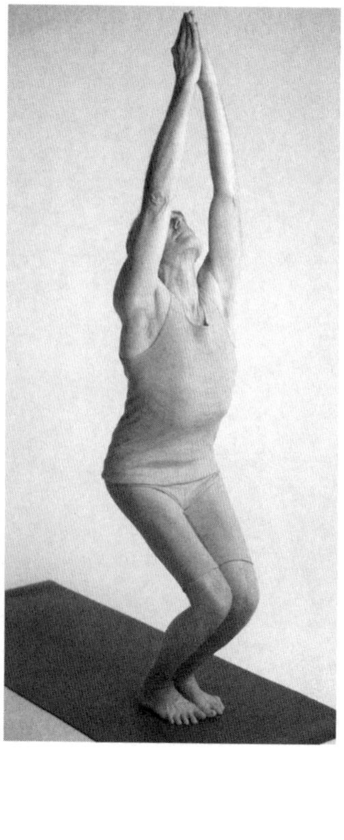

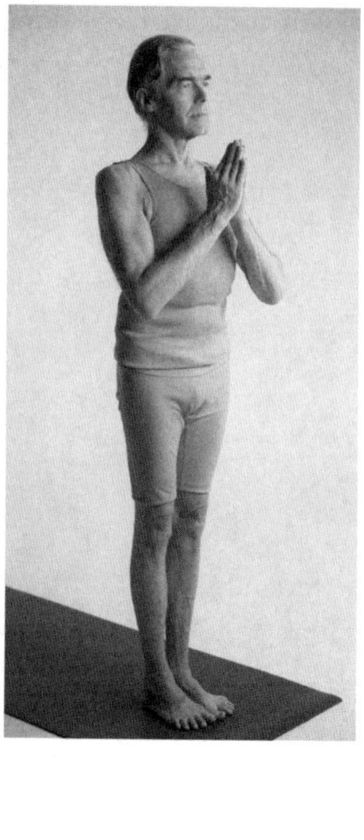

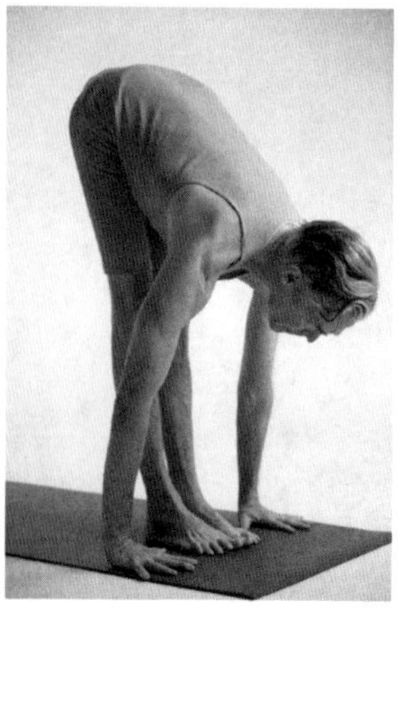

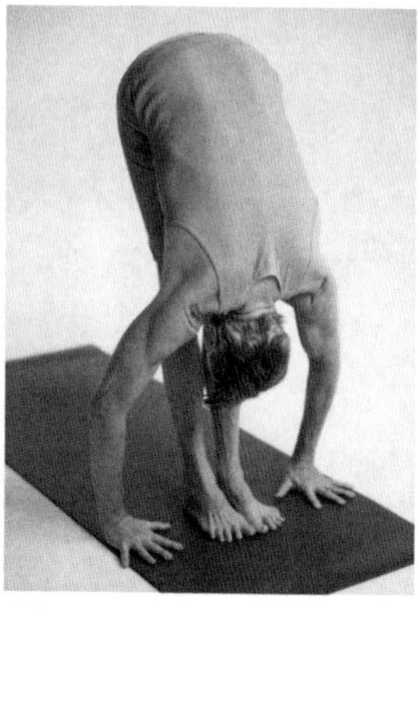

Index

Note: This index does not include all the information in the appendices.

abdominal muscles, 87–88, 89, 204, 236, 256
abduction and adduction, 159–60
abhiniveśa, 42–43
abhyāsa, 79
accuate line, 88
acetabular notch, 91
acromion, 94
Adho Mukha Śvānāsana (Downward Facing Dog), 70, 90, 114–15, 116, 119, 122, 123
Adho Mukha Vṛkṣāsana (Downward Facing Tree Pose), 274
Adiśeṣa, 34
Advanced A Series, 226, 242, 266
agonist, 84
ahiṃsā, 36–37
Air Vehicle Pose. *See* Vatayanāsana
ajñā cakra, 30, 57
alignment
- balance and, 245
- cultivating inner, 143
- in forward bends, 161
- skin flow and, 72, 73
- in twists, 230
- ujjāyī and, 13
- using imagery for, 7–8, 51–55
- whole-body patterns of, 52, 80–81

amṛta, 18–19, 59, 286, 294
amṛta plavana, 32
anal sphincter muscles, 55–56, 74
anatomy, 8–9, 82–95
Añjali Mudrā, 101, 131, 141–42, 147, 197, 250
antagonist, 84
anterior cruciate ligament (ACL), 93
apāna, 12, 14, 15, 74, 147
- in backbends, 202–5, 224
- in forward bends, 158–59, 161, 187, 195, 198
- in Mūlabandha, 21
- in twists, 231
- *See also under* prāṇa

aparigraha, 38–39
Aparokṣānubhuti, 45, 55
appendicular skeleton, 82–83
apuṇya, 44–45
arches of feet, 76, 128, 143, 154
Ardha Baddha Padma Paśchimottānāsana (Half-Bound Lotus Forward Bend Pose), 163
Ardha Baddha Padmottānāsana (Half-Bound Lotus Forward Bend Pose), 151–52
Ardha Matsyendrāsana (Half Spinal Twist Pose), 242–43, 244
Ardha Nāvāsana (Half Boat Pose), 187–88
Art of Happiness (Dali Lama XIV), 41
āsana
- ahiṃsā in, 37
- dṛṣṭi and, 17–18
- internal forms and, 10
- Mūlabandha, importance of in, 21
- plumb line, importance of to, 78
- prāna and apāna in, 77
- Prāṇa and citta in, 51
- ujjāyī in, 14–15

Aṣṭa, 118, 122
Aṣṭāṅga tradition, 35, 265, 275
Aṣṭāṅga Vinyāsa, 10, 98
- breath in, 13, 16
- criticism of, 157–58
- Downward Facing Dog in, 114
- finishing poses, importance of to, 275–76
- standing sequence in, 129, 154
- Sūrya Namaskāra, role of in, 99
  - *See also* Intermediate Series; Primary Series

asmitā, 42
asteya, 37
asymmetry, 230, 232
Avalokiteśvara, 7–8

avidyā, 41
axial skeleton, 82–83

backbends, 147–48, 202–6, 206–7, 213, 216, 224, 284, 307
Baddha Hasta Śīrṣāsana (Bound Hand Headstand Pose), 271–73
Baddha Koṇāsana (Bound Angle Pose), 161, 176–78
Baddha Padmāsana, 293–94
Bakāsana A, B (Crane Pose), 252–53, 256
balancing poses, 245–46
Balāsana (Child's Pose), 275, 290–92
Bali, 64
bandhas, 10, 19–20, 23, 25, 28–29, 32, 123, 276–77. *See also individual bandha*
Bharadvājāsana (Bharadhvāja's Pose), 239–40
Bhekāsana (Frog Pose), 210, 211–13
Bhujaṅgāsana (Cobra Pose), 111, 113, 212
Bhujapīḍāsana (Arm Squeezing Pose), 250–52, 258
biceps, 90
biceps femoris, 92
Big Toe Pose. *See* Pādāṅguṣṭhāsana
bindu dhāraṇa, 32
Boat Pose. *See* Nāvāsana
bodhisattva vow, 43
Bound Angle Pose. *See* Baddha Koṇāsana
Bound Hand Headstand Pose. *See* Baddha Hasta Śīrṣāsana
Brahmā, 34
Brahmā nāḍī, 38, 70
Brahmacarya, 38
breath, 10
  in backbends, 203–4, 206, 216, 219
  listening to, 282, 295–96
  movement and, 107, 193
  in Mūlabandha, 57
  preferences in, 12–13
  psoas buttons for training, 67–68
  in psoas line, 61
  in Reclining Angle Pose, 181
  retention, 13, 21, 22, 23, 27
  riding, 77, 78, 124–25
  in Samasthitiḥ, 100–101
  skeletal system and, 83
  in Sūrya Namaskāra, 119
  trusting, 191
  in twists, 242–43
Bridge Poses. *See* Dhanurāsana; Setu Bandhāsana
Bridge Shoulderstand. *See* Setu Bandha Sarvāṅgāsana

Cakorāsana (Moonbeam-Drinking Bird Pose), 198–99
cakras, 30, 57
Cakrāsana (Wheel Pose), 123, 125–26, 222
Calf Face Pose. *See* Gomukhāsana
Camel Pose. *See* Uṣṭrāsana
Caturdaśa, 122
Catvāri and variations, 109–10, 113, 119, 122, 123, 253
celibacy, 38
central channel (suṣumnā nāḍī), 29, 78
  in backbends, 204, 206
  bandhas and, 23
  cakras and, 31
  in Downward Facing Dog, 115
  Gaṇeśa and, 68–69
  in headstands, 287
  internal forms and, 11
  in Khecarī Mudrā, 25
  in kidney wings, 66
  in Mūlabandha, 56, 57
  palate and, 57–58
  paramātman in, 15–16
  prāṇa and apāna in, 79
  in Samasthitiḥ, 100
  ujjāyī and, 13, 14
  umbilical breathing and, 34
cervical spine, 160, 204, 205–6
Child's Pose. *See* Balāsana
circulatory system, 29
cit, 32
citta, 10, 12, 46–47, 49, 51, 55
clavicle, 94
cobra hood, 23, 70–72, 103, 225, 315
Cobra Pose. *See* Bhujaṅgāsana
coccygeus, 74, 86
coccyx
  apāna and, 66, 177
  in backbends, 204, 205, 224
  in Downward Facing Dog, 117
  in holding serpent's tail, 73–74
  in Mūlabandha, 57
  pelvic floor and, 86, 198
  sacrum and, 64, 91
  in Samasthitiḥ, 100
  in twists, 231
Cock Pose. *See* Kukkuṭāsana
co-contraction, 84, 128
Compass Pose. *See* Dikāsana
compassion
  as amṛta, 32, 59, 294
  in boundless abodes, 43
  discriminating awareness and, 46, 50
  ego and, 42
  ethics and, 36
  in Khecarī Mudrā, 26
  in Mūlabandha, 56
  in releasing palate, 18–19
  for suffering of others, 44
  visualization and, 60
contemplative practices, 8, 46–47, 49–50
Corpse Pose. *See* Śavāsana
costal cartilage, 87
counternutation, 87
Crane Poses. *See* Bakāsana; Karandavāsana
Crocodile Pose. *See* Nakrāsana

Daṇḍāsana (Staff Pose), 20, 209, 246–47
Daśa, 122
death, 42–43
deep six, 91
deity visualization, 8, 9, 10, 56–57, 66, 128, 287
Dhanurāsana (Bridge Pose), 213–14
diaphragm, 23–24, 60, 65–66, 88–89, 102, 204, 205, 206, 230–32, 236
Difficult Pose. *See* Utkaṭāsana
digestion, 211, 232
Dikāsana (Compass Pose), 266–68
discriminating awareness, 18–19, 45, 50
divine sound (nāda), 69
Downward Facing Dog. *See* Adho Mukha Śvānāsana
dṛṣṭi, 10, 16–17, 164, 177, 206
  in finishing poses, 276
  in Khecarī Mudrā, 26
  in psoas line, 62
  in Samasthitiḥ, 100
  traditional, list of, 17–18
  ujjāyī and, 13
  as view, 18
  See also gaze
duḥkha, 41, 44
Dvādaśa, 122
Dve, 77, 84, 102, 104, 106, 109, 118, 119
dveṣa, 42

Dvi Pāda Śīrṣāsana (Two Feet Behind the Head Pose), 161, 196, 199–200
Dvi Pāda Viparīta Daṇḍāsana (Two-Footed Inverted Staff Pose), 226–27

eccentric contraction, 84
Eka Pāda family, 195, 196, 198
Eka Pāda Rāja Kapotāsana (One-Footed King Pigeon Pose), 228–29
Eka Pāda Śīrṣāsana (One Foot Behind the Head Pose), 196–98
Eka Pāda Viparīta Daṇḍāsana (One-Footed Inverted Staff Pose), 227
Ekādaśa, 122
Ekam, 101–2, 103, 104, 107, 118, 119
embodiment, 46–47, 52, 71–72, 80, 91
emotions, 43, 58, 60, 68, 80, 151, 161, 203, 265
erector spinae, 84, 89, 187, 206
ethics, 35–37

fascia, 76, 83
fear, 12, 31–32, 42–43, 125, 150–51, 158, 202–3, 222, 232, 276
feet, general placement of, 90, 129–30, 136, 160
femoroacetabular impingement, 140
femurs, 90, 93, 160, 170, 188
fibula, 90
finishing poses, 275–77, 307
Fish Pose. *See* Matsyāsana
Forward Bend to the Side Pose. *See* Pārśvottānāsana
Forward Bend with Feet Spread Pose. *See* Prasārita Pādottānāsana A, B, C, D
forward bends, 157–62, 258, 259
four boundless abodes, 43–45
foveal ligament, 91
Full Vinyāsa, 123, 154, 161–62, 256

Gaṇeśa, 9, 68–69, 237
Gaṇeśa Belly, 68–70, 88
Garbha Piṇḍāsana, 191–93
Garuda, 9
gaze, 59, 107, 123. *See also* dṛṣṭi
gemellus inferior and superior, 91
glenoid fossa, 94
gluteus maximus, 91, 92, 204
Gomukhāsana (Calf Face Pose), 265–66
granthis (energy blockages), 122

Halāsana (Plough Pose), 181, 278, 281–82, 284
Half Padmāsana, 166–67, 175–76
Half Vinyāsa, 123, 161–62
Half Vīrāsana, 167
Half-Bound Lotus Forward Bend Pose. *See* Ardha Baddha Padmottānāsana
hamstrings, 84, 90, 91, 92
  in backbends, 204, 208–9, 224
  in forward bends, 157, 158, 160–61
Hand and Foot Pose. *See* Pādahastāsana
Handstand. *See* Adho Mukha Vṛkṣāsana (Downward Facing Tree Pose)
Hanumanāsana (Hanuman's Pose), 248–50
hard palate, 59, 85
hatha yoga, 23, 32, 65
Haṭha Yoga Pradīpikā, 35, 70
Headstand. *See* Śirṣāsana
Head-to-Knee Pose, A, B, C. *See* Jānuśīrṣāsana
heart
  in backbends, 203, 205, 206, 284
  in cobra hood, 71, 72
  in forward bends, 157–58, 159–61, 198
  in Jālandhara Bandha, 20
  in nauli, 25
  prāṇa and, 12, 14, 177
  in psoas line, 61
  in Samasthitiḥ, 101, 130, 131
  scalenes and, 89
  in Utkaṭāsana, 153
Hero Pose. *See* Vīrāsana
Hinge Pose. *See* Parighāsana
hip flexors, 61, 66, 75, 91, 92, 204
hips, 90–91, 128
  in forward bends, 158, 160, 171, 176
  in twists, 230–32, 236
holding serpent's tail, 73–75, 144, 208–9
humerus, 90, 94, 95

idā nāḍī (moon channel), 30, 61
iliacus, 91
iliococcygeus, 74, 86
iliopsoas muscle, 91
ilium, 86–87, 90–91
imagination and imagery, 51–53
  in animal pose names, 194, 252, 253, 258, 262
  central channel and, 29
  Prāṇa and, 10–11
  in psoas line, 60–61

impermanence, 9, 31, 203, 276
Indian mythology and iconography, 34, 194, 237
infraspinatus, 94
insertion of muscle, 84–85, 92
insight, 9, 49–50, 60, 80–81
integration, 21, 56, 89, 99, 123, 157, 203–4, 265, 297
intention, 3, 14, 44, 130, 141
interconnectedness, 12, 33, 45, 61, 203
intercostal muscles, external and internal, 88–89
interdependence, 48, 60
Intermediate Series, 98, 169, 309–11
  backbends in, 207, 210, 211, 213, 214, 216
  balances in, 256, 263
  headstands in, 268
  twists in, 236, 239, 242
internal forms, 243
  alignment and, 9
  in backbends, 202, 205, 218
  defining, 10–11
  in forward bends, importance of, 157
  in headstand, 287
  importance of, 31–32, 47
  as sādhanā bhāṣā, 54–55
  in standing poses, 127
  in Sūrya Namaskāra, 107
invocations, 101
iṣṭa devatā, 40, 57
Īśvara-praṇidhāna, 40

Jālandhara Bandha, 19, 20–21, 247, 294, 295
Jānuśīrṣāsana A, B, C (Head-to-Knee Pose), 159, 167, 170–73
Jihvā Bandha, 26
Jñāna Mudrā, 295
joints
  acetabulofemoral, 91
  atlanto-axial, 231
  atlanto-occipital, 206
  ball-and-socket, 90
  glenohumeral, 94, 95
  hinge, 90
  sternoclavicular, 94
  synovial hinge, 93, 94
  See also sacroilian (SI) joints
Jois, Sri K. Pattabhi, 149, 246, 296
Jumping Back, 123, 124

Kapotāsana (Pigeon Pose), 217, 218–20, 228
Karandavāsana (Crane Pose), 255–56
Karṇa Pīḍāsana (Squeezing the Ears Pose), 282–83
Khecarī Mudrā, 25–26, 27
kidney wings, 65–66, 71, 89, 204, 205, 206, 314
kindness, 59, 66, 237
  boundless, 43
  Prāṇa and, 16
  toward oneself, 31–32
  in yamas and niyamas, 36, 37, 39
kleśas, 41–43
knees, 90, 93, 147, 153
Krauñcha, 169, 237
Krauñchāsana, 169–70
kriya practices, 65
Kukkuṭāsana (Cock Pose), 193–94
Kuṇḍalinī, 29, 70
Kūrma Purāṇa, 71
Kūrmāsana (Turtle Pose), 161, 194–95, 196, 258

labrum, 94, 160
Laghu Vajrāsana (Light Thunderbolt Pose), 217–18
lateral collateral ligament (LCL), 93
life breath. *See* Prāṇa
Light Thunderbolt Pose. *See* Laghu Vajrāsana
linea alba, 87
lineage, 52
Locust Pose. *See* Śalabhāsana A, B
lotus, symbolism of, 34. *See also* sahasrāra (thousand-petaled lotus)
Lotus Pose. *See* Padmāsana
lumbar spine, 60, 85, 204, 205, 231, 284

maitrī, 43–44
maṇipūra cakra. *See* nābhi cakra
mantra, 14, 15–16
Marīchyāsana (Marīchi's Pose)
  A, B, 174–76
  C, D, 232, 233–36
Matsyāsana (Fish Pose), 220, 222, 223, 224, 275, 284–86
Mayūrāsana (Peacock Pose), 256–57
medial collateral ligament (MCL), 93
meditation (meditative states)
  asana and, 15, 51
  in cave of sacrum, 65
  embodiment and, 80–81
  finishing poses and, 275–77, 282, 287
  internal forms and, 10
  nāḍīs and, 30
  name and form in, 50
  in Padmāsana, 293
  in Sūrya Namaskāra, 99–100
  Vīrāsana for, 211
  viveka khyātiḥ in, 45–46
meniscus, 93
mind
  altered states of, 81
  in balancing poses, 245
  discursive, 80–81
  dṛṣṭi and, 18
  mantra and, 15–16
  in mudrās, 28–29
  pelvis floor and, 12
  Prāṇa and, 60
  resetting, 123
  role of, 49
  symbols and, 47
  wandering, 18, 40, 41, 66, 68, 191
moon channel. *See* idā nāḍī
muditā, 44
mudrā, 10, 25, 28, 32, 123. *See also individual mudrās*
Mukta Hasta Śīrṣāsana A, B, C (Unbound Hand Headstand Pose), 268–71
mūla, 11, 23, 26, 56
Mūlabandha, 19, 21, 70, 313
  in backbends, 204–5, 224, 225
  in Downward Facing Dog, 115
  feet and pelvic floor in, 76
  in finishing poses, 282, 283, 289, 293, 294, 297
  in forward bends, 142, 143, 171, 182
  Gaṇeśa and, 69
  hip joints and, 262
  imagery for, 55–57, 313
  importance of, 32
  other bandhas and, 22, 23
  palate in, 86
  pelvic floor in, 86
  psoas and, 62, 66, 68
  sacrum and, 64
  in Samasthitiḥ, 131
  serpent's tail in, 74, 75
  in Sun Salutation, 103
  in twists, 237
  Yoni Mudrā and, 26, 27
muscles, origin of, 84–85
muscular system, 83
myofascia, 49, 72, 276
mystical experiences, 48

nābhi cakra, 34, 69–70
nāḍīs (internal channels), 29–31, 32, 49, 59, 61, 69. *See also* central channel (suṣumnā nāḍī)
nagas, 71
Nakrāsana (Crocodile Pose), 262–63
nasal septum, 18, 57, 59
nauli, 23–25, 88
Nava, 118, 122
Nāvāsana (Boat Pose), 186–87, 274
nectar, 59, 286, 294
nervous system
  cobra hood and, 71
  impact of matrī on, 43–44
  integrating, 265, 297
  nāḍīs and, 29
  palate release and, 158–59
  pattern sensations in, 11
  plumb line in, 79
  reciprocal inhibition in, 85
  resetting, 123
  twists, effect of on, 230–31
  whole-body patterns in, 53, 54
nirodha, 47, 78, 79
niyamas, 39–40
nonattachment, 45, 72, 79
Noose Pose. *See* Paśāsana
nutation, 87

oblique muscles, internal and external, 88, 147, 167
obturator externus and internus, 91
Old Dog Pose, 115–17
One Foot Behind the Head Pose. *See* Eka Pāda Śīrṣāsana
One-Footed Inverted Staff Pose. *See* Eka Pāda Viparīta Daṇḍāsana
One-Footed King Pigeon Pose. *See* Eka Pāda Rāja Kapotāsana
One Leg Reversed Forward Bend Pose. *See* Tiryang Mukha Eka Pāda Paśchimottānāsana

Pādahastāsana (Hand and Foot Pose), 131, 133
Pādāṅguṣṭhāsana (Big Toe Pose), 131–33, 159

Padmāsana (Lotus Pose), 20, 93, 191, 235, 236, 244, 256, 284, 292–93
Padmāsana with Ujjāyī Prāṇāyāma (Lotus Pose Variation), 295
palate, 85
  in Jālandhara Bandha, 20, 21
  in Mūlabandha, 57
  in nauli, 25
  opening of, 222
  releasing, 18, 57–60, 62, 73, 101, 158–59
  root of, 86, 286, 289, 294
palate-perineum reflex, 77–78, 79, 294
Pañca and variations, 110–13, 119
Pañcadaśa, 122
paramātman, 15–16
Parighāsana (Hinge Pose), 231, 236–37
Parivṛtta Pārśvakoṇāsana (Twisted Side-Angle Pose), 140–42
Parivṛtta Trikoṇāsana (Revolving Triangle Pose), 128, 134, 136–38
Pārśva Dhanurāsana (Side-Angle Bridge Pose), 214–15
Pārśvakoṇāsana (Side-Angle Pose), 138–44
Pārśvottānāsana (Forward Bend to the Side Pose), 129, 147–48
Paśāsana (Noose Pose), 231, 237–39
Paśchimottānāsana A, B, C (Upward-Facing Forward Bend), 157, 160, 161, 162–66, 172, 208
Paśchimottānāsana and variations (Tuning Up the Back Pose), 277–78
patella, 93
patience, 31–32, 149, 163, 185
Peacock Feather Pose. *See* Piñcha Mayūrāsana
pelvic diaphragm. *See* pelvic floor
pelvic floor, 86
  apāna and, 12, 14
  in backbends, 203–5
  balance in, 265
  feet reflecting, 75–76, 128
  in finishing poses, 276–77, 283
  in forward bends, 158, 198
  in holding serpent's tail, 73–75
  in Mūlabandha, 21, 56, 57
  nauli and, 23–24
  palate and, 86, 159, 230
  psoas and, 61, 68
  respiratory diaphragm and, 89
  sacrum and, 64
  in Samasthitiḥ, 100
  skeletal system and, 83
  in standing poses, 128
  in twists, 240–41
  ujjāyī and, 13
  visualizing, 11
  Yoni Mudrā and, 26–27
pelvic nostril, 61
pelvis, 60, 90–91, 131, 135, 158, 160, 188, 232
perception, 11–12, 47, 48, 50
pieriformis, 91
Pigeon Pose. *See* Kapotāsana
Piñcha Mayūrāsana (Peacock Feather Pose), 76, 253–54
Piṇḍāsana (Embryo Pose), 284
piṅgālā nāḍī (sun channel), 30, 61
pituitary gland, 18, 86
Plough Pose. *See* Halāsana
plumb line, 13, 78–79
  in balancing poses, 246, 264, 266
  in headstands, 287, 288
  scalenes and, 89
  in skeletal system, 83
  in standing poses, 128
  See also central channel (suṣumnā nāḍī)
Pond Mudra. *See* Tāḍāgī Mudrā
posterior cruciate ligament (PCL), 93
prāṇa, 12, 14
  and apāna, integration of, 23, 26, 32, 69–70, 123, 231, 234, 242–43, 246
  in backbends, 202–5
  in forward bends, 158–59, 161
  separation from apāna, 66, 68
Prāṇa, 11–12
  in backbends, 206
  in bandhas, 19–20
  in central channel, 25
  citta and, 46–47, 51
  finishing poses and, 282
  in integrating body and mind, 16
  movement and, 129
  nāḍīs and, 29
  in psoas line, 61
  in releasing palate, 18
  seed sound for, 15
  skin and, 73
  during Yoni Mudrā, 27
prāṇāyāma, 10, 14, 77, 87, 101, 277, 293
Prasārita Pādottānāsana A, B, C, D, 142–47, 160, 178
Primary Series, 98, 308–9
  forward bends in, 157, 162, 167, 169, 174, 178, 191, 195, 196
  twists in, 233, 238
Proust, Marcel, 48–49
psoas (*psoas major*), 91–92
  awakening, 75
  in backbends, 204
  buttons, 66–68, 144
  kidney wings and, 65, 66
  line of, 60–62, 225
  in Mini Uḍḍīyāna Bandha, 23
  stretch, 62–64
  in Ūrdhvā Dhanurāsana, 84
pubic bone, 57, 91, 100, 116, 159, 177
pubic crest, 87
pubic symphysis, 87, 90–91
pubococcygeus (PC) muscle, 68, 74, 86, 88, 143, 231, 283
puṇya, 44
Puppy Pose, 100, 115, 117
Pūrṇa Matsyendrāsana (Full Spinal Twist Pose), 244
Pūrvottanāsana (Stretching Up the Front Pose), 208–10

quadratus femoris, 91, 93
quadratus lumborum (QL), 23, 62, 65, 66, 88
quadriceps, 75–76, 84, 85, 90, 210, 212

radius bone, 90
rāga, 42
range of motion, 82, 83, 90, 94, 159
rasa, 58
reciprocal inhibition, 85
Reclining Angle Pose. *See* Supta Koṇāsana
Reclining Feet Up Thunderbolt Pose. *See* Supta Ūrdhva Pāda Vajrāsana
Reclining Hand-to-Big-Toe Pose. *See* Supta Hasta Pādāṅguṣṭhāsana
Reclining Lightning Bolt Pose. *See* Supta Vajrāsana
Reclining Turtle Pose. *See* Supta Kūrmāsana
rectus abdominis, 84, 87–88, 124, 198, 257
rectus femoris, 91
Remembrance of Things Past (Proust), 48–49
resistance, 31–32, 80, 161

respiratory system, 65, 83
Revolving Triangle Pose. *See* Parivṛtta Trikoṇāsana
rhomboid muscle, 73, 95
rib cage, 60, 65, 72–73, 83, 232
rotator cuff, 94–95

SA- HAṂ mantra, 15–16
sacroilian (SI) joints, 64, 75, 86–87, 91, 187, 205, 230–32, 236
sacrum, 64–65, 73–74, 86–87, 91
sādhanā bhāṣā (practice language), 53–54
sahasrāra (thousand-petaled lotus), 18, 57, 59
Śalabhāsana A, B (Locust Pose), 207–8, 213–14
samāna vāyu, 12, 69–70
Samasthitiḥ, 76, 79, 127, 130–31
  as quintessential balance, 245, 246
  in Sūrya Namaskāra, 99, 100–101, 107, 118–19, 123
  ujjāyī in, 14
saṃskāras, 48–49
saṃtoṣa, 39
Sanskrit counting, 100
Sapta, 118, 119
Saptadaśa, 122
sartorius muscle, 91
Sarvāṅgāsana (Shoulderstand), 76, 183, 275, 278–80, 282, 284
sattva, 39, 58
satyam, 37, 40
śauca, 39
Śavāsana (Corpse Pose), 27, 275, 296–97
scalene muscles, 68, 89
scapula, 94–95
Seated Angle Pose. *See* Upaviṣṭha Koṇāsana A, B
semimembranosus muscle, 92
semitendinosus muscle, 92
serratus anterior, 95, 147, 167, 212, 253
Setu Bandha Sarvāṅgāsana (Bridge Shoulderstand), 223–24, 280–81
Setu Bandhāsana (Bridge Pose), 222–24
ṣaṭ and variations, 114–17, 119
ṣodaśa, 122
shoulders, 62, 90, 94–95, 114, 115, 205, 212, 253, 274, 287
Shoulderstand. *See* Sarvāṅgāsana
Side-Angle Bridge Pose. *See* Pārśva Dhanurāsana
Side-Angle Pose. *See* Pārśvakoṇāsana
Śirṣāsana (Headstand), 76, 253, 275, 287–90
sitting bone (ischial tuberosity), 61, 91, 92
  in forward bends, 161, 174
  in Mūlabandha, 57
  nutation and counternutation of, 87
  origin and insertion, examples of, 84–85
  in twists, 232
  in Utkaṭāsana, 153
Śiva and Śakti, 32
Śiva Saṃhitā, 26, 57
skeletal system, 82–83
skin flow, 72–73
Small Water Bird Pose. *See* Ṭiṭṭibhāsana
soft palate, 59, 85
sphenoid sinus, 25–26
Sphinx Pose, 111–13, 212
spine/spinal column, 85, 160
  in backbends, 204–6, 228
  in finishing poses, 276–77
  in forward bends, 158, 160, 195, 196–97
  pelvic floor and, 75
  psoas and, 92
  respiratory diaphragm and, 89
  in twists, 140, 230–32
Squeezing the Ears Pose. *See* Karṇa Pīḍāsana
Staff Pose. *See* Daṇḍāsana
standing poses, 75–76, 127–30, 157, 306
sternocleidomastoid muscles, 89
Stretching Up the Front Pose. *See* Pūrvottanāsana
suboccipital muscles, 206
subscapularis, 94, 95
subtle body
  anatomy of, 10–11, 53–54
  balance in, 128, 129
  encountering, 49
  patterns in, 52
  Prāṇa and citta in, 46–47
  psoas in, 91
  purification of, 48
  working with, 81
suffering, 36, 41, 51–52. *See also* duḥkha
sukha, 43
sun channel. *See* piṅgālā nāḍī
Sun Salutation. *See* Sūrya Namaskāra
supraspinatus, 94
Supta Hasta Pādāṅguṣṭhāsana (Reclining Hand-to-Big-Toe Pose), 188–91
Supta Koṇāsana (Reclining Angle Pose), 181–83
Supta Kūrmāsana (Reclining Turtle Pose), 195–96
Supta Ūrdhva Pāda Vajrāsana (Reclining Feet Up Thunderbolt Pose), 239, 240–42
Supta Vajrāsana (Reclining Lightning Bolt Pose), 220–22
Supta Vīrāsana (Reclining Hero Pose), 210–11
Sūrya Namaskāra (Sun Salutation), 99–100, 122–23, 157
  dṛṣṭi during, 17, 101, 103, 107, 110, 111–12
  origin and insertion in, 84
  palate-perineum reflex in, 77
  transitioning in, 117–18
Sūrya Namaskāra A, 107–19, 122, 316
Sūrya Namaskāra B, 119–22, 317–18
suṣumnā nāḍī. *See* central channel
svādhyāya (self-inquiry), 40

Tāḍāgī Mudrā (Pond Mudra), 27, 275, 297
tail tucking, 74, 204
tamas, 157, 276
tapas, 39–40
Tenzin Gyatso, H. H. Dalai Lama XIV, 41
teres minor, 94, 95
ṬHAṂ mantra, 57
thighbone, 60
thoracic spine, 85, 204, 205, 206, 212, 229, 231, 284
throat, 12, 19, 21, 73, 265
tibia, 90, 92, 93
Tiryang Mukha Eka Pāda Paśchimottānāsana (One Leg Reversed Forward Bend Pose), 167–69
Ṭiṭṭibhāsana (Small Water Bird Pose) A, B, C, D, 200, 258–60
tongue, 25–26, 59, 86
transversus abdominis, 23, 67, 88
trapezius, upper, 73
Trayodaśa, 122
Triangle Pose. *See* Trikoṇāsana
triceps, 90

Trikoṇāsana (Triangle Pose), 127, 129, 130, 134–36, 231
Trīṇi, 102, 104, 106, 109, 118, 119
Trivikrama, 64
trochanters, greater and lesser, 90, 91
trust, 31–32, 72, 191, 287
Turning Up the Back Pose. *See* Paśchimottānāsana and variations
Turtle Pose. *See* Kūrmāsana
Twisted Side-Angle Pose. *See* Parivṛtta Pārśvakoṇāsana
twists, 136, 140, 147, 169, 230–33
Two Big Toes Pose. *See* Ubhaya Pādāṅguṣṭhāsana
Two Feet Behind the Head Pose. *See* Dvi Pāda Śīrṣāsana

Ubhaya Pādāṅguṣṭhāsana (Two Big Toes Pose), 183–84, 185
udāna, 12
Udāna Vāyu, 265
Uḍḍīyāna Bandha, 19, 21, 22
  in finishing poses, 282, 283, 293, 294
  in forward bends, 143, 158, 159, 167, 182
  Mini, 23
  nauli in, 24–25
  psoas in, 68
  sacrum and, 64
  in Staff Pose, 247
  Tāḍāgī Mudrā and, 27
  in Utkaṭāsana, 153
ujjāyī, 13–14, 16, 19–20, 27, 31, 102, 123
Ujjāyī Prāṇāyāma, 13, 14
ulna, 90
umbilical breathing, 34–35
Unbound Hand Headstand Pose A, B, C. *See* Mukta Hasta Śīrṣāsana
union of opposites, 41, 154
Upaniṣads, 35
Upaviṣṭha Koṇāsana A, B (Seated Angle Pose), 159, 178–81, 182
upekṣā, 45
Uprooting Pose. *See* Utplutiḥ (Ūrdhvā Padmāsana)
Upward Bow Pose. *See* Ūrdhvā Dhanurāsana
Upward Facing Dog. *See* Ūrdhvā Mukha Śvānāsana
Upward-Facing Forward Bend. *See* Paśchimottānāsana
Upward-Facing Forward Bend Pose. *See* Ūrdhvā Mukha Paśchimottānāsana
Upwardly Stretched Legs Pose. *See* Uttāna Pādāsana
Ūrdhvā Dhanurāsana (Upward Bow Pose), 70, 84, 205, 207, 224–26, 277
Ūrdhvā Mukha Paśchimottānāsana (Upward-Facing Forward Bend Pose), 183, 185
Ūrdhvā Mukha Śvānāsana (Upward Facing Dog), 89, 110–11, 114, 119, 122, 123, 202–3
Ūrdhvā Padmāsana (Upturned Lotus Pose), 283
Uṣṭrāsana (Camel Pose), 216–17
Utkaṭāsana (Difficult Pose), 119, 122, 153, 154
Utplutiḥ (Uprooting Pose), 296
Uttāna Pādāsana (Upwardly Stretched Legs Pose), 286–87
Utthita Hasta Pādāṅguṣṭhāsana (Standing Hand-to-Big-Toe Pose), 149–51, 245
uvula, 59, 85
vairāgyam, 45, 79, 276
Vāsiṣṭhāsana (Vāsiṣṭha's Pose), 260–62
Vatayanāsana (Air Vehicle Pose), 263–65
vinyāsa
  cobra hood image and, 70
  complementary movement in, 83
  definitions of, 28–29
  deity visualization and, 9
  flow of poses in, 122–23
  Prāṇa and citta in, 47, 50
  visualization in, 52–53
Vīrabhadrāsana A, B (Warrior Pose), 119, 122, 130, 154–56
Vīrāsana (Hero Pose), 93, 210
Viṣṇu, 34, 64
visualizations, 8–11, 19–20, 27, 34–35, 52–53, 60, 80–81. *See also* deity visualization
viveka khyātiḥ, 45–46
vṛtti, 47, 49–50
vyāna vāyu, 12, 173

Warrior Pose. *See* Vīrabhadrāsana A, B
Wheel Pose. *See* Cakrāsana
whole-body patterns, 19, 52–53, 62–64, 77–78, 80–81

xiphoid process, 87

yamas, 35–39
Yoga Mudrā (Seal of Yoga), 275, 294–95
Yoga Nidrāsana (Yoga Sleeping Pose), 161, 200–201
Yoga Sūtra, 35, 41, 43, 47, 79
Yoni Mudrā, 26–27

About the Authors

Richard Freeman has been a student of yoga since 1968. He has studied and taught a variety of yoga and contemplative traditions, which he synthesizes in his approach to the Aṣṭāṅga Vinyāsa methodology as taught by his principal teacher, the late Sri K. Pattabhi Jois of Mysore, India. He remains an avid student fascinated by the linking points between different traditions and cultures. He is the cofounder of the Yoga Workshop in Boulder, Colorado, and author of the *Mirror of Yoga* (Shambhala).

Mary Taylor began studying yoga in 1972, but it was not until 1988 and finding her primary teacher, Sri K. Pattabhi Jois, and the Aṣṭāṅga Vinyāsa system that she felt the profound and transformative impact that a dedicated and daily practice can have. She continues to study and practice, incorporating the residue that is produced on the mat into other aspects of her life, training as a professional chef, and applying a contemplative approach to caregiving within hospital settings through her teaching. She cofounded with Richard the Yoga Workshop and is the author of several books.

For more information, please visit richardfreemanyoga.com.